The *AIRWAY●CAM*™
Guide to Intubation
&
Practical
Emergency Airway Management

Richard M. Levitan, MD

Assistant Professor
Department of Emergency Medicine
The University of Pennsylvania School of Medicine

Attending Physician
Department of Emergency Medicine
The Hospital of the University of Pennsylvania
Philadelphia Pennsylvania

Airway Cam Technologies, Inc.
Wayne Pennsylvania
© 2004

Publisher:

Airway Cam Technologies, Inc.
PO Box 337
Wayne PA 19087
610-341-9560 (voice)
610-341-1866 (fax)
www.airwaycam.com

Printed in the Unites States of America. Apple Press Inc., Exton, Pennsylvania.

The Airway Cam Guide to Intubation and Practical Emergency Airway Management / Richard M. Levitan

Library of Congress Control Number: 2004111858

ISBN 192901812-6

Table of Contents

Acknowledgements . . . . *v*

Foreword. . . . . *vii*

Introduction *1*

Chapter 1. A Practical Approach to Emergency Airway Management. *3*

Chapter 2. Above the RSI Line and RSI Decison Making. *11*

Chapter 3. The Limitations of Difficult Airway Prediction in Emergency Airways . . . *27*

Chapter 4. Crossing the RSI Line: Skydiving as a Metaphor for Patient Safety in
Emergency Airway Management *43*

Chapter 5. Mask Ventilation, Rescue Ventilation, and Rescue Intubation *49*

Chapter 6. Laryngoscopy Overview. *71*

Chapter 7. Curved Blade Laryngoscopy. *99*

Chapter 8. Passing the Tracheal Tube. *147*

Chapter 9. Straight Blade Laryngoscopy: Paraglossal Technique. *161*

Chapter 10. Advanced Concepts in Laryngoscope Blade Design. *185*

Chapter 11. Putting it All Together: A Pre-planned Laryngoscopy Strategy
for First Pass Success. *195*

Chapter 12. Pediatric Laryngoscopy *201*

Chapter 13. Blind Nasal Intubation *217*

Chapter 14. Alternative Intubation Devices. *225*

Chapter 15. Surgical Airways. *243*

Chapter 16. Special Clinical Challenges. *259*

Chapter 17. Confirmation of Tracheal Tube Placement. *273*

Chapter 18. Airway Equipment Kits for Emergency Settings *279*

References. *283*

Index *317*

Acknowledgements

I am very grateful to my colleagues—the physicians, nurses, and paramedics—that I have worked with at Bellevue Hospital (1986-1996), Lincoln Hospital (1994-1996), and the Hospital of the University of Pennsylvania (HUP, 1996-present).

I am indebted to my teachers and fellow residents at Bellevue who supported me when direct laryngoscopy imaging was just an idea in 1994. Susi Vassallo, Katherine Delaney, and Robert Hessler were exceptional teachers who shared with me their love of procedures. Robert Hoffman and Lewis Goldfrank have been supportive of me throughout my career.

Andrew Ochroch, from the Department of Anesthesiology at HUP, and Scott Cook-Sather, Department of Anesthesiology at the Children's Hospital of Philadelphia, helped obtain the Airway Cam recordings that I have used for the laryngoscopy images in this textbook.

I am especially appreciative of Dr. Ochroch's friendship and collaboration over the years.

Judd Hollander has been an effective mentor and a valued friend.

Dwayne Hallman provided assistance with cadaver studies and procedure labs at Penn. Ronald Wade made possible my cadaver based airway courses at the University of Maryland. William J. Levin (Metropolitan Hospital, NYC) has been a co-instructor of these courses and helped obtain the images of surgical procedures that are included in this text.

William Kinkle (HUP) has been essential to the success of my cadaver courses and numerous Airway Cam projects. I thank him for his technical expertise, hard work, and enthusiasm.

Past and present residents in the emergency medicine training program at the University of Pennsylvania assisted with acquiring numerous photographs for this text, and have also helped out at my cadaver courses. A dozen residents reviewed a rough draft of this text and their input is greatly appreciated.

Worth Everett (HUP) and John Henderson (Western Infirmary, Glasgow) gave me important feedback about sections of the book. I have also benefited tremendously from the insights about airway management from other physicians within my own department, particularly Edward Dickinson, as well as academicians from across the country and around the world. It would be impossible to name them all. They have written the references cited in this text and authored the books that I have listed for additional reading.

The prototypes of the Airway Cam were made with technical assistance from Mitchell Wagenberg, StreeTVisions Remote, New York City. The device was built by Peter Guasti at the Peter Lisand Machine Corporation, Edgewater NJ.

The production of the book itself was a result of enormous efforts by Daniel Stegeman (Apple Press, Exton PA). Sue Cole (copy editing) and Liz Otwell (cover design) were also integral to making the project come together.

Finally, I have to thank my father, for exemplifying persistence and hard work, my wife, for her support and keeping together everything of value in my life, and my children, for giving me great pride and joy.

–RML

Foreword

Richard Levitan was a New York University medical student and entered the first class of Emergency Medicine residents at New York University and Bellevue Hospital Center in 1990. As a student and resident he was recognized for his passion, keen intellect, probing questions and frustration at the lack of adequate equipment, education and cooperation in our clinical environment. The first years of our emergency medicine residency proved challenging for faculty and residents alike. Richard had many interests during those years, but nothing equaled his quest to understand airway management, to improve airway management education and to achieve collaborative efforts among the specialties in the establishment of the airway. These were difficult tasks that only a motivated and scientifically rigorous clinician could accomplish. Richard's great battles and successes at Bellevue and New York University subsequently led him to the emergency departments of Lincoln Hospital in the South Bronx and the University of Pennsylvania in Philadelphia.

Richard Levitan has continued to investigate, educate and advance the field of airway management in a uniquely rigorous manner. He invented his own airway camera. He has studied his own airway. He has developed innovative strategies allowing us to improve airway management education and care in the clinical arena. This broadly focused text is like many of Richard's efforts – done compulsively and with a clear vision and sustained passion. The depth and breadth of knowledge presented in this text are remarkable.

This book is indicative of Richard's commitment to clinicians and patients. Throughout the text I can see evidence of Richard's clinical experience and devotion to detail. This text is a testimony to the fact that emergency medicine has matured, the care is dramatically improved from many perspectives and collaboration is evident in so many areas where it was previously absent. This book will help us feel more secure when facing a critically ill or injured patient with a compromised airway, provide better care and be better teachers. This book traces the creative investigative efforts of a committed physician's attempt to improve emergency care, increase patient safety, and decrease clinical risk. Richard has answered many critical questions, solved organizational and technological issues and enhanced our intellectual environment. Our patients, our students and all who care for those in need of airway evaluation and support will be better for his efforts.

Lewis R. Goldfrank, MD
Professor and Chair, Emergency Medicine
New York University School of Medicine
Director, Emergency Medicine
Bellevue Hospital/NYU Hospitals/VA Medical Center
Medical Director, New York City Poison Center

Introduction

The goal of this text is to provide a practical approach to emergency airway management and laryngoscopy. The emphasis is on effective techniques that function well in the emergency setting. The text has been written with the emergency provider in mind, not as an abstract academic reference, but for practical clinical use. Emergency airway management has tremendous impact on patient outcomes; this text will make you more confident handling this weighty responsibility.

The solutions to emergency airway management almost always involve the fundamentals, laryngoscopy and ventilation. Laryngoscopy is the mainstay of emergency airway management. This text provides a new look at the subtleties of laryngeal anatomy and the optical issues of laryngeal sighting and target visualization. Images from the Airway Cam Direct Laryngoscopy Video System are used to demonstrate critical landmarks as seen by the operator. The result is a visual guide to the procedure that has never before been available.

Coupled with unique imaging, this text defines the novel concept of a pre-planned "laryngoscopy strategy." This involves a specific set of rapidly applicable interventions designed to result in first pass intubation success.

Many airway management algorithms suggest: 1) patient safety can be improved by prediction of difficult laryngoscopy; 2) awake laryngoscopy (as opposed to rapid sequence intubation, i.e., RSI) should be used in instances of predicted difficulty; 3) complicated and rarely used devices should be used for rescuing failed airways; and 4) surgical airways are rescue airways.

It is the author's opinion that prediction of the difficult airway has limited utility in emergency patients. Pre-procedural airway assessment cannot be appropriately done in the vast majority of emergency airways and even when feasible, such tests perform poorly. In patients without evident anatomic abnormalities, laryngoscopy using muscle relaxation (RSI) has a success rate exceeding 99%. With rare exception, RSI is the approach most likely to result in first pass success in emergency situations. When patients have obvious anatomic abnormalities, suggesting that laryngoscopy will be very difficult or impossible, it is counterintuitive to expect that sub-optimal conditions using an awake approach will result in success. The best choice in such situations is often not awake laryngoscopy (and the associated risks of vomiting, regurgitation, trauma, etc.), but rather an approach through the nose or the neck. This text reviews nasal and surgical airway approaches in detail, emphasizing practical techniques that can be readily used in emergency settings.

Although there are numerous alternative intubation devices now available, the utility and role of these devices in emergency settings is largely undefined. "Difficult airway" texts and courses give a review of every available intubation device on the market even though no practitioner can realistically acquire expertise with so many devices. Likewise, complicated algorithms that involve dozens of steps cannot be remembered, let alone applied, by most practitioners in real clinical settings. Practical emergency airway management mandates easily applied algorithms and a very selective approach to alternative devices and techniques.

This text will present a more applicable and simpler approach to the emergency airway based on the route of intubation and the predominant reliance on RSI augmented laryngoscopy. A conceptual framework for patient safety in RSI is presented using metaphorical lessons from skydiving, an activity with tremendous inherent risk. Specific metaphorical lessons applicable to RSI are: 1) a redundancy of safety; 2) a step-wise and methodical approach to primary chute deployment; 3) a back-up chute that is fast, simple, and easy to deploy; 4) attention to monitoring; and 5) equipment vigilance. These lessons will be applied to RSI where the primary chute is laryngoscopy, the back-up chute is rescue ventilation, and monitoring involves pulse oximetry.

In order to understand the array of new airway devices now available and their potential utility in emergency settings, this text categorizes alternative devices into rescue intubation devices and rescue ventilation devices. Rescue intubation devices should not be the immediate response to failed RSI and laryngoscopy. The immediate need following failed laryngoscopy is ventilation. Proper mask ventilation, and if needed, rescue ventilation devices (the laryngeal mask airway and the tracheal-esophageal Combitube), are critical for ensuring patient safety when using RSI. Alternative intubation devices designed for elective use, particularly flexible bronchoscopes, have a very limited role in the emergency situation. This text reviews alternative intubation devices and evaluates their appropriateness for emergency providers in the conditions common to emergency airways.

This text also reviews specific clinical challenges emergency providers are likely to encounter, ranging from traumatic facial injuries to intrinsic laryngo-tracheal pathology. Finally, guidelines are provided for selecting equipment and creating effective airway kits for emergency settings.

Chapter 1

A Practical Approach to Emergency Airway Management

Background and the American Society of Anesthesiology Difficult Airway Algorithm

Emergency airway management has changed dramatically in the last twenty years. Twenty years ago oral intubations in emergency settings were performed without the use of induction agents and muscle relaxants. The only drugs in common use for assisting laryngoscopy were sedatives, such as diazepam, and many oral intubations involved significant force to open the patient's mouth. Nasal intubation and cricothyrotomy were common, particularly in trauma patients, because it was believed that oral intubation was contraindicated in known or suspected cervical spine injury. Twenty years ago the routine solution to failed laryngoscopy was cricothyrotomy. In the operating room, failed airway management and unrecognized esophageal intubation were common causes of anesthesia related morbidity and mortality.

Many things have changed over the last two decades. Neuromuscular blocking agents, once restricted to the operating room, are now commonly used in the emergency department and pre-hospital setting. Rapid sequence intubation is now used in the vast majority of emergency department intubations, and RSI is also commonly used by most helicopter services and many ground paramedic units. Cricothyrotomy and nasal intubation combined now occur in less than 1% of ED cases. Patient monitoring technology, such as pulse oximetry and end-tidal CO_2 detection, once found only in the OR, is now the standard of care in all settings.

In 1993 the American Society of Anesthesiology (ASA) proposed an algorithm for management of the difficult airway in the operating room (Figure 1-1). This created a new perspective on the problem and fundamentally altered OR airway management. According to these guidelines for management of the difficult airway, failed airway management was not an unpredictable "accident" but rather a phenomenon that was destined to occur on rare occasion. The ASA recommended that clinicians prepare and train for such events. In addition to emphasizing pre-procedural patient assessment, the guidelines outlined which alternative ventilation and intubation devices could be used to prevent hypoxic injury and provide intubation when laryngoscopy was difficult or impossible.

The "difficult airway" is now a well-recognized concept. Workshops on the topic have become commonplace for anesthesiologists, emergency medicine physicians, and EMS providers. Dozens of devices have been developed as alternative means of intubation and a handful of devices provide an alternative means of ventilation. In the OR, the laryngeal mask airway (LMA) is now commonly used for routine anesthetic care and it has become the de facto means of rescue ventilation for failed laryngoscopy. Coupled with a flexible fiberscope the LMA has also become a standard means of rescue intubation. Prediction of difficult laryngoscopy, comprised of checking the mouth, jaw, and neck, is a commonly accepted aspect of pre-anesthetic evaluation. Anticipated difficult laryngoscopy is routinely managed in the OR setting with awake fiberoptic intubation.

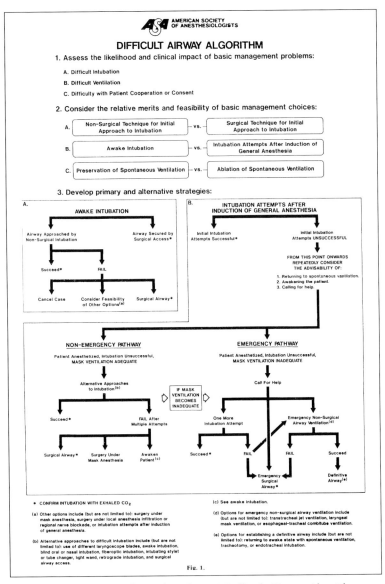

DIFFICULT AIRWAY ALGORITHM

1. Assess the likelihood and clinical impact of basic management problems:

   A. Difficult Intubation

   B. Difficult Ventilation

   C. Difficulty with Patient Cooperation or Consent

2. Consider the relative merits and feasibility of basic management choices:

   A. Non-Surgical Technique for Initial Approach to Intubation — vs. — Surgical Technique for Initial Approach to Intubation

   B. Awake Intubation — vs. — Intubation Attempts After Induction of General Anesthesia

   C. Preservation of Spontaneous Ventilation — vs. — Ablation of Spontaneous Ventilation

3. Develop primary and alternative strategies:

A. AWAKE INTUBATION

Airway Approached by Non-Surgical Intubation   Airway Secured by Surgical Access*

Succeed*   FAIL

Cancel Case   Consider Feasibility of Other Options(a)   Surgical Airway*

B. INTUBATION ATTEMPTS AFTER INDUCTION OF GENERAL ANESTHESIA

Initial Intubation Attempts Successful*   Initial Intubation Attempts UNSUCCESSFUL

FROM THIS POINT ONWARDS REPEATEDLY CONSIDER THE ADVISABILITY OF:

1. Returning to spontaneous ventilation.
2. Awakening the patient.
3. Calling for help.

NON-EMERGENCY PATHWAY
Patient Anesthetized, Intubation Unsuccessful, MASK VENTILATION ADEQUATE

Alternative Approaches to Intubation(b)

Succeed*   FAIL After Multiple Attempts

Surgical Airway*   Surgery Under Mask Anesthesia   Awaken Patient(c)

IF MASK VENTILATION BECOMES INADEQUATE

EMERGENCY PATHWAY
Patient Anesthetized, Intubation Unsuccessful, MASK VENTILATION INADEQUATE

Call For Help

One More Intubation Attempt   Emergency Non-Surgical Airway Ventilation(d)

Succeed*   FAIL   FAIL   Succeed

Emergency Surgical Airway*   Definitive Airway(e)

* CONFIRM INTUBATION WITH EXHALED CO₂

(a) Other options include (but are not limited to): surgery under mask anesthesia, surgery under local anesthesia infiltration or regional nerve blockade, or intubation attempts after induction of general anesthesia.

(b) Alternative approaches to difficult intubation include (but are not limited to): use of different laryngoscope blades, awake intubation, blind oral or nasal intubation, fiberoptic intubation, intubating stylet or tube changer, light wand, retrograde intubation, and surgical airway access.

(c) See awake intubation.

(d) Options for emergency non-surgical airway ventilation include (but are not limited to): transtracheal jet ventilation, laryngeal mask ventilation, or esophageal-tracheal combitube ventilation.

(e) Options for establishing a definitive airway include (but are not limited to): returning to awake state with spontaneous ventilation, tracheotomy, or endotracheal intubation.

Fig. 1.

1-1 *American Society of Anesthesiologists' Difficult Airway Algorithm. (From Anesthesiology 78:597, 1993. Used with permission.)*

The ASA difficult airway algorithm was designed for the OR. Options within the algorithm, such as allowing the patient to wake up or canceling the surgery are obviously not relevant to the emergency setting. Awake intubation techniques, such as flexible fiberoptic intubation, generally work poorly in emergency situations for a variety of reasons. Blood, secretions, and vomitus are the rule in emergency cases, and patients are frequently hypoxic, agitated, or combative. The ASA algorithm does mention options for the emergency airway, but its focus is primarily on elective cases in which a difficult airway is anticipated, or on elective cases which progress to an emergency situation. Critics have also pointed out that it is actually a "difficult algorithm of the airway" because of the scope and complexity of the pathways.

Emergency Airway Management Issues

There is no agreed upon standard for airway management outside of the OR. Emergency medicine organizations have no standards specifying appropriate airway equipment, let alone algorithms, for emergency departments or pre-hospital settings. Protocols, procedures, and equipment vary widely between institutions and different localities.

Airway management in the emergency department or pre-hospital setting is different than in the OR for many reasons. Multiple factors either prevent or limit the ability to do pre-procedural airway evaluation similar to what normally occurs in the elective setting. Evaluating the mouth, jaw, and neck, as is done in elective settings, is very dependent on patient cooperation and effort. These tests can be difficult to correctly perform under elective circumstances and overall they have poor interobserver agreement. Obtaining patient cooperation and applying the correct technique in the emergency situation is frequently impossible. Patients are having their airway "managed" for a reason, and this often involves respiratory distress, major trauma, shock, significant neurologic injury or other impairment that precludes following even simple commands. Other physiognomic assessments done for predicting difficult laryngoscopy require neck mobility and are also positioning dependent. This is a problem in trauma patients who are immobilized because of cervical spine precautions. Neck mobility testing is often either limited or impossible in other emergency patients as well (agitation, altered mental status, meningismus, etc.).

Even when proper pre-procedural evaluation may be possible, the purpose and end-point of performing such an evaluation is different in emergency scenarios. As an example of this difference, consider a morbidly obese man with a bull neck, short chin, and large tongue who is scheduled for elective removal of his gallbladder. A conservative approach to managing this airway in the OR would involve an awake intubation using a fiberoptic bronchoscope via the nasal route. The risk of aspiration would be minimized by having the patient brought to the OR with an empty stomach, and by the administration of medications to minimize salivation, to inhibit vomiting, and to reduce gastric acidity. Other complications of using the nasal route would be minimized by proper topicalization of the nasal mucosa with a vasoconstrictant and topical anesthetic. Muscle relaxation or high concentrations of inhalational anesthesia would be avoided until the tracheal tube was conclusively placed into the trachea and a definitive airway established.

Another potential approach in this elective situation might be a single look with a laryngoscope using topical agents or upper airway nerve blocks. The risk of regurgitation is minimal, and with effective anesthesia, a cooperative patient might permit a reasonable effort at awake laryngoscopy.

Now imagine the same morbidly obese patient with a potentially difficult laryngoscopy arriving in the ED having been shot four times in the chest. He arrives hypoxic, hypotensive and agitated. His mouth contains blood and vomitus. An awake intubation, either via laryngoscopy or a blind nasal approach, is going to be very difficult and potentially dangerous for many reasons. Laryngoscopy in an agitated patient with muscular tone has a high likelihood of causing patient injury and will very likely not succeed. It may also trigger more emesis and bleeding. Topicalization of the airway with sprays is not likely to be effective given the blood, vomit and secretions. Blind nasal intubation might be better tolerated, but does not permit oxygen administration during attempts, and will probably still be a wrestling match requiring many persons to hold the patient down. Awake fiberoptic guided intubation techniques would be impossible, not only because of the lack of cooperation and agitation, but also because of the blood and vomitus obstructing visualization through the scope.

Apart from the obvious technical differences in these two scenarios, the balance between need for an immediate airway and risk of failed laryngoscopy changes dramatically. In the elective setting there is no immediate need for a definitive airway and there is a small but real risk of failed laryngoscopy (somewhere between 2 and 35 in 10,000). Although failed laryngoscopy may not become clinically dangerous if mask ventilation (or LMA ventilation) is possible, the safest approach, given the lack of time constraint, may be to secure the airway awake and then to put the patient to sleep. In the situation of multiple gunshot wounds there is an immediate need for oxygenation and an immediate need to protect the patient from aspiration. There is also an immediate need to control the patient so that diagnostic studies and life saving therapeutic interventions can occur. The real risks and immediate dangers to the patient now substantially outweigh the very small risk of failed laryngoscopy. It is likely that the safest, fastest, and overall best approach to securing this airway is with rapid sequence intubation, even though it may be a difficult laryngoscopy. In the remote chance that laryngoscopy with RSI and optimal technique fails, it is exceedingly unlikely that mask ventilation could not be done. Should this occur the Combitube or LMA can be used as a temporizing measure while a surgical airway is performed.

As the above case illustrates, the method and route of securing the airway can vary depending upon the clinical status of the patient. Emergency airway providers should not practice with the same approaches and algorithms as anesthesiologists functioning in the elective setting. Not only is there a fundamental difference from a patient perspective, there is a fundamental difference from a provider perspective. The emergency setting is a difficult environment for providers to acquire confidence and competence with rarely performed and technically difficult procedures.

Overestimation of laryngoscopy difficulty and the selection of alternative means of intubation may be patient endangering if the practitioner is not comfortable or competent with the alternative technique. Fiberoptic intubation, for example, requires complex hand-eye coordination, an appreciation of how hand movement translates into scope movement, and the ability to recognize landmarks as seen through the scope. Unless done routinely it is unlikely that it will be successfully accomplished in the emergency setting under adverse circumstances. Even in a busy emergency department, the need for fiberoptic intubation will be less than a handful of cases per year, so any individual practitioner will practice the skill very infrequently. ED physicians can attain proficiency with fiberoptic scopes, not through intubation opportunities, but rather through frequent performance of diagnostic rhinolaryngoscopy.

For some ED practitioners in major centers, the availability of ENT or anesthesia back up in house will obviate the need for competence with a fiberoptic scope in the urgent but not truly emergent airway. Practitioner competence and comfort are extremely important factors in selecting the most appropriate means of securing an airway in a given case.

Not only is direct laryngoscopy the technique that is most appropriate in almost all emergency airway scenarios, it is also the intubation technique most familiar to emergency care providers. Except when rapid sequence intubation is contraindicated or unnecessary, most emergency airways are performed with rapid sequence intubation. Any algorithm of emergency airway management must provide a rapid, step-wise approach for determining when RSI is appropriate and when it should be avoided. An emergency airway algorithm should also quickly identify the unusual instances when a surgical or nasal approach is indicated as a primary technique. Finally, since failed RSI laryngoscopy will occur, albeit very infrequently, it is also necessary to plan a response to this situation.

A Practical Approach to Emergency Airway Management

An overview of emergency airway management is provided in Figure 1-2. It involves a series of four steps designed to determine when RSI should be used or avoided, followed by management options in the event of failed laryngoscopy. The focus of this algorithm is on the approach to intubation, and it is divided into two parts by the heavy dashed line that represents RSI administration. Above the line is the decision making process of choosing RSI or an awake approach. Above the RSI line the patient is awake; no muscle relaxants are needed or they have been deliberately avoided. Below the line represents what happens after RSI drugs have been given. Below the RSI line, in the red zone of the diagram, the focus is on laryngoscopy and ventilation.

The significance of the decision to use RSI cannot be overstated. The administration of a muscle relaxant means that you are stopping the patient's respiratory drive and abolishing all protective laryngeal reflexes. It also means that you must ensure either successful intubation or successful rescue ventilation until a definitive airway is secured. Moreover, this must be accomplished while continuously monitoring the patient, ensuring adequate oxygenation, and preventing regurgitation and aspiration. The procedure can not be considered a success if a tracheal tube is correctly placed but the patient has suffered a hypoxic injury.

The primary purpose of RSI is to facilitate direct laryngoscopy by optimizing laryngoscopy conditions. Specifically, neuromuscular blocking agents prevent the gagging and muscular resistance that occurs upon laryngoscope insertion in the patient with intact reflexes and muscular tone. In cardiac arrest or near arrest, patients are flaccid and lack gag reflexes. RSI is not necessary to augment laryngoscopy in these situations and it is contraindicated.

The second contraindication to RSI is when the oral route of intubation is mechanically impossible. Giving a muscle relaxant in this situation does not facilitate laryngoscopy because muscular relaxation about the jaw is not the problem. Mechanical obstruction that prevents laryngoscopy will also make it difficult or impossible to insert an oral airway or other device (LMA or Combitube) and create a patent upper airway. Combined with the cessation of spontaneous respiration, the inability to ventilate following RSI in such situations can be catastrophic.

The third potential contraindication to using RSI involves intrinsic laryngo-tracheal pathology. Problems intrinsic to the larynx or trachea, like evident mechanical problems about the mouth, adversely affect both intubation and ventilation.

The first three steps of the algorithm (Figure 1-2) are understandable in light of the considerations just mentioned. Step 1: Is the patient in cardiac arrest or imminent arrest? If the patient is in cardio-pulmonary arrest RSI is not necessary; proceed directly to laryngoscopy or rescue ventilation, either with a supraglottic ventilatory device (LMA or Combitube), or less preferably, with a facemask. The LMA and Combitube are preferable to a facemask because they provide a better seal and are more likely to supply effective ventilation while at the same time minimizing gastric distention.

Apply 100% oxygen.   Mask ventilate as needed. . .

1. Cardiac arrest or near arrest?

2. Is the oral route impossible? ➡️

> NASAL
> SURGICAL

3. Is there intrinsic laryngo-tracheal pathology? ➡️

> FIBEROPTIC
> TRACHEOTOMY

4. The four Ds of difficult laryngoscopy?

> A. Laryngoscopy
> B. Combitube
> C. Laryngeal Mask
> D. Mask Ventilation

Distortion
Disproportion
Dysmobility
Dentition

> LARYNGOSCOPY
> NASAL
> SURGICAL
> Alternative Device

RAPID SEQUENCE INTUBATION

OPTIMAL LARYNGOSCOPY
Pre-planned strategy for first pass success

> Alternative
> Oral
> Intubation
> Device

MASK VENTILATION
RESCUE VENTILATION
LMA / Intubating LMA / Combitube

RESCUE INTUBATION
Alternative Device / Intubating LMA / Surgical Airway

1-2 *A Practical Approach to Emergency Airway Management based on the route of intubation and RSI decision making. The colored arrows (blue and green) represent contraindications to RSI at step 1 (cardiac arrest, blue arrow), step 2 (oral route impossible, green arrow), and step 3 (intrinsic laryngo-tracheal pathology, green arrow). Blue box shows management choices in cardiac arrest. Green boxes show approaches to intubation with the patient breathing spontaneously. At step 4, the decision to use RSI is a matter of judgment, not a strict contraindication. RSI is represented by the heavy dotted lines. Management after RSI is shown in the red area in the bottom half of the image.*

Unlike the Combitube or LMA, surgical airways do not provide effective rescue ventilation in cardiac arrest because the time to ventilation with a surgical approach is generally too long. There is nothing therapeutic per se about a plastic tube within the trachea. The therapeutic intervention is the oxygen being delivered to the lungs. Simply stated, surgical airways begun on dead patients do not improve outcome. The immediate priority in cardiac arrest is to prevent brain injury from hypoxia; this requires immediate ventilation and oxygenation. Apart from ventricular fibrillation or pulseless ventricular tachycardia, when immediate defibrillation precedes airway management, establishing a patent airway and initiating ventilation supersedes all other interventions in cardiac resuscitation.

Immediately proceeding to direct laryngoscopy is indicated in imminent arrest just as it is in actual cardiac arrest. The profoundly hypotensive patient, making agonal or no respirations, who is non-responsive to painful stimuli and who has no muscular tone or protective laryngeal reflexes (i.e., is tolerating an oral airway without resistance), clearly does not need supplemental medications to facilitate intubation. In fact, the patient is frequently deteriorating so rapidly that there is no time to draw and administer medications. Agents typically used in rapid sequence intubation will likely cause immediate hemodynamic collapse by blunting the patient's catecholamine response and by affecting muscular tone and cardiac afterload.

Step 2 in the algorithm asks "Is the oral route impossible?" This does not mean "Is laryngoscopy difficult", but rather is the mouth obviously a problem. Is there evident anatomic abnormality? Examples of evident anatomical problems involving the mouth include massive angioedema, advanced Ludwig's angina, wired jaw, or any mechanical situation in which the mouth cannot be opened (see Figure 1-3a). In these situations the airway will need to be secured via the nose or through the neck and RSI should not be used. Patients in such situations present with nose breathing, impaired phonation, and often refuse to lay flat. It is safest to allow the patient to keep breathing on his or her own while the airway is secured via the nasal or surgical route.

Step 3 in the algorithm asks, "Is there intrinsic laryngo-tracheal pathology?" This is really an extension of the same reasoning for avoiding RSI when the oral route is obviously impossible. Examples include traumatic injuries that violate the larynx or trachea, or obstruction at the level of the larynx or below. RSI will permit laryngoscopy, but the problem is not the insertion of the laryngoscope, the problem is that a tracheal tube may not be passable into the trachea. Moreover, once the patient has stopped breathing, it may be impossible to provide ventilation due to obstruction or air leak.

A classic example of intrinsic laryngo-tracheal pathology affecting intubation is a large neck wound that violates the trachea. RSI in these cases permits insertion of the tube through the vocal

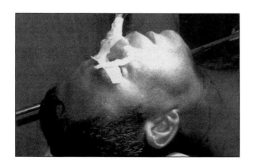

1-3 *Arrow impaled through the floor of the mouth and exiting skull. Tongue is pinned to hard palate. (From Joly LM, et al. Difficult endotracheal intubation as a result of penetrating cranio-facial injury. Anesth Analg. 2002; 94: 231-232. Used with permission.)*

cords, but the anterior curvature of the tube causes the tip to pass out of the violated trachea when inserted. Mask ventilation creates a blow hole with the bulk of each ventilation passing out the front of the neck. In such situations, when access to the trachea already exists as a consequence of the wound, the tracheal tube should be directly inserted into the hole that already exists. Obliteration of the patient's respiratory drive should only occur in these cases after a cuffed tube has been definitively placed into the trachea.

Additional examples of intrinsic laryngo-tracheal pathology are laryngeal fractures and obstructing lesions caused by neoplasm or infection. High-grade laryngeal fractures are associated with false passages that may prevent tube passage into the trachea. The mechanical action of passing a tube from above may precipitate complete laryngeal tracheal disruption. In practice, some of these patients are found in cardiac arrest in the field and intubated orally. In the setting of cardiac arrest or near arrest this is appropriate, but if the patient arrives at the hospital relatively stable and a laryngeal fracture is suspected, RSI should be avoided because the combination of failed intubation with impossible ventilation may be catastrophic. Similar concerns exist with obstructing lesions at the level of the larynx or below; it may be easy to perform laryngoscopy and yet impossible to advance the tracheal tube past the obstruction. Lesions that are do not cause airway obstruction when the patient is upright and awake may progress to complete obstruction and inability to ventilate after the loss of muscular tone with RSI.

Laryngo-tracheal injury is often obvious in penetrating trauma based upon proximity and trajectory. With blunt laryngeal trauma there may be ecchymosis across the neck or crepitus caused by subcutaneous emphysema. Patients with high-grade laryngeal trauma or obstructing lesions present with stridor, dyspnea, and the inability to lay flat. These clinical signs should never be ignored. If time permits, these patients should receive a surgical airway below the level of the lesion, i.e., a tracheotomy. This is an inevitable part of their definitive care and the safest way to manage the airway. For the patient with less severe laryngeal injury, and who is relatively stable, fiberoptic examination can occur via the nasal route with intubation over the fiberoptic scope as needed.

Occasionally in cardiac arrest or near arrest situations, intubation will be done emergently from above (with laryngoscopy), either before intrinsic pathology is appreciated or as a dire effort to avert imminent demise, but always without RSI. If the patient is relatively stable and only has a low-grade injury, elective intubation with laryngoscopy from above may potentially be feasible, but this option should only be done after advanced studies, i.e., fiberoptic evaluation and or CT scanning, have demonstrated it will be feasible.

The 4th step in the algorithm and the last step prior to choosing RSI is an evaluation of the airway in terms of laryngoscopy difficulty. The four "Ds" refer to distortion, disproportion, dysmobility, and dentition. Each of these factors can influence laryngoscopy difficulty. Frequently in emergency situations, even if laryngoscopy difficulty is a possibility, RSI will still be the best choice for securing the airway. In the prior steps within the algorithm, i.e., cardiac arrest (blue arrow in Figure 1-2), obvious impossibility of the oral route and intrinsic laryngo-tracheal pathology (green arrows in Figure 1-2), RSI is a contraindication. At this 4th step, the decision whether to use RSI is a matter of judgment. Other options include awake direct laryngoscopy, awake nasal intubation (with or without a fiberscope), and awake surgical approaches. In the author's opinion, if the first three steps of the algorithm have been addressed and there is no evident anatomic abnormality, RSI is almost always the best option. Aggressive use of RSI, however, requires a thorough understanding of patient safety issues coupled with a pre-planned laryngoscopy strategy for first pass success.

Chapter 2

Above the RSI Line and RSI Decision Making

Determining When Neuromuscular Agents are Not Needed

RSI is frequently not necessary in emergency situations because the neurologic or hemodynamic status of the patient has already created unconsciousness without muscular tone. Such patients have no response to laryngoscope insertion, making RSI unnecessary. Common examples include cardiac arrest and near arrest, but this also occasionally occurs in massive sedative hypnotic overdose and some neurological catastrophes.

Determining which patients need no pharmacologic adjuncts for oral intubation is best ascertained by an overall assessment of the patient, not through tongue blade insertion or other gag testing. Gag testing may induce emesis, and a tongue blade will not reach the base of the tongue and perilaryngeal structures. The larynx is heavily innervated and laryngeal reflexes are amongst the last protective reflexes to be abolished as the patient deteriorates. Signs that the patient may tolerate laryngoscope insertion without response include flaccidity, easy jaw opening, no response to painful stimuli (intravenous lines and sternal rub), and a presentation consistent with a significant pathologic process. Often these patients present with signs of airway obstruction as the tongue and soft tissues of the hypopharynx collapse. Sonorous respirations, poor air exchange, and tolerance of an oral airway without response are all suggestive that laryngoscopy can be done without pharmacologic adjuncts. Instead of gag testing patients who are flaccid and non-responsive, laryngoscopy should be attempted with suction immediately available. If the patient indeed has no response, the tracheal tube can be immediately placed. If it is clear the patient is resisting mouth opening or responding to laryngoscope insertion, the blade should be withdrawn and RSI initiated if no contraindications exist.

In situations where RSI is deliberately being avoided, either because of concern about difficult laryngoscopy or for other reasons, there are two other pharmacological options that can be used to facilitate success without obliterating the patient's respiratory drive with neuromuscular blockers. The first of these is the use of local anesthetics, and the second is intravenous administration of sedative hypnotic agents.

Laryngoscopy with Topical, Injected and Nebulized Anesthesia

The most commonly used local anesthetic for topical application in the upper airway is lidocaine but benzocaine is also widely available. Absorption through the mucosa is rapid and toxicity can occur if the clinician loses track of the cumulative dose. A 4% topical solution of lidocaine contains 4 grams per deciliter or 40 milligrams per milliliter. Total dose should not exceed 3 mg/kg body weight, or approximately 5 ml in a normal 70 kg adult (Figure 2-1). Mucosal absorption is limited by secretions, blood, and vomitus. Assuming the mouth can be opened, anesthetic can be sprayed at the posterior pharynx and the base of the tongue. Prepackaged aerosolized lidocaine sprays work well, or alternatively, the 4% topical solution can be applied with

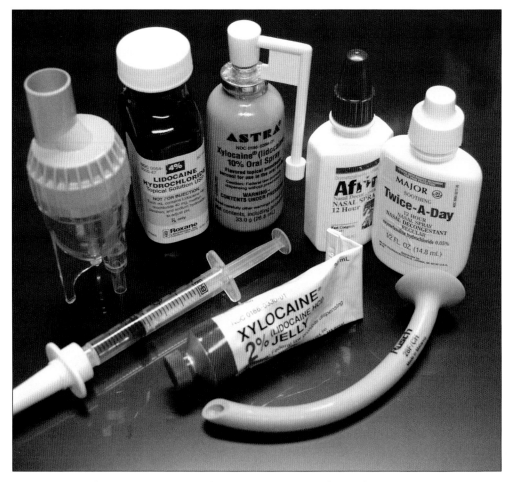

2-1 *Equipment for topical anesthesia of the mouth and nose (from left to right). Foreground: Mucosal Atomizer Device (Wolfe Tory Medical, Salt Lake City UT) on syringe, 2% lidocaine ointment, nasal trumpet. Background: acorn nebulizer, 4% topical lidocaine solution, 10% Xylocaine aerosol spray, Afrin brand oxymetazoline, generic oxymetazoline.*

a disposable single patient use atomizer. The Wolfe Tory (Salt Lake City UT) Mucosal Atomizer Device (Figure 2-2) is very effective for this purpose and comes with a long malleable plastic tube for directing the spray around the curvature of the tongue. If the epiglottis is visible even without a neuromuscular agent, it is very likely laryngoscopy can be successfully achieved, especially if RSI is used. The risk of initially attempting laryngoscopy without a neuromuscular blocker is that the patient may buck, cough, or vomit. Subsequent laryngoscopy can be made more challenging because of blood or vomitus. As a general rule, the first attempt at laryngoscopy is usually the most favorable.

To create full laryngeal anesthesia requires much more than a quick spray from above. Laryngeal anesthesia involves anesthetizing the larynx and perilaryngeal structures. This will not compromise respiratory drive but it may compromise the patient's ability to prevent aspiration. The benefit of effective laryngeal anesthesia is that the patient will have a decreased response to laryngoscope insertion and tube placement. True laryngeal anesthesia requires blocking the

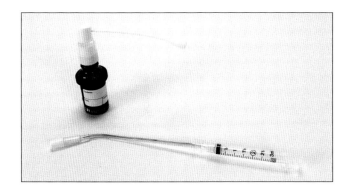

2-2 *Mucosal Atomizer Device (Wolfe Tory Medical, Salt Lake City UT) with long malleable tube and spray bottle.*

glossopharyngeal nerves and superior laryngeal nerves bilaterally, as well as administering anesthesia into the trachea, either through inhaled nebulized agents or via trans-tracheal injection.

In emergency scenarios multiple factors argue against using complete laryngeal anesthesia. Unlike in the operating room or the bronchoscopy setting, where such techniques are commonly used, emergency patients are presumed to have a full stomach and hence are at risk for regurgitation. Also, emergency patients are usually unable to cooperate with placement of pledgets or deep sprays into the mouth. Trans-tracheal injection and superior laryngeal nerve blocks are also difficult to do in non-cooperative patients. Nerve blocks are performed in the OR for awake fiberoptic intubation, but even in this setting they are used infrequently and they have no proven benefit over topical approaches. In the ED or pre-hospital setting nerve blocks are almost never done, due to the technical challenges already mentioned, and also because they are outside most physicians' or paramedics' routine practices. Probably the most effective and accessible technique in the emergency setting for creating effective oral and laryngeal anesthesia involves the use of nebulized lidocaine. To mix the solution, add 3 milliliters of 4% topical lidocaine solution to 3 milliliters of normal saline in a standard acorn nebulizer. The nebulized solution can be administered via a standard mouthpiece set-up, or through a facemask.

Pharmacologic Assisted Laryngoscopy (Laryngoscopy with Sedation Only)

Another means to facilitate oral laryngoscopy without the use of neuromuscular blockers is pharmacologic assisted laryngoscopy (PAL) using sedative agents. Despite sedation, the patient is still able to breathe and presumably protect his or her airway. This becomes a tricky slope; as you increase the dose of a sedative and improve laryngoscopy conditions, you also increase the risk of respiratory insufficiency and compromised protective reflexes. Many sedative agents in high doses are also associated with hypotension. Even if the patient retains respiratory efforts after a failed attempt with PAL, the underlying issues of respiratory insufficiency, hypoxia, and inability to protect the airway still exist.

It is worth noting that the PAL approach was historically used in emergency departments in the past, a.k.a. "benzos and brutane," with relatively poor outcomes. If there is resistance to mouth and jaw opening, such attempts may worsen subsequent laryngoscopy efforts and cause resultant trauma and bleeding. Patients may actively vomit or regurgitate. The presence of vomitus in the upper airway in a patient who has been chemically sedated increases the risk of aspiration, and sedative doses high enough to facilitate laryngoscopy will likely impede respiratory drive.

In the author's opinion, PAL is rarely the best way to secure airways in the ED, especially airways that may involve difficult laryngoscopy. A multi-center ED study has shown that the most common means of rescuing failed intubation in the emergency department is the subsequent use of RSI. Laryngoscopy without muscle relaxants is not optimal laryngoscopy, and in cases of evident difficult laryngoscopy, suboptimal conditions are unlikely to result in success. Ultimately, the provider must weigh the risks. Does the risk of RSI, namely provider inability to intubate and ventilate, exceed the risks of sub-optimal laryngoscopy, emesis, and clinical deterioration that can occur with PAL?

The risk of RSI is provider inability to intubate and provider inability to ventilate. The laryngoscopy and ventilation skills of the provider are major factors in this decision, as are anatomic characteristics and pathologic processes specific to a given patient. For patients with evident anatomic abnormality, or a combination of the four Ds (distortion, disproportion, dysmobility, and dentition) unfavorable to both laryngoscopy and ventilation, RSI should be avoided. In such patients, when RSI is considered a significant risk because of failed laryngoscopy, PAL is fraught with a higher risk of failure, plus the added risks of vomiting and clinical deterioration. The best choice when laryngoscopy is such a concern is to bypass the oral approach altogether.

Although the author prefers to avoid PAL in most emergency situations, a brief mention of different agents used for this purpose is warranted. A wide variety of sedative agents and other medications have been used for laryngoscopy without muscle relaxation. Each has risks and benefits, and although a review of RSI pharmacology is beyond the scope of this text, several agents, including ketamine, midazolam, and etomidate deserve special mention because these drugs are sometimes advocated for use in potentially difficult laryngoscopy.

Ketamine is a unique dissociative anesthetic (not actually a sedative) that does not obliterate respiratory drive or protective laryngeal reflexes. The patient becomes non-responsive and does not feel pain or make purposeful movements. The problem with ketamine is that it does not consistently create muscular relaxation. It is known to cause massetter spasm, creating clenching of the teeth, and can render laryngoscope insertion very difficult. Ketamine can also cause increased salivation. In addition, ketamine accentuates the gag reflex so stimulation from a laryngoscope is likely to cause gagging and active vomiting. Furthermore, it is unproven that ketamine assisted laryngoscopy in ED situations creates better laryngoscopy conditions than other non-RSI regimens, and the risks are significant. Ketamine is considered contraindicated in patients with head injury and increased intracranial pressure. It increases heart rate, blood pressure, and myocardial oxygen demand and should be avoided in the setting of cardiac ischemia. Ketamine is also associated with emergence reactions, particularly in adults and in those with psychiatric disorders. These reactions, however, can be prevented or minimized by pre-procedural suggestion (having the patient think of pleasant places and situations) and by use of benzodiazepines for both sedation and amnesia. Overall, it is the author's recommendation to avoid ketamine for PAL.

The best pharmacologic agents for PAL in emergency settings are benzodiazepines and etomidate. Etomidate is a barbiturate-like agent that has minimal hemodynamic effects. Both midazolam and etomidate have been used as sole agents for laryngoscopy in the EMS setting with moderate success (roughly 80%), but far higher intubation success rates result from RSI. Propofol and inhalational agents have also been used for laryngoscopy in anesthesia settings without neuromuscular blockers. Their use in ED and EMS settings has not been reported.

Midazolam is a benzodiazepine that is widely used in emergency settings for short painful procedures and is commonly used to augment laryngoscopy in pre-hospital settings. It is very effective for creating amnesia, but often does not effectively create muscular relaxation like other benzodiazepines, such as diazepam, for example. True induction doses of midazolam, between 10 and 20 mg IV push, would render the patient deeply unconscious and are never used because of the risks of hypotension and apnea. Commonly used doses, such as 2 to 4 mg, create very effective amnesia but are often inadequate to facilitate jaw relaxation and laryngoscope blade insertion.

Etomidate in true induction doses (0.3 mg/kg) can cause apnea, though it is much less of a respiratory depressant than other true induction agents (sodium thiopental), and its clinical effect is brief (minutes). Etomidate as a single agent may precipitate an airway crisis by impeding respiratory drive enough to make the patient critically hypoxic and yet not creating enough muscular relaxation of the mouth and jaw to permit successful laryngoscopy. The patient may also actively vomit with the stimulus of laryngoscopy. Etomidate is being increasingly used at half or one third the induction dose (0.1 or 0.15 mg/kg) for short painful procedures in the emergency department. This dosing is now being tested in pre-hospital settings for laryngoscopy, with initial results similar to midazolam.

The ease of laryngoscopy with etomidate or other sedative agents is a function of dose, body size, underlying pathology, and other factors. In the frail elderly person or a neuromuscular disease patient with minimal muscle mass, sedatives alone can achieve excellent muscular relaxation for laryngoscopy. Conversely, in an agitated muscular man with seizures and head injury, a neuromuscular blocking agent will likely be needed to permit effective laryngoscopy.

Numerous ED and pre-hospital studies have shown increased intubation success and fewer complications with the use of neuromuscular blockers. In addition to the technical advantages of laryngoscopy with full muscle relaxation, the other benefit of RSI derives from the concomitant administration of an appropriate dose of an induction agent. Laryngoscopy is strong stimulus that will induce hypertension, tachycardia, and increased intracranial pressure unless these responses are blunted with pharmacologic agents. When intubation is attempted with midazolam or etomidate at the low doses commonly used for PAL, the hemodynamic responses may be detrimental to the patient's underlying disease process that necessitated intubation. This may be particularly detrimental in the setting of head injury or intracranial bleeding, or in cardiac patients with active ischemia.

Nasal and Surgical Airways (Bypassing Problems with the Oral Route)

When RSI is deliberately avoided because of evident anatomic problems about the mouth, instead of attempting suboptimal laryngoscopy (using topical anesthetics or PAL) it makes the most sense to select a means of intubation that bypasses the problem altogether. This means going through the nose or neck, either of which is performed with the patient breathing spontaneously. Judicious use of topical and injected anesthetics can make the patient more comfortable during these procedures, as can careful use of amnestic agents (midazolam), pain medications (fentanyl), and sedatives. When used in these circumstances, the doses necessary are not the same doses needed to create jaw relaxation for laryngoscopy, and there is minimal risk of creating respiratory depression.

Nasal Intubation

Nasal intubation is the author's preferred method of handling emergent intubation when there are evident anatomic problems with an oral approach. As will be discussed, blind nasal intubation should not be used when there is a question of intrinsic laryngo-tracheal pathology or hypopharyngeal pathology. Fiberoptic visualization is necessary in these circumstances.

In the past, nasal intubation was frequently used in the emergency department, although with the widespread use of RSI it now represents less than 1% of all ED intubations. Nasal intubation has lower success rates than RSI. It is difficult to oxygenate the patient during the procedure and bleeding is a common immediate complication. Apart from patients in whom there are obvious problems with the oral route, nasal intubation is less desirable than oral intubation in most emergency situations.

Factors that contribute to difficulty with nasal intubation are generally different than those that contribute to laryngoscopy difficulty. This is important to consider whenever selecting an alternative means of intubation. It makes little sense to avoid one approach because of certain patient characteristics or anatomic features, and then to select an alternative technique that is also made more challenging by the very same issues.

Passage of a tracheal tube from the nares to the larynx requires a patent passageway through the nasopharynx, posterior pharynx, and hypopharynx that is at least as large as the tracheal tube. The nasopharynx can be somewhat assessed by observation or feel of air movement through the nares, but actual turbinate anatomy cannot be assessed externally. High-grade obstruction of the pharynx or larynx is usually manifested by stridor, inability to lay flat, and difficulty with phonation. Depending upon the location and characteristics of the pathology, in these circumstances a nasal approach may be possible, but it is best done under direct fiberoptic visualization. With blind nasal intubation, vigorous spontaneous ventilation helps to identify the location of the tube as the tube is advanced towards the trachea, and often patients will literally inhale the tube into their larynx.

Surgical Airways

Surgical airways comprise any approach in which the neck is cut or accessed in order to place a trachea tube. Surgical airways have already been mentioned in situations where the oral route is impossible or when there is intrinsic laryngo-tracheal pathology. For some patients with the 4 Ds of difficult laryngoscopy, a surgical airway is an inevitable aspect of definitive hospital care. It is these patients with an inevitable surgical airway for whom emergency providers should consider a surgical approach as an initial means of airway control. The patient is heading in that direction anyway. Why take the chance of losing the airway through either RSI or PAL? Conversely, a surgical airway is to be avoided when intubation is likely to be brief and when other options exist.

Surgical airways have considerably more immediate and long term complications compared to laryngoscopy and nasal intubation. Incisional bleeding is to be expected in any patient with a pulse and may be significant. Fractures and other injuries of the thyroid and cricoid cartilage can also occur. Even if there are no immediate complications there is a risk of delayed tracheal stenosis. These risks are not warranted unless there is no other effective option.

Some patients with anticipated difficult laryngoscopy due to obesity and a short neck will also have difficult surgical airways because of problems locating landmarks and working through the fat of the anterior neck.

In emergency settings, a surgical airway most commonly involves cricothyrotomy, where a direct incision is made through the cricothyroid membrane between the thyroid cartilage and the cricoid cartilage. Tracheotomy, i.e., cutting a hole through the tracheal rings (usually the 2nd and 3rd), is sometimes necessary when the problem is actually intrinsic to the larynx or high up within the trachea itself.

Cricothyrotomy is much less technically difficult than tracheotomy for several reasons. The incision site for a cricothyrotomy is relatively avascular and easily palpable, and in most situations, it is more easily exposed than the tracheotomy site. Adjacent to the trachea at the level of a tracheotomy is the thyroid gland and its associated blood vessels. Bleeding is a significant issue with tracheotomies, and under elective circumstances is prevented by ligation of the thyroid isthmus, and clamping and cauterization of the divided thyroid tissue. Finally, the trachea is simply deeper in the neck at the level of the second and third tracheal ring, compared to its location at the cricothyroid membrane. Elective tracheotomy may take 30-45 minutes, whereas cricothyrotomy can usually be done in two minutes or less under emergency conditions. "Slash" tracheotomies, in which the thyroid tissue is not specifically ligated and clamped, can be performed much more quickly, but in any event are still significantly slower and more complicated than a cricothyrotomy.

Whether performing a cricothyrotomy or a tracheotomy, the ideal patient position is with the patient supine, the head maximally extended backward and towels or other support under the neck and shoulders. The patient should be as flat as she or he can tolerate. In situations of upper airway bleeding and obstruction, however, having the head somewhat elevated helps with drainage and secretion management. Of note, arching the shoulders backward and maximally extending the head is contraindicated in cervical spine precautions and may be difficult in the morbidly obese, two groups of patients in whom laryngoscopy is also challenging.

Case Examples in RSI Decision Making and Considering an Awake Approach

Actual patient presentations best illustrate the clinical decision making issues commonly faced by emergency care providers. The choice in each of these cases is whether to attempt or avoid RSI, and if RSI is avoided, to decide between awake laryngoscopy, nasal intubation, or a surgical airway.

Case 1: Explosive blast to lower face (Figure 2-3a–c)

A young man in an apparent suicide effort swallows a small explosive and is found ambulatory at home with massive lower facial trauma. The supportive structures of the upper airway, namely the mandible, tongue, and hyoid are all disrupted. Unless sitting upright, the patient cannot maintain a patent airway.

Laryngoscopy in massive lower facial trauma is sometimes feasible if the mandible has been disrupted enough to permit unrestricted forward displacement and if the bleeding can be managed.

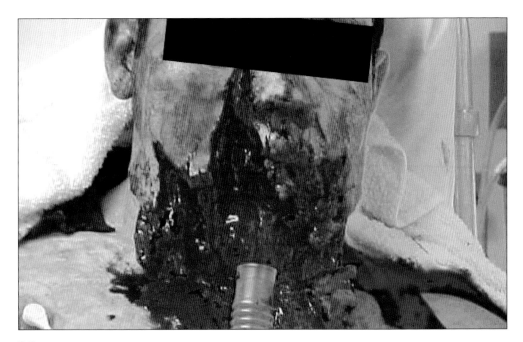

2-3a

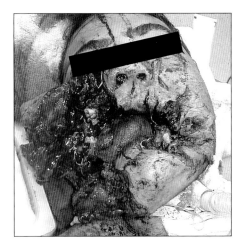

2-3b

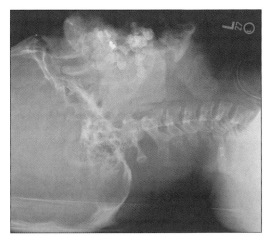

2-3c

2-3a *Initial presentation with patient upright and blow by oxygen (blue tubing).*
2-3b *Subsequent photograph in supine position after tracheotomy.* **2-3c** *Radiograph shows fragmentation of mandible and midface with complete upper airway collapse.*

In this case, the injury has destroyed any predictable relationship between the tongue and epiglottis, and the laryngoscope cannot be advanced down the tongue because the bulk of the tongue has been blown apart. Ventilation with a mask will be impossible due to inability to form a face seal and because supportive structures are so disrupted that even oral and nasal airways will not create a patent passage.

In this type of extreme distorted anatomy and evident problems with oral intubation, PAL is no safer than RSI. By attempting laryngoscopy in a supine position, airway obstruction will occur, and the addition of a sedative is detrimental for both respiratory drive and airway protection.

If the patient were in cardiac arrest it might be appropriate to use a hand and a laryngoscope to move tissue out of the way and try to identify the larynx. With the patient spontaneously breathing and hemodynamically stable, laying the patient backwards to attempt oral intubation (with or without neuromuscular agents) will cause immediate airway collapse and is unimaginable. Having decided the oral route is not appropriate, the other options are nasal intubation or a surgical airway. The injury to the nasopharynx and posterior pharynx precludes a nasal approach, leaving surgical airway as the only option.

Decision-making in this case is quick with our 4 step algorithm. RSI is contraindicated as determined by Step 2, evident anatomic problems about the mouth. Laryngoscopy is not an option if the answer at Step 2 is yes. A nasal approach is eliminated because of the evident pathology here as well, and only a surgical approach remains.

Case 2: Self-inflicted gunshot wound to floor of mouth (Figure 2-4a–d)

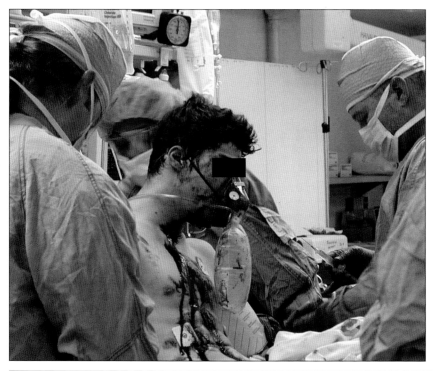

2-4a

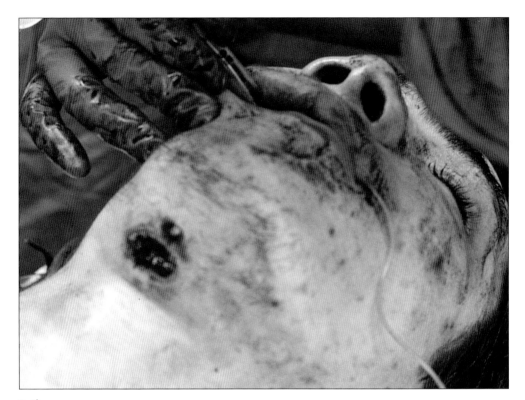

2-4b

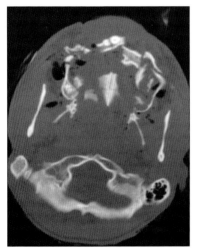

2-4c

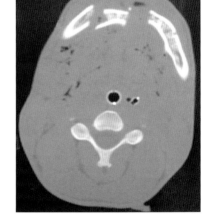

2-4d

2-4b *Post-intubation, bullet hole entrance in floor of mouth very close to chin. Tenting of skin above nose represents subcutaneous bullet in mid-forehead.* **2-4c–d** *CT scans of maxilla and mandible, respectively.*

This self-inflicted injury with a handgun involves the floor of the mouth and raises some of the same issues as the previous example. The trajectory of the bullet is upward and the bullet is palpable in the middle of the forehead (Figure 2-4b). Subcutaneous emphysema and swelling suggest extensive injury to the bony structures of the midface. This degree of midface injury probably makes mask ventilation impossible (Figure 2-4c–d). The patient is also bleeding extensively and is uncooperative, a result of shock, airway compromise, and intoxicants.

Given the trajectory, a nasal approach is out of the question. An immediate surgical airway would be entirely appropriate. As in the last example, this is a surgically inevitable airway. The problem with doing a surgical airway in this patient was that he was agitated and uncooperative, and given the degree of bleeding into his airway, he was also unable to extend his head or lean backward to any extent. Unlike the prior case, the entire injury is anterior to the hyoid bone, so the base of the tongue and epiglottis are not affected. Laryngoscopy is potentially feasible in this case, unlike in the blast injury, but bleeding will still be a problem. If laryngoscopy fails, mask ventilation cannot be expected to work, and an immediate surgical airway will be required to prevent hypoxic injury.

After deciding that an attempt at laryngoscopy was worthwhile because of the logistical issues with a surgical airway, the question became whether to try it with or without RSI. Topicalizing the airway was not an option. The degree of bleeding would have prevented any absorption. Given the patient's lack of cooperation and the technical difficulties of laryngoscopy, attempting laryngoscopy without optimal conditions (RSI) was ascertained to be too dangerous. Prolonged laryngoscopy would certainly create critical hypoxia, as the patient is already anemic and agitated and poorly compliant with efforts at pre-procedural oxygenation. Without neuromuscular blockers the patient may vomit with the laryngoscopy stimulus, since he has already swallowed a significant amount of blood.

In this instance, despite the possibility of laryngoscopy difficulty, the decision was made to perform RSI. Understanding the limitations of mask ventilation, the plan was that if a single attempt at laryngoscopy failed, the patient would be ventilated with a LMA while the cricothyrotomy was performed. The neck was marked prior to laryngoscopy and equipment and personnel for cricothyrotomy were at the bedside with a scalpel ready. Following RSI and extensive suctioning it was easy to follow the tongue downward to the epiglottis and laryngeal exposure was excellent permitting first pass success. Subsequent CT showed the mandible was broken in two places making forward distraction of the lower jaw and tongue easy (Figure 2-4d). Under controlled circumstances in the operating room, the airway was converted to a tracheotomy.

As this case proved, RSI in patients with significant facial trauma may be an appropriate choice as long as the practitioner anticipates potential problems with rescue ventilation and the possibility that an immediate surgical airway may be needed.

In terms of our algorithm, because the mouth could open and because the tissue disruption was so anterior to the base of the tongue and epiglottis, we did not eliminate laryngoscopy at Step 2. There was no laryngo-tracheal pathology (Step 3), so we came to Step 4. The nasal option did not exist because of evident trauma in this area (maxilla fractures, disruption of the floor of the nasopharynx). The options of laryngoscopy or a surgical airway remain, and for the reasons already mentioned, RSI was chosen with a surgical airway as an immediate backup if laryngoscopy had failed.

Case 3: Massive obesity and hypercarbic respiratory failure

A massively obese man with a remarkably large tongue, a small mouth, and full dentition (fixed implants) is brought to the ED minimally responsive. The patient is strikingly large; a fire company was needed to evacuate him from the house (>600 pounds). Rolls of adipose tissue exist between the chin and the chest. For all intents and purposes, the neck does not exist. Surgical landmarks, even the thyroid cartilage, cannot be identified. Neck extension is not possible because a thick roll of adipose is palpable at the base of the occiput. The patient has sleep apnea and now presents with hypercarbic respiratory failure, with borderline hypoxia (92% saturation), and is responsive only to painful stimuli. Various permutations of CPAP, BiPAP and adjustments of FiO2 failed to improve the hypercarbia.

Laryngoscopy difficulty was an obvious concern in this case, not because of trauma, but because of a combination of the patient's incredible size and degree of obesity along with the characteristics of his mouth and limited neck mobility. Also similar to the other case examples, mask ventilation in such a patient may be impossible. His history of sleep apnea points to the fact that he has trouble maintaining a patent airway during sleep, even prior to the narcotizing effects of hypercarbia or added pharmacological agents.

This case comes down to Step 4, the four Ds of difficult laryngoscopy. The patient did not have obvious anatomic problems about the mouth (Step 2 contraindication) or intrinsic laryngo-tracheal pathology (Step 3 contraindication). When taken collectively, however, the four Ds of laryngoscopy are overwhelming. RSI in this situation is potentially dangerous because of foreseeable problems with both laryngoscopy and ventilation. The likelihood of laryngoscopy success in this patient is low with or without RSI, but the odds are even worse with PAL. Any deterioration in respiratory status or vomiting could be disastrous. Remaining options include nasal intubation or a surgical airway. The surgical approach without neck landmarks was unappealing. The nasal route was chosen and the patient was easily intubated using a blind technique. Several days later, in the medical intensive care unit, the patient was extubated but hypercarbic respiratory failure recurred. Laryngoscopy proved impossible as did fiberoptic efforts because of secretions, bleeding, and redundant tissue. The patient was ventilated by facemask and a LMA and a surgical airway was eventually achieved with great difficulty.

Case 4: Pulmonary edema and potentially difficult laryngoscopy (Figure 2-5a–b)

The last case example involves an obese woman with pulmonary edema. She presents with a saturation of 50% on a non-rebreather and can speak only single words. Blood pressure is 250/150 and she is tachycardic to 150. She is restless and pulling at the oxygen mask.

In terms of airway assessment, she has full dental implants and a small mouth (Figure 2-5b), but not the degree of obesity or neck characteristics of the prior case. In elective circumstances she might be considered a potentially difficult airway.

Unlike the prior three cases, this patient is in immediate respiratory distress and critically hypoxic.

Her need for airway management is expected to be brief, as most etiologies of pulmonary edema are rapidly reversible. Her body habitus and bolt upright positioning are additional reasons

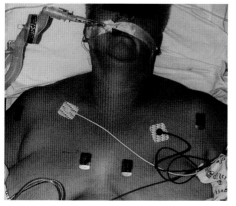
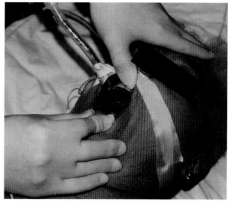

2-5a   **2-5b**

2-5a *Large woman with acute pulmonary edema, severe respiratory distress, and critical hypoxia.* **2-5b** *Small mouth, large tongue, and full dental implants. Despite potentially difficult laryngoscopy, successful oral intubation was accomplished by intern on first pass.*

to avoid a surgical approach. Nasal intubation could have been attempted, but there was concern about the time required, the hypoxia during the attempt, and what would happen if it failed. Fiberoptic assistance was not an option as she had frothy material at both nares and mouth.

In this case, access through the mouth is an option but difficult laryngoscopy is also a concern. She is too agitated to permit an awake look and will not lay flat. If laryngoscopy is attempted, she will likely tolerate only one attempt. Without sedation the stimulus of laryngoscopy may further worsen her congestive heart failure and hemodynamic status. As with the patient with the submental gunshot wound, even in the face of potentially difficult laryngoscopy, the decision was made to use RSI. With RSI she received ventilation while the succinylcholine produced muscular relaxation. Rescue ventilation devices were available if needed, but they were not, and she was effectively ventilated. With careful laryngoscopy she was intubated on first pass, despite a poor view of laryngeal structures.

In terms of our algorithm, there were no Step 2 or Step 3 contraindications to RSI in this case. We were again at Step 4, and PAL had a high risk of failure and clinical deterioration. She was not a surgically inevitable airway, so the options were reduced to RSI laryngoscopy or nasal intubation.

Alternative Devices for Awake Intubation

The above cases illustrate some of the logistical and technical issues involved in managing emergency airways. A final option listed above the RSI line in our algorithm (Figure 2-1) is the use of an alternative intubation device that can bypass the potential problems of direct laryngoscopy.

Flexible Fiberoptic Devices

The role of alternative devices in emergency settings is very limited compared to the elective setting where fiberoptic intubation is the most commonly used alternative intubation device. Awake fiberoptic intubation, whether through the mouth or nose, becomes impossible in the combative patient. Bleeding, secretions, emesis, and distorted tissue all add significantly to the logistical challenges. Patients in emergent settings often begin the procedure hypoxic or quickly deteriorating, and do not tolerate prolonged intubation efforts. For all these reasons, flexible fiberoptics would not have been feasible or beneficial in the cases presented above.

Apart from flexible fiberoptic intubation, other alternative techniques include rigid optical devices, trans-illumination with a lighted stylet and retrograde intubation. The detailed use of these devices is separately reviewed elsewhere in the text, but the appropriateness of their use above the RSI line is discussed below.

Alternative Oral Intubation Devices: Rigid Fiberoptic Devices (Bullard, Wu, Upsher Scopes), Glidescope Video Laryngoscope

The Bullard laryngoscope, Wu-scope and Upsher scope have different shapes than a standard laryngoscope, but are similar in general construction, i.e., curved stainless steel blades attached to a handle with built in light sources. They all employ a fiberoptic viewing element that runs from the blade out to an eyepiece or monitor, and a means to guide the tracheal tube into the larynx. The Shikani Stylet is a malleable stainless steel optical stylet coupled with a small lens element and a light source. Another new oral optical intubation device is the Glidescope video laryngoscope. It has a miniature black and white video camera embedded in the curvature of a plastic blade.

As is the case with a standard laryngoscope, the use of these oral devices in spontaneously breathing patients with muscular tone requires anesthetizing the upper airway or pharmacologic adjuncts. Compared to the flexible fiberoptic scope, rigid optical devices have the potential to be used much more quickly, though they are still slower than standard laryngoscopy. As with the flexible scope, their use can be compromised by secretions, blood, or emesis obscuring the lens element. The degree of difficulty seeing the larynx with these devices is unrelated to direct laryngoscopy difficulty since the optical path (via the fiberoptic element or video camera) is not dependent on a direct line of sight. Some patients who may be difficult to intubate with a rigid optical device may have an easy direct laryngoscopy and vice a versa. All of these devices still depend on visualization and mechanics at the base of the tongue and epiglottis, variables that cannot be predicted externally.

Alternative Oral Device: Lighted Stylet

Unlike the instruments involving optical elements noted above, lighted stylet intubation uses trans-illumination of the neck to achieve intubation. When the tube and stylet combination are properly directed past the vocal cords, a bright, well-circumscribed glow is seen in the anterior neck, first at the level of the cricothyroid and then in the trachea. Trans-illumination works best in thin patients with light skin pigmentation. Bright ambient light, obesity, and dark skin make visualization of the light glow more difficult. Trans-illumination is not a good choice in many patients who also have difficult laryngoscopy, namely large patients with short, thick necks. Conversely, it can be useful in situations of poor neck mobility, short thyromental distance, and relatively small mouth opening.

When compared to all other alternative means of oral intubation, only trans-illumination with a lighted stylet is comparable in speed to direct laryngoscopy.

It remains to be seen what role, if any, these alternative oral devices will have in emergency settings. Given the problems of inserting these devices into patients with an intact gag response and resistance to mouth opening, they add little to emergency airway management above the RSI line. None of the patients presented in the above cases, for example, would have tolerated their insertion. Following RSI, alternative oral intubation devices exchange the variables and pitfalls of laryngoscopy with a different set of variables and pitfalls. Visualization with any of these optical devices would be expected to be poor or impossible in the cases previously presented.

Alternative Intubation Approach Using a Retrograde Placed Wire

Retrograde intubation is a semi-surgical approach that potentially can be done as an awake technique. "Retrograde intubation" is somewhat of a misnomer, however, because the technique involves retrograde passage of wire through the cricothyroid membrane and out through the nose or mouth, followed by anterograde passage of a tracheal tube over the wire. Like open surgical airway techniques, this procedure generally takes several minutes. Accordingly, it is best done on patients who are spontaneously ventilating, or easily ventilated, and who are not critically hypoxic.

Retrograde intubation is a hybrid technique that uses the neck for wire placement and either the mouth or nose for tube passage. Unlike traditional surgical approaches through the neck, retrograde intubation does not bypass the upper airway, and therefore may not be appropriate with pathology in this area. In non-cooperative patients wire placement and retrieval can be difficult. Although there are specific tricks for facilitating tracheal tube passage over the wire, this too is problematic, especially in a patient with intact laryngeal reflexes. Lastly, in the awake patient, tube passage through the nose or mouth requires topicalization. In practical application, retrograde intubation has little advantage over either nasal intubation or a direct surgical approach and it is rarely used.

Conclusions

With the exception of awake direct laryngoscopy, blind nasal intubation, or traditional open surgical techniques, each of the potential alternative means of awake intubation require special devices that may not be available in all settings. Multiple factors discourage the use of alternative devices in emergency cases; there are educational and skill acquisition issues, logistical considerations regarding acquisition costs and maintenance, and most significantly, the effective use or implementation of these rarely needed devices under challenging conditions common to emergency airways (Figure 2-6).

Practically speaking, very few emergency care providers will have the need or opportunity to use an alternative device with any frequency. In large multi-center studies, alternative devices are used in less than one in one thousand emergency department cases. Providers must assess their own confidence and competence with a given alternative device as they consider abandoning their standard approach, namely RSI with a laryngoscope. With the availability of effective rescue ventilation devices, specifically the LMA and the Combitube, the risk of failed intubation and failed ventilation is exceedingly small using optimal laryngoscopy (with RSI and a pre-planned strategy for first pass success).

In the author's experience, the most valuable and commonly used of the awake techniques are the ones that are simplest and do not involve special devices, i.e. blind nasal intubation and direct laryngoscopy. The techniques are complementary in that they tend to work best in different types of patients. Blind nasal intubation is easiest when the patient is making strong respiratory efforts and positioned at least somewhat upright. Laryngoscopy without pharmacological adjuncts is easiest on patients lying supine, profoundly obtunded, usually making agonal or shallow respirations, and in whom the mouth is easy to open. With careful patient selection and appropriate use of topical anesthesia as needed, a "quick look" with a laryngoscope permits determination of whether RSI is in fact required, or if immediate awake intubation can be accomplished without pharmacological adjuncts. Blind nasal intubation can generally be done quickly and easily and with very high success rates if attention is paid to the subtleties of proper topicalization and insertion technique.

Educational Considerations
1. Initial training requirements to obtain proficiency
2. Frequency of use required to maintain proficiency
3. Expected frequency of use for intubation unless alternative indication
4. Manikin, cadaver, animal, or virtual reality model for additional practice
5. Success rates of infrequent users in critical situations
6. Potential for supervisor assistance and targeted feedback
7. Secondary educational benefits

Logistical considerations
1. Initial purchase price and/or per-use expenses
2. Expected repair costs
3. Setup and preparation time/labor
4. Re-sterilization time/labor
5. Maintenance/cleaning requirement
6. Mobility/maneuverability
7. Cable connection required to light source and/or electrical supply
8. Breakage/accidental disposal/theft risks
9. Backup unit availability

Clinical considerations
1. Time to tracheal tube placement among infrequent users
2. Oxygenation and/or ventilation concurrent with use
3. Potential for significant complications
4. Immediate confirmation of correct tube placement
5. Airway examination/inspection
6. Use with distorted anatomy
7. Use with secretions, blood, vomitus
8. Option for use in non-paralyzed patient
9. Option to use with patient in sitting position
10. Option for nasal tube placement
11. Integration with consultant services
12. Integration with current clinical practice

Additional considerations specific to ventilation devices
1. Time to oxygenation/ventilation
2. Adequacy of oxygenation/ventilation
3. Aspiration protection
4. Option to convert to endotracheal intubation
5. Ability to oxygenate/ventilate when oral route obstructed

2-6 *Considerations for selection and use of alternative intubation and ventilation devices in the emergency setting. (Reprinted from Levitan RM, Kush S, Hollander JE. Devices for difficult airway management in academic emergency departments: results of a national survey. Ann Emerg Med. 1999: 33: 694-8, with permission from the American College of Emergency Physicians.)*

Chapter 3

The Limitations of Difficult Airway Prediction in Emergency Airways

Should RSI be used in emergency cases with the potential for difficult laryngoscopy? The preceding chapters proposed that the aggressive use of RSI may enhance patient safety even when the possibility of difficult laryngoscopy exists. This runs counter to an approach that emphasizes physiognomic assessment with the intention to avoid RSI in cases of potential difficulty. Physiognomic tests assess the visible parameters of the patient's mouth, mandible, and neck with a consideration of what characteristics are most likely to negatively impact on laryngoscopy.

If failed laryngoscopy could be accurately predicted, avoiding RSI in these instances would prevent "cannot intubate," "cannot ventilate" situations. Empowering providers with predictive powers is very appealing and consistent with the goal of patient safety. In practice, however, difficult airway prediction through specific physiognomic testing is neither feasible nor effective in the vast majority of emergency cases.

Physiognomic testing is often reduced to the Mallampati score, thyromental distance measurement, and neck mobility testing. This chapter will address the feasibility and potential utility of these three tests in emergency airways, and explain why their use cannot significantly enhance patient safety.

Determinants of Laryngoscopy Success or Failure

The ability to successfully perform direct laryngoscopy and intubation on a given patient involves many variables that can be divided into five different areas: 1) physical features of the patient's airway that can be externally assessed (a.k.a. physiognomic assessment); 2) physical features of the patient's airway that cannot be externally assessed; 3) laryngoscopy technique; 4) equipment; and 5) the degree of muscular relaxation.

The potential utility of physiognomic testing is inversely related to the contribution made by the other determinants of laryngoscopy success or failure. If other determinants are commonly influencing outcome, then the contribution of physiognomic testing will be very limited.

Physical Features of the Patient That Cannot Be Externally Assessed

To expose the larynx, it is necessary to control the epiglottis at least to some degree. This is accomplished indirectly with a curved blade at the vallecula (by pressure on the hyoepiglottic ligament), or through direct elevation with the tip of a straight blade. Regardless of blade type, the mechanical interaction of the blade tip at the base of the tongue and epiglottis critically influences laryngeal exposure. This area of the tongue and epiglottis cannot be visually examined without special instrumentation, such as a nasoendoscope or a laryngeal mirror. The mechanical response of the hyoepiglottic ligament and epiglottis also cannot be predicted through external assessment.

Unrecognized epiglottic or supraglottic pathology can cause unanticipated laryngoscopy failure despite normal external physiognomic assessment (Figure 3-1a–c). Through endoscopic examination and MRI imaging, supraglottic pathology as a cause of laryngoscopy failure is being increasingly recognized within elective anesthesia. Ovassapian recently described 33 cases of failed laryngoscopy secondary to lingual tonsillar hyperplasia, and none of the patients had an airway examination that suggested a difficult intubation (Ovassapian A, Glassenberg R, Randel GI, et al. The unexpected difficult airway and lingual tonsil hyperplasia: A case series and a review of the literature. *Anesthesiology.* 2002; 97:124-32.)

The incidence of lingual tonsillar hyperplasia and other unrecognized problems in this region is not defined. Nonetheless, its existence precludes achieving 100% sensitivity for difficult airway prediction using external parameters. In short, no physiognomic tests can accurately predict all laryngoscopy failures.

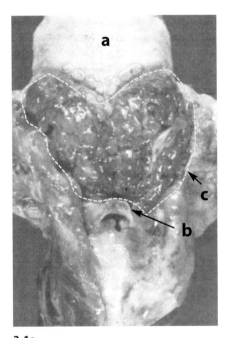

3-1a–c *Autopsy specimen of lingual tonsillar hyperplasia in patient who died following rapid sequence intubation and inability to intubate, inability to ventilate. 3-1a. View from above. 3-1b. Side view. 3-1c. Side view of normal larynx and trachea for comparison. (Reprinted from Coble SD, Jones DH, Puri S. Lingual tonsillar hypertrophy causing failed intubation and cerebral anoxia. Am J Forensic Med & Path. 1993; 14:158-61. Used with permission.)*

a = Tongue
b = Epiglottis
c = Lingual tonsillar hyperplasia
d = Trachea

3-1a

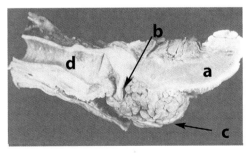

3-1b

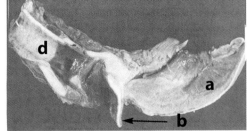

3-1c

Laryngoscopy Technique

Novice laryngoscopists taught with traditional instruction methods, including practice on plastic mannequins, have initial intubation success rates below 50%. Experienced intubators succeed in 99.6+% of cases, even in emergency settings. The skill of the clinician holding the laryngoscope is the single biggest determinant of success or failure in any intubation. Even for experienced intubators, Schmitt, in an OR study with anesthesiologists, found that simple modifications in technique, i.e., external laryngeal manipulation and increasing head elevation, reduced the incidence of epiglottis-only views from 10% to less than 0.2% (Schmitt HJ, Mang H. Head and neck elevation beyond the sniffing position improves laryngeal view in cases of difficult direct laryngoscopy. *J Clin Anesth.* 2002;14(5):335-8.).

The contribution of laryngoscopy technique cannot be overstated. Most cases of "difficult" laryngoscopy (multiple attempts) in emergency settings are not truly difficult but instead, poorly performed at first and then subsequently managed with better technique. This assertion is supported by the fact that more than 90% of cases involving 3 or more laryngoscopy attempts in the ED setting are ultimately successfully intubated using a laryngoscope.

Laryngoscopy Equipment Variables

A bulb is loose and flickers off and on, the light seems dim, and the electrical contact between the blade and handle works intermittently; these are all commonly experienced problems with laryngoscopes. However, they represent only a small fraction of equipment variables.

Design differences in laryngoscope blades can significantly influence performance of the blade and the quality of illumination. Although standard equipment includes a Macintosh and Miller blade, not all Macintosh or Miller blades are equivalent.

Two parameters that demonstrably influence performance of a curved blade include the size and shape of the proximal flange and the distance from the light to the blade tip. The large proximal square shaped flange on Macintosh blades can be difficult to fully insert and will prevent proper placement of the tip into the vallecula. The location of the light is also important, since the epiglottis is suspended between the light source and the larynx during curved blade laryngoscopy. Additionally, light sources set too far back on the flange will create poor illumination.

With Miller blades, illumination is also significantly affected by the location of the light. The tongue commonly blocks a light source located on the leading left edge of the flange (when viewed down the lumen from the handle connection), compared to a right-sided light source that performs much better. Flange shape and height also impact on target visualization and tube passage.

Apart from the design itself, blade material can also affect performance. While not all plastic blades have noticeable shortcomings, some widely distributed plastic blades are too flexible and too slippery for effective placement or epiglottis elevation.

Illumination of laryngoscope blades is itself a multi-variable phenomenon, dependent upon the type of blade (fiberoptic or conventional), the type of bulb (xenon, halogen, etc.), the size of the illumination bundle on a fiberoptic blade, and battery performance (number and type of batteries, as well as charge level).

Beyond the laryngoscope, other equipment variables influence intubation outcome. The author believes a malleable stylet should be used in all emergency cases, and the manner in which it is shaped is critical for successful visualization and tube passage. The bougie, or tube introducer, is considered standard equipment in much of the world, but it is not commonly used in the United States.

Few studies have examined how equipment variables affect outcomes. Despite the lack of comparative research studies, providers with any degree of experience quickly learn that equipment variables have real impact on patient care.

Degree of Muscular Relaxation

It is not surprising that the highest intubation success rates in pre-hospital airway management occur in patients with cardiac arrest. Conversely, in the head injured patient with clenched teeth or seizures, laryngoscopy without muscular relaxation generally fails. The patient's intrinsic muscular tone is probably the major determinant of oral intubation success in systems that do not use neuromuscular blockers. Numerous studies have demonstrated much higher intubation success rates when RSI is added into an ED or EMS system.

Especially in cases of potential laryngoscopy difficulty, the lack of muscular relaxation adds an enormous additional challenge. Converting from an awake approach to RSI is the most commonly used means of rescuing initial failed intubation in the ED.

Physical Features That Can Be Externally Assessed: The Challenges of Creating A Screening Program for Emergency Airways Using Physiognomic Assessment

Assuming there are no hidden issues about the base of the tongue and epiglottis, and assuming laryngoscopy is performed with optimal technique, that is, with the best available equipment and complete muscular relaxation, can physiognomic assessment positively influence patient outcomes?

The first challenge of creating an effective screening program using physiognomic assessment is to start with the correct goal. Physiognomic tests are screening tests for identifying patients at risk for RSI-associated laryngoscopy failure. In emergency settings, the real concern should be failure to intubate, not difficulty with laryngoscopy. If the tube can be placed successfully, without critical hypoxia, aspiration, or other clinical consequence during the attempt, it does not matter if only a small portion of the glottic opening is seen at laryngoscopy. Because intubation failure is such a rare event, many studies use surrogate markers of laryngoscopy difficulty, like poor laryngeal view or multiple attempts, instead of failed laryngoscopy (cannot intubate). Poor laryngeal view and the need for multiple attempts may have minimal clinical significance and each is dependent on laryngoscopy technique and operator skill. Taken to the other extreme, it could be argued that a screening program should focus on combined intubation and ventilation failure, because patients who can be ventilated may also have no consequence from failed laryngoscopy. The inability to perform rescue ventilation (with a facemask, the laryngeal mask, or Combitube) is orders of magnitude lower than the risk of failed laryngoscopy and involves numerous other variables unrelated to laryngoscopy. In clinical practice the major decision point in emergency airways involves the use of RSI, and patient safety is often compromised when laryngoscopy fails. It is therefore appropriate that screening tests identify laryngoscopy failure, not simply difficulty as characterized by parameters that have no clinical significance.

To justify physiognomic testing in emergency airways, a screening program using these tests must be both feasible and effective. Feasibility is a reflection of actual performance when a screening test with a given set of test characteristics (sensitivity, specificity, and reliability), is applied to a specific population of patients. Tests with excellent sensitivity and specificity may not be feasible if they are not tolerated by patients or easily applied by clinicians.

Another measure of feasibility is the yield, or the proportion of cases accurately identified by a screening test. Yield is now commonly referred to as predictive value. Positive predictive value is the ratio of true positive cases to all test positive cases. In situations when the disease prevalence is low, as in failed laryngoscopy, many predicted positives are false positives, and the positive predictive value may be very poor despite good sensitivity and specificity.

The ultimate goal of a screening program is to positively influence clinical management and reduce morbidity and mortality. In statistical terms this is termed effectiveness. In emergency airway management, this involves using the test results from physiognomic screening to alter intubation strategy (specifically to avoid RSI) and to somehow improve patient outcomes.

Now that we have introduced the terminology and major components of a screening program we can present specific physiognomic tests and fully address their performance, feasibility, and effectiveness.

Specific Physiognomic Tests

Dozens of physiognomic tests have been described for predicting laryngoscopy difficulty. Mallampati scoring, thyromental distance measurement and neck mobility testing are the most commonly cited, and many other tests are indirectly represented by these three tests. In essence, these three tests represent: 1) what is seen when looking inside the mouth; 2) the area under the mandible; and 3) how well the neck moves.

Looking Inside the Mouth: Mallampati Scoring

Since the tongue is the main structure that fills the oral cavity, the size of the tongue in relationship to the oral cavity can impact on how easy it is to accommodate the laryngoscope and expose deeper structures. Mallampati described a three-tiered scoring system based on the visible structures of the palate and pharynx, a.k.a. the Mallampati score (Figure 3-2). The test is supposed to be done on a cooperative patient, sitting upright, leaning forward, with the mouth maximally opened, and the tongue protruded without phonation. A Mallampati class I means that the uvula and tonsils are visible, i.e., there is plenty of room and laryngoscopy should be easy. A class II Mallampati score describes when the base of the tongue obscures the uvula but the tonsils are still seen. With a Mallampati class III, only the soft palate can be seen. Subsequent clinicians have described the Mallampati class 0, where even the epiglottis is visible, and a Mallampati class IV, in which even the soft palate is not visible (Figure 3-3a–b).

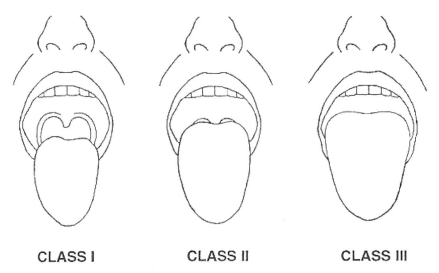

CLASS I   CLASS II   CLASS III

3-2 *Original Mallampati classification. Class I: Tonsils and uvula visible. Class II: Uvula and soft palate visible. Class III: Only soft palate visible. (Reprinted from Samsoon GLT, Young JRB. Difficult tracheal intubation: a retrospective study. Anaesthesia. 1987; 42: 487-90. Used with permission.)*

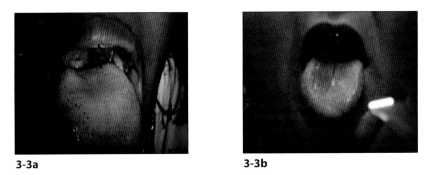

3-3a   3-3b

3-3a–b *Extreme examples of Mallampati classification: Class 0 (epiglottis seen) and Mallampati III (soft palate only).*

The interdental gap, or the specific measured distance between the teeth (or alveolar ridge), when the mouth is maximally opened, is one of the tests indirectly assessed by the Mallampati score. If the interdental gap is small (<35 millimeters), pharyngeal structures will be poorly visible. Conversely, in almost all cases, when the gap is large the Mallampati score will be good. The possibility does exist that pharyngeal visibility can be very poor despite decent mouth opening, which occurs, for instance, with macroglossia (congenital large tongue), tongue masses, or angioedema.

If the mouth cannot open direct laryngoscopy cannot be done. Mouth opening (and Mallampati scoring) is mechanically affected by the temporomandibular joint (TMJ), the integrity of the mandible, and as previously noted, the masseter muscles. Wiring of the jaw and other types of mechanical fixation and TMJ dysmobility, e.g., condylar fractures and dislocations, create the most severe limitation of mouth opening. Space occupying lesions and those that spread within the musculature, like Ludwig's angina or neoplasms of the tongue and oropharynx, can create trismus and limit mouth opening as well as intraoral visualization.

Beyond the dimensions of the patient's tongue and oropharynx, Mallampati scoring is affected by many other variables: patient effort, patient positioning, mechanical issues affecting mouth opening, and pathology about the floor of the mouth. Unless there are evident mechanical problems (wired jaw), or evident pathology about the tongue or floor of the mouth (angioedema, Ludwig's angina, mandible fracture with hematoma), the Mallampati score becomes very dependent on positioning and patient effort (Figure 3-4a–c). In clinical use, this is especially problematic in emergency situations when patients are in a supine position and often have altered mental status. In this instance, the tongue falls backward and all patients have a very poor Mallampati score.

In respiratory distress, even if sitting upright with an open mouth, patients do not naturally expend effort to maximally open their mouth or protrude their tongue. Imagine how difficult this effort becomes in patients with profound hypercarbia or critical hypoxia. It has been sarcastically noted that if a patient can cooperate and perform a proper Mallampati test (upright with the mouth maximally opened and the tongue protruded without phonation) the patient probably does not need emergent intubation.

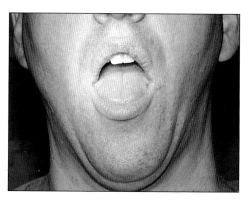

3-4a

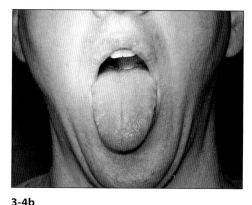

3-4b

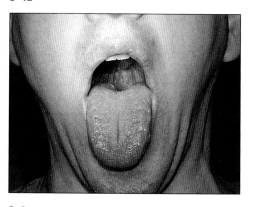

3-4c

3-4a–c *Minimal mouth opening and effort causing a Mallampati class IV. 3-4b. With slight effort a Mallampati class II is achieved. 3-4c. Maximum effort yields a Mallampati class I.*

The significance of a given Mallampati score is dependent to some degree on the type of laryngoscope blade used. Curved blades, especially Macintosh blades with an American flange (a large, square shaped proximal flange), have the greatest volume dimensions of commonly used blades. Straight blades, especially Miller designs, have the smallest. When the Mallampati score is poor, there is relatively less space for tongue and blade in the mouth, and from a volume perspective alone it makes sense that a straight blade is a better choice.

The Space Under the Mandible: Thyromental Distance

The laryngoscope displaces the tongue and must fit within the floor of the mouth so it makes sense that a small displacement space, as measured by the thyromental distance (from the bony chin to the prominence of the thyroid cartilage), might impact on the ease of laryngoscopy. A short thyromental distance in adult patients was originally defined by Frerk as less than 7 centimeters, but some predictive studies have lowered this criterion to 6 centimeters. Children normally have small thyromental distances since the mandible and chin are underdeveloped. Severe micrognathia (small jaw) occurs in some congenital syndromes that are also associated with macroglossia. The combination of micrognathia and macroglossia makes laryngoscopy impossible, for example, in Pierre-Robbin and Treacher-Collins syndromes.

It can be readily appreciated that the thyromental distance is affected by neck positioning and specifically atlanto-occipital extension. If the head is maximally extended at the atlanto-occipital joint, the distance from the chin to the thyroid is increased. Conversely, the thyromental distance is lessened when the head is held in neutral position with the chin not protruding (Figure 3-5a–b). Just as the ability to follow complex commands is integral to proper Mallampati scoring, atlanto-occipital extension is integral to proper measurement of thyromental distance. Accordingly, this is a real limitation in emergency care, where many patients are cervical spine immobilized.

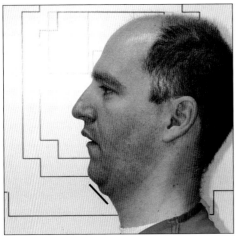
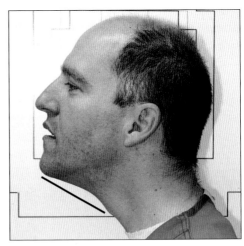

3-5a

3-5b

3-5a *With head and neck straight, thyromental distance is approximately 5 cm.*
3-5b *With neck flexion and jaw protrusion, thyromental distance is almost 12 cm.*

Two other tests that involve mandible length and mobility are indirectly related to thyromental distance. One is the patient's ability to prognath, or jutting the jaw forward so the lower teeth can advance forward of the upper teeth. Another is the upper lip bite test, or the ability to bite the upper lip using the lower teeth.

As with Mallampati scoring, the choice of blade influences the significance of a short thyromental distance in a given patient. Straight blades, with their smaller volume, generally work better in situations of a small displacement space. For this reason, as well as for better control of the relatively long pediatric epiglottis, straight blades are generally used in small children.

Neck Mobility

The third commonly used screening test for laryngoscopy difficulty involves neck mobility. Optimal laryngoscopy positioning involves flexion of the head on the chest (i.e., elevating the head when the patient is supine), and tilting the head backward, i.e., atlanto-occipital extension. Patients with cervical spine precautions, or those with a halo immobilization device, cannot be optimally positioned. This can also be a factor in other patients who have intrinsic spine disease, such as ankylosing spondylitis, severe cervical kyphosis, neck contractures, and degenerative changes that affect mobility. Occasionally, in extreme obesity, neck mobility may be limited by excessive adipose tissue at the base of the head.

Neck mobility by itself, even if completely limited, rarely precludes successful laryngoscopy. Almost all major trauma cases are successfully intubated using direct laryngoscopy with cervical spine in-line stabilization. Neck flexion is much more critical to laryngeal exposure than atlanto-occipital extension. Successful laryngoscopy has been reported even in situations of marked fixed kyphosis from ankylosing spondylitis.

Applying Mallampati Scoring, Thyromental Distance Measurement, and Neck Mobility Testing to ED Intubated Patients

As we cited above, feasibility is a function of how well a screening test can be applied in addition to the test's sensitivity, specificity and reliability. Even if a screening test has excellent sensitivity and specificity, if it cannot be widely applied, it will not influence outcomes, i.e., it will not be effective. Physiognomic tests for difficult laryngoscopy were originally conceived for elective anesthesia use, and their potential use in the emergency setting has never been assessed or validated.

The author recently investigated the feasibility of using predictive screening tests in emergency patients by retrospectively examining all intubations in his ED (Levitan RM, Everett WW, Ochroch AE. Limitations of difficult airway prediction in emergency department intubated patients, *Ann Emerg Med*. 2004; 44: 307-13.). The setting is a level-one trauma center with approximately 50,000 ED visits per year. All non-cardiac arrest ED intubated patients were included for analysis. Eight hundred fifty intubations met the inclusion criteria and 838 patients underwent RSI.

To decide when the tests could theoretically have been applied, Mallampati scoring was deemed unobtainable only if patients could not follow simple commands, and neck mobility and thyromental measurement were deemed unobtainable only with cervical spine precautions.

Laryngoscopy failed in 3 of the 838 patients who underwent RSI. Eight patients had awake nasal intubation and four oral intubations were done without RSI. Four hundred fifty-two (53%) patients could not follow simple commands and C-spine immobilization was present in 370 (44%). Only 32% of patients could follow simple commands and were not C-spine immobilized. Among the 3 RSI laryngoscopy failures, none were following commands. Collectively, Mallampati scoring, thyromental distance measurement, and neck mobility testing could not have been used in 2/3 of the ED intubated patients.

Regardless of the sensitivity and specificity of these tests in ideal circumstances (elective anesthesia) it is apparent that physiognomic screening has very limited applicability in patients requiring emergent airway management.

Sensitivity, Specificity, and Reliability

After applicability, the second component of feasibility is the ability of a screening test to do what it is supposed to do. For our purposes, this means correctly categorizing patients in whom intubation by direct laryngoscopy will fail versus those patients in whom intubation will succeed. A positive screening test in this situation is a prediction of failed intubation. A negative screening test is the prediction that laryngoscopy will result in successful intubation (Figure 3-6).

Sensitivity is the probability of testing positive if the disease is truly present (test positives/true positives). Specificity is the probability of testing negative if the disease is truly absent (test negatives/true negatives) (Figure 3-6). A test that is 95% sensitive for detecting laryngoscopy failure correctly identifies 95 out of 100 patients who cannot be intubated with a laryngoscope. Ninety percent specificity means that the test detects 90 out of 100 of the true negatives, or in our case, 90% of those who can in fact be intubated using a laryngoscope.

For a screening test to have both high sensitivity and specificity there must be a significant difference between the true negatives and the true positives and the screening test has to somehow detect that distinction. Usually, the groups overlap and the consequence is that sensitivity and specificity are a trade off. In order to capture as many as possible intubation failures, i.e., to increase the sensitivity, the threshold for a positive screening test must be lowered. Lowering the criterion of a positive test causes the test to erroneously identify persons who can in fact be intubated as positive, i.e., lowering the specificity.

The sensitivity, specificity, and predictive value of screening tests has been extensively studied in elective settings, but the results are skewed by differences in outcome measures. Many studies use poor laryngeal view or other soft end points as positive test results rather than intubation failure. An excellent literature review of this information is summarized by Yentis, an anesthesiologist who has questioned the role of physiognomic testing in elective settings (Yentis SM. Predicting difficult intubation–worthwhile exercise or pointless ritual? (Editorial) *Anaesthesia*, 2002; 57: 105–109.). Yentis pointed out that the best studies of these tests have been applied to a group of patients separate from those in whom the tests were originally derived. Focusing on these validation studies (which used poor laryngeal view or need for a bougie as end points), Mallampati scoring has reported sensitivity ranging from 42–60% and specificity from 53–82%; thyromental

Sensitivity, specificity, and positive predictive value applied to prediction of the failed airway

a = the number of individuals for whom the screening test is positive (predicted failed intubation) and the individual actually has failed intubation with laryngoscopy *(true positive)*

b = the number for whom the screening test is positive (predicted failed intubation) but the individual can be intubated with laryngoscopy *(false positive)*

c = the number of individuals for whom the screening test is negative (intubation success predicted) but the individual actually has failed laryngoscopy with intubation *(false negative)*

d = the number of individuals for whom the screening test is negative (intubation success predicted) and the individual is able to be intubated with laryngoscopy *(true negative)*

SCREEENING TEST	*OUTCOME* Intubation Failure	*OUTCOME* Intubation Success	TOTAL
Failure Predicted (screening test +)	a	b	a + b
Success Predicted (screening test -)	c	d	c + d
TOTAL	a + c	b + d	

Sensitivity = a / a + c
Specificity = d / b + d
Positive predictive value (PV+) = a / a + b

3-6 *Sensitivity, specificity, and positive predictive value applied to prediction of the failed airway.*

distance measurement has sensitivity ranging from 7–91% and specificity from 25–99%; and neck mobility testing has sensitivity ranging from 10–17% with a specificity of 98%. Sensitivity and specificity in these studies are clearly a trade off. The studies yielding the best sensitivity did not have the best specificity, and those with the highest specificity did not have the best sensitivity.

One approach to deal with the trade off between sensitivity and specificity is to use a combination of screening tests. This has been done with physiognomic testing, but this approach does not yield significantly better results. Combinations of screening tests in Yentis' review had sensitivity ranging from 42–81% and specificity from 92–98%.

The performance of screening tests in clinical settings is influenced by reliability and reproducibility in addition to sensitivity and specificity. Reliability and reproducibility refer to the consistency of results when used by different clinicians and upon repeat examinations. A significant issue with airway assessment is interobserver reliability, or how consistently two different observers come up with the same result when using the same test. Interobserver reliability is better when there are well-defined and quantifiable end points, and when there are fewer categories of test results. Karkouti has examined the interobserver reliability of Mallampati scoring, thyromental distance measurement, and atlanto-occipital extension in an elective setting when evaluated by two different anesthesiologists (Karkouti K, Rose DK, Ferris LE, Wigglesworth DF, Meisami-Fard T, Lee H. Inter-observer reliability of ten tests used for predicting difficult tracheal intubation. *Can J Anaesthesia.* 1996; 43: 554-9.). Mallampati scoring had poor interobserver reliability (K= 0.31), while thyromental distance and atlanto-occipital extension had only moderate reliability (K=.74 and .66, respectively). Karkouti concluded that this could explain the poor performance of laryngoscopy difficulty screening tests.

Physiognomic screening, even in elective settings by anesthesiologists, performs poorly and has questionable significance for influencing airway management. As explained below, in the emergency setting, the ability of physiognomic screening to influence patient care is even more limited.

Predictive Value of Physiognomic Testing: Statistical Limitations

Beyond problems with applicability (the tests cannot be applied in as many as 2/3 of ED patients who receive RSI) and poor sensitivity and specificity, the last aspect of feasibility that also argues against using such tests in emergency airways is the yield, or the positive predictive value. Unlike sensitivity and specificity, positive predictive value is greatly impacted by the prevalence of the disease in the population being studied. If RSI laryngoscopy rarely fails, and the specificity of a screening test is less than 100%, the test will have very low positive predictive value because almost all the predicted positive cases will be false positives.

Case examples best illustrate the importance of prevalence on positive predictive value (Figure 3-7). If laryngoscopy failed in 100 out of every 1,000 patients this would create a prevalence of 10% (see Figure 3-7, example A). If the sensitivity of a screening test for failed laryngoscopy is 90%, then the test will correctly predict 90 out of the 100 cases in which laryngoscopy will fail. If the specificity is 80%, then 80% of those who in fact can be intubated (1,000-100 = 900) will test negative, or 0.8 x 900 = 720. Twenty percent of the 900 who can in fact be intubated will be incorrectly predicted to have laryngoscopy failure (.20 x 900 = 180). The likelihood that a positive test actually means the patient cannot be intubated is 90 true positives divided by the true and false positives, or 90 + 180 for 270 total. The positive predictive value is the ratio of the actual laryngoscopy failures to all those who were predicted to have intubation failure (true positives and false positives), in this case 90/270, or 33%.

Now imagine the same test, (same sensitivity and specificity), applied to a second population where the prevalence of failed laryngoscopy is only 10 in 1,000 or 1% (Figure 3-7, example B). With a sensitivity of 90%, 9 of the 10 actual failed laryngoscopies will be accurately predicted. With a specificity of 80%, 792 of the 990 who can in fact be intubated are predicted correctly. The false positives, those who have a positive screening test but can actually be intubated (198), now comprise

Example A: PV+ = 33%

Prevalence Failed Intubation 10%	OUTCOME	OUTCOME	TOTAL
SCREENING TEST	Intubation Failure	Intubation Success	
Failure Predicted (screening test +)	90	180	270
Success Predicted (screening test -)	10	720	730
TOTAL	100	900	1000

Sensitivity = a / a + c   90%
Specificity = d / b + d   80%
Positive predictive value (PV+) = a / a + b   90 / 90 + 180 = 33%

Example B: PV+ = 4.3%

Prevalence Failed Intubation 1%	OUTCOME	OUTCOME	TOTAL
SCREENING TEST	Intubation Failure	Intubation Success	
Failure Predicted (screening test +)	9	198	207
Success Predicted (screening test -)	1	792	793
TOTAL	10	990	1000

Sensitivity = a / a + c   90%
Specificity = d / b + d   80%
Positive predictive value (PV+) = a / a + b   9 / 9 + 198 = 4.3%

Example C: PV+ = 15.5%

Prevalence Failed Intubation 1%	OUTCOME	OUTCOME	TOTAL
SCREENING TEST	Intubation Failure	Intubation Success	
Failure Predicted (screening test +)	9	49	58
Success Predicted (screening test -)	1	941	942
TOTAL	10	990	1000

Sensitivity = a / a + c   90%
Specificity = d / b + d   95%
Positive predictive value (PV+) = a / a + b   9 / 9 + 49 = 15.5%

Example D: PV+ = 1.5%

Prevalence Failed Intubation 0.4%	OUTCOME	OUTCOME	TOTAL
SCREENING TEST	Intubation Failure	Intubation Success	
Failure Predicted (screening test +)	3	199	202
Success Predicted (screening test -)	1	797	798
TOTAL	4	996	1000

Sensitivity = a / a + c   75%
Specificity = d / b + d   80%
Positive predictive value (PV+) = a / a + b   3 / 3 + 199 = 1.5%

3-7, examples A–D *The effect of sensitivity, specificity, and prevalence on positive predictive value.*

a much larger number relative to the true laryngoscopy failures. The positive predictive value, the true positives (9) divided by the true and false positives (9 + 198 = 207), is only 9/207 or 4.3%. In the first population, a positive screening test (predicted failure) means there is a 1 in 3 chance of actual laryngoscopy failure; in the second population, a positive screening test (predicted failure) means there is less than a 1 in 20 chance of actual laryngoscopy failure.

As should be evident from these examples, when screening for a rare disease (or event), it is the specificity that has a much greater impact on the positive predictive value. In such situations, even if the sensitivity and specificity are excellent, i.e., 90% and 95% respectively, most of the test positives will still be false positives (see Figure 3-7, example C). With a prevalence of 1%, even if the test were 95% specific, 5% (49) of the true negatives (total 990) is still a relatively large number, and the positive predictive value would be 9 divided by 9 + 49 (9/58) or 15.5%. Even at this high sensitivity (90%) and specificity (95%), the ratio of actual laryngoscopy failures to those patients erroneously predicted to have failed laryngoscopy is almost 1:6 (Figure 3-7, example C).

The statistical problem with physiognomic screening becomes even more apparent when realistic numbers for sensitivity and specificity are applied to the very low incidence of failed laryngoscopy in clinical practice. Sensitivity and specificity in many studies do not reflect numbers of failed laryngoscopy, but instead some measure of "difficulty." For example, in one study that combined Mallampati scoring and thyromental distance, the sensitivity was 82% and the specificity 98% (the best overall numbers found in Yentis's review), but there were zero intubation failures in 244 laryngoscopies. All patients in this study had the screening tests applied, a completely unrealistic goal in the emergency setting.

What numbers should be used to realistically estimate the potential positive predictive values of physiognomic testing in an ED setting? If we generously assume 75% sensitivity and 80% specificity, when this is applied to an actual incidence of failed RSI laryngoscopy of 0.4%, the positive predictive value falls to 1.5% (Figure 3-3, example D). For every case of laryngoscopy failure we accurately predict (true positive), we would erroneously predict 65 failures (false positives).

Effectiveness of Physiognomic Screening for Predicting Laryngoscopy Failure and Influencing ED Airway Management

Feasibility of physiognomic screening for laryngoscopy failure in the emergency setting is a problematic for many reasons. But what about effectiveness? What should happen in the emergency patient in whom laryngoscopy failure is predicted when it is understood that the actual risk of RSI laryngoscopy failure is one in 65 cases?

As already mentioned, choosing an awake technique instead of RSI is almost always available in the elective OR setting, but frequently not an option in emergency situations. Laryngoscopy with RSI has numerous advantages in the emergency setting including speed, simplicity, and universal availability without the need for special equipment. It does not require patient cooperation and is effective at dealing with problems common to emergency airways such as secretions, vomitus or bleeding.

The clinical decision to select an alternative means of intubation instead of RSI has much greater ramifications for the patient who needs an emergency airway than for the person who needs an elective airway. Prolonged intubation efforts and delaying the time to intubation places the emergent, unstable patient at risk. Depending upon the reason the patient is being intubated, the risks to the patient include delaying therapeutic or diagnostic interventions, delaying effective oxygenation and ventilation, and prolonging the risk of aspiration.

In terms of effectiveness, the application of pre-procedural Mallampati scoring, thyromental distance measurement, and neck mobility testing–and avoidance of RSI based on the results– holds little promise for influencing patient outcome in emergency airways.

Conclusions: The Role of External Assessment in Emergency Airways

Ironically, as a growing number of anesthesiologists are beginning to realize the limitations of predicting the difficult airway, there is much more attention to this effort being directed to emergency care providers. Mallampati scores now occupy the third page of emergency medicine's major reference text, and evaluation of the difficult airway using finger width measurements of thyromental space have been recommended for all ED airways.

The enthusiasm for difficult airway prediction began with the 1993 ASA Difficult Airway Algorithm. Many anesthesiologists have come to appreciate that physiognomic testing is a ritual that adds little to patient safety even in elective settings, where the applicability of testing is not an issue. Such tests over-predict laryngoscopy difficulty and fail to predict all instances of laryngoscopy failure. The 2002 Updated Report of the ASA Practice Guidelines for Management of the Difficult Airway states, "In patients with no gross upper airway pathology or anatomic anomaly, there is insufficient published evidence to evaluate the effect of a physical examination on predicting the presence of a difficult airway."

In the author's experience, specific Mallampati scoring, measuring thyromental distance, or measuring neck mobility is a waste of valuable time immediately before intubation. Even though Mallampati scoring itself is not useful, the importance of checking the mouth prior to RSI cannot be overstated. The whole point is to optimize laryngoscopy. If it is clear that the oral route is impossible, RSI is contraindicated. Checking the mouth also makes the clinician aware of removable dental devices and dental gaps that can impact on blade selection and expected performance. Likewise, the tongue and mandible warrant examination, especially in trauma cases. While actual measurement of thyromental distance is not recommended, the mandible, submandibular space, and neck should be carefully checked for masses and other pathology, especially in clinical situations when intubation is being done because of upper airway pathology.

Checking the mouth and the submandibular space and inspecting the neck are part of steps 2, 3, and 4 in the Practical Approach to the Emergency Airway. At step 2, obvious impossibility of the oral route is a contraindication to RSI. Step 3 is about intrinsic laryngo-tracheal pathology, and if present, is a contraindication to RSI. At step 4 in the algorithm the four Ds of distortion, disproportion, dysmobility and dentition should contribute to an overall judgment about the likelihood of laryngoscopy success. When the four Ds of difficult laryngoscopy are so evidently present and in combination, a non-RSI approach should be carefully considered. This approach is in line with the terminology in the ASA 2002 Updated Report that mentions "gross pathology and anatomic anomaly."

Chapter 4

Crossing the RSI Line: Skydiving as a Metaphor for Patient Safety in Emergency Airway Management

Rapid sequence intubation (RSI) is the fastest and most effective means of controlling the emergency airway. RSI creates optimal laryngoscopy conditions, but the cessation of spontaneous ventilation involves considerable patient risk if intubation or ventilation is not achieved in a timely manner. Patient safety in RSI is about managing the inherent risk involved with the cessation of spontaneous ventilation.

Skydiving, the combination of jumping out of an airplane and then using a parachute to land, is undeniably an inherently dangerous activity. The sport is the ultimate paradigm of managing inherent risk. In skydiving, the combination of free fall and parachute deployment is the fastest direct way to the ground. The free fall is what permits the rapid descent, but the resultant terminal velocity becomes incompatible with survival unless a parachute opens with enough time to allow a safe landing. In RSI, the muscle relaxation that provides optimal laryngoscopy conditions also causes the cessation of spontaneous ventilation. This situation becomes incompatible with survival unless intubation or ventilation is achieved rapidly enough to prevent hypoxic injury.

The time to functional recovery of spontaneous respiration following succinylcholine (given intravenously at a dose of 1.0 mg/kg) is about 9 minutes. The time to onset of critical hypoxia with absent ventilation varies among different patients and is affected by initial alveolar oxygen concentration, hemoglobin, metabolic state, and other factors. Using physiologic modeling, Benumof has calculated the time to critical hypoxia (80% saturation), in different patient scenarios and reported results varying from 8.7 to 3.1 minutes. This is well short of the time spontaneous ventilation will resume following succinylcholine administration (Figure 4-1). In emergency

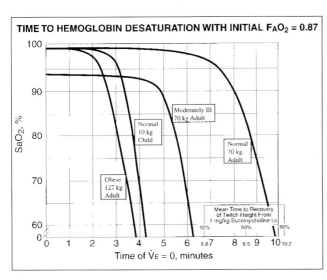

4-1 *SaO2 versus time of apnea for a healthy 70-kg adult, the moderately ill 70-kg adult, a healthy 10-kg child, and an obese 127-kg adult. SaO2 = 80% is reached after 8.7, 5.5, 3.7, and 3.1 minutes, respectively, and SaO2 = 60% is reached at 9.9, 6.2, 4.3, and 3.8 minutes, respectively. (From Benumof JL. Dagg R. Benumof R. Critical hemoglobin desaturation will occur before return to an unparalyzed state following 1 mg/kg intravenous succinylcholine. Anesthesiology. 1997; 87:979-82. Used with permission.)*

situations, when hypoxia and pulmonary pathology are major reasons for intubation, critical hypoxia following RSI is sometimes measured in seconds. If intubation and ventilation both fail, neurologic injury and death will result. Returning to our skydiving analogy, this is analogous to a low altitude dive. The safe period in which to deploy a parachute before ground impact is very brief.

A Redundancy of Safety

There are five lessons from skydiving about managing inherent risk that are applicable to RSI (Figure 4-2). The first metaphorical lesson of skydiving is a redundancy of safety. There is a primary chute and a back-up chute. One does not jump out of a plane unless both are functional. In RSI the primary chute is laryngoscopy. The back-up chute is rescue ventilation.

The back-up chute in RSI is rescue ventilation, provided either by facemask, laryngeal mask airway, or esophageal-tracheal Combitube. All rescue ventilation devices require both an effective seal and a non-obstructed airway. For the facemask, the seal involves the skin and the supporting bony structures of the midface and mandible. For the LMA and the Combitube, the seal involves the hypopharynx, the structures about the laryngeal inlet, and the upper esophagus. Severely traumatized or distorted anatomy of the face and upper airway can prevent an effective seal, and hypopharyngeal or laryngo-tracheal pathology can prevent effective ventilation.

As a general rule, obliterating the patient's respiratory drive with RSI should not be done if it is clear that the back-up chute of rescue ventilation would not work. In such situations failed laryngoscopy means the patient can be critically injured or killed; there is no redundancy of safety and we should be very reluctant to jump out of the plane. If an awake surgical airway cannot be performed in a combative trauma patient with massive lower facial trauma, RSI may be required to get control of the situation. This should be done with careful pre-planning and awareness that the airway must be secured either with laryngoscopy or a surgical airway very rapidly after drug delivery.

It is not surprising that surgical airways following failed RSI are most likely in ED patients with facial, neck, and head trauma. That said, a surgical airway may be the first and best choice in

---

1. **A redundancy of safety (2 parachutes)**

2. **A methodical approach to primary chute deployment**

3. **Back-up chutes that are fast, simple and easy to deploy**

4. **Attention to monitoring**

5. **Equipment vigilance**

4-2 *Metaphorical lessons from skydiving about managing inherent risk.*

---

such patients, as many patients with massive lower face and airway trauma will inevitably receive a surgical airway at some point. In these and other instances of the "surgically inevitable" airway, when rescue ventilation is not an option, the safest approach, if feasible, is a surgical technique with avoidance of RSI.

RSI is specifically done to optimize laryngoscopy conditions and permit oral intubation. As we noted in the prior chapter on predicting laryngoscopy failure, if it is apparent that the oral route is impossible, not merely difficult, but truly impossible, RSI should never be considered. When the oral route is truly impossible, intubation will need to take place through the nose or neck, and this should be done with the patient breathing spontaneously. Examples include massive angioedema, advanced Ludwig's angina, wired jaw, or readily apparent combinations of airway distortion, disproportion, and dysmobility (cervical spine and mandible), that preclude oral intubation.

A Methodical Approach to Primary Chute Deployment

The second metaphorical lesson skydiving can teach us about RSI is to use a pre-planned, step-wise approach to deployment of the primary chute. Skydivers go through a specific series of steps for primary chute deployment that includes proper positioning and body orientation. Failing to do this series of steps in proper order risks immediate injury, chute failure, or a hazardous landing.

With RSI we should have a laryngoscopy strategy that involves a methodical progressive visualization of landmarks as well as a pre-planned series of simple maneuvers in response to poor laryngeal view.

Use of Back-Up Chutes that are Fast, Simple, and Easy to Deploy

The third metaphorical lesson skydiving can teach us about RSI is that our back-up chute must be fast, simple, and easy to use if it is to work in the crisis situation where it will be required. If the primary chute fails, the skydiver will have a very limited time to deploy the back-up chute. Considering the rare incidence of primary chute failure, it is likely that the skydiver has never previously needed to deploy a back-up chute. With the ground coming up quickly, many persons in this predicament will panic. The same is true in RSI associated failed laryngoscopy and failed mask ventilation.

The traditional approach to RSI associated failed laryngoscopy and failed mask ventilation has been immediate cricothyrotomy. The problem with surgical airways, as well as with retrograde intubation or flexible fiberoptic devices, is that they do not meet the time requirements of a back-up chute. They are not rescue ventilation devices per se, but rather rescue intubation devices. They may ultimately achieve intubation and subsequently ventilation, but they are generally too slow to prevent critical hypoxia. Many clinicians are reluctant to preemptively perform a surgical airway. The result is that surgical airways are often initiated after the patient has already become critically hypoxic and hemodynamically unstable. Cricothyrotomy, whether using an open or percutaneous technique, has an average time requirement ranging from 75 to 100+ seconds. Fiberoptic intubation done by experienced practitioners under ideal OR conditions averages 60 to 200+ seconds. Retrograde intubation averages 150 seconds. For many patients who require emergent intubation, critical hypoxia will already be present after the initial failed laryngoscopy attempt. An additional 1-2 minute delay before ventilation may be intolerable. By contrast, the LMA and Combitube provide ventilation in less than 20 seconds. Medical personnel with no prior airway skills and a brief manikin demonstration of the devices can effectively provide ventilation with either device in less than 45 seconds.

Surgical approaches, retrograde intubation, and fiberoptic devices also do not meet the simplicity and ease of use requirements of a back-up chute. They are too technically complex for most clinicians under duress with infrequent or no experience using the procedure or device on actual patients. Also, these approaches work poorly in patients most likely to have failed laryngoscopy. Surgical airways are very difficult in obese patients with short, thick necks, and in those who cannot have their necks fully extended. Fiberoptic devices are especially difficult to use in the presence of the blood, secretions, and edema that follow failed laryngoscopy. Visualization of structures and navigation with a flexible scope are much more challenging with the patient supine and flaccid. Common conditions that make laryngoscopy difficult, such as a large tongue to pharynx ratio and lingual tonsil hyperplasia, also make fiberoptic intubation difficult. In the setting of failed laryngoscopy, the combination of inadequate prior experience, psychological stress, and technical difficulty makes any complicated intubation method a poor means of rescue ventilation.

Ironically, the widespread use of RSI in emergency medicine has made laryngoscopy failure a very rare event, and this has contributed to markedly decreased clinical experience with cricothyrotomy, the traditional back-up technique in an emergency situation. Unlike fiberoptic devices or surgical airways, the LMA and the Combitube have been shown to have very high rates of success, even when used by inexperienced users. Both devices have been extensively used in the setting of RSI and failed laryngoscopy. Their effectiveness is generally independent of laryngoscopy difficulty and the issues that make surgical and fiberoptic techniques challenging. Anecdotally, in a handful of cases in the author's ED during the last four years, the LMA and the Combitube provided effective ventilation in every instance each device was used. The routine approach to laryngoscopy difficulty in the anesthesia department of the author's hospital has become insertion of the LMA as a bridging device, followed by rescue intubation (most commonly fiberoptic intubation via the LMA).

Following rescue ventilation, possible solutions for rescue intubation in any specific situation depend upon the patient, the clinician, and the setting. Not all ED patients with failed laryngoscopy have the same appropriateness for a surgical airway. For instance, an immediate surgical airway may be an appropriate first choice in a major trauma patient who needs prolonged airway management, but in a teenager with an alcohol overdose who needs airway protection for only 16 hours it would be an unfortunate outcome. Additionally, the response to failed RSI may not be the same for a single physician coverage ED in a community hospital as for a tertiary care center with immediate availability of advanced devices and specialty consultants. While there are many different acceptable approaches to solving failed laryngoscopy, unacceptable outcomes for any provider using RSI are hypoxic injury and death. In any scenario, it is rescue ventilation that prevents hypoxic injury and provides the time to pursue rescue intubation.

Attention to Monitoring

A fourth metaphorical lesson that skydiving can teach us about RSI has to do with monitoring and how it factors into critical decision making. If the skydiver persists too long at trying to open the primary chute, even if it eventually opens, it will not open in enough time to sufficiently slow the fall. An altimeter dictates when the back-up chute must be deployed. Automatic activator devices have been developed that automatically deploy the back-up chute if the skydiver is falling above a certain speed and below an altitude necessary for a safe landing.

In RSI, pulse oximetry should dictate when efforts at laryngoscopy must be suspended and rescue ventilation deployed. The slope of the oxygen-hemoglobin dissociation curve falls precipitously below SpO2 values of 90 - 92%. Pulse oximetry readings falling to this level in a patient previously in the high 90s suggest impending disaster unless ventilation is achieved quickly. The pulse oximetry on a distal extremity has a time lag of 60 to 90 seconds, so it is important to follow oxygen saturation closely and proactively begin rescue ventilation before critical hypoxia occurs. Repeat laryngoscopy efforts should not be initiated with the patient critically hypoxic, otherwise, if laryngoscopy fails, there may not be sufficient time to prevent hypoxic injury and hemodynamic instability. Mask ventilation between laryngoscopy efforts however, especially with high bag volumes and pressures, can increase gastric distention and the risk of regurgitation. To minimize aspiration risk associated with repeat bagging and the risk of hypoxia from prolonged laryngoscopy, first pass laryngoscopy success is critical with emergency RSI, particularly in unstable patients.

If mask ventilation is necessary it should be done at low volumes (4-6 ml/kg), low pressure (less than 20 cm H20), and with slow inflation (1-2 seconds). The focus should be on upper airway patency and not on squeezing the bag harder or pushing the facemask onto the face in a manner that causes the mandible to be pushed downward, (and the airway obstructed). It is critical to lift upward on the mandible and the submandibular tissues and to use oral and/or nasal airways. As the first line technique of rescue ventilation, especially between laryngoscopy attempts, the importance of mask ventilation in RSI patient safety cannot be overstated. In the very rare event that mask ventilation fails, the LMA or Combitube should be immediately placed. Compared to the facemask, the LMA and Combitube cause less gastric distention (and probably less aspiration), and create a better seal and more effective ventilation.

Monitoring of altitude is essential not only for deployment of the back-up chute, but also for determining when it is safe to jump out of the plane in the first place. Without sufficient altitude there may not be enough time to open the primary chute (let alone a back-up chute) and sufficiently slow the descent. In RSI, without sufficient preoxygenation the onset of critical hypoxia will be precipitously fast. By maximizing oxygen concentration in the alveoli, blood, and tissues, the clinician extends the time the patient will tolerate apnea before becoming dangerously hypoxic. Pulse oximetry in RSI is not completely analogous to an altimeter used in skydiving, however. Because of the shape of the oxygen-hemoglobin curve, pulse oximetry does not accurately reflect oxygen tension at higher SpO2 values. A PaO2 value of 100 can correlate with 100% saturation, though a PaO2 value in excess of 600 might be achievable in the same patient and also display a pulse oximetry saturation of 100%. This difference can be a clinically significant margin of safety if difficult laryngoscopy and mask ventilation are encountered. To truly maximize preoxygenation, the pulmonary space, tissues, venous, and arterial compartments of the body all need time to fill with oxygen. The best means of achieving maximal preoxygenation is the application of a well fitting, non-rebreather mask for four minutes prior to RSI. Optimal pre-oxygenation for patients not making adequate respiratory effort requires mechanical assistance with a bag and facemask.

Equipment Vigilance

The fifth and final metaphorical lesson skydiving can teach us about RSI has to do with equipment vigilance. For skydiving, it is not difficult to appreciate the need for the most reliable equipment. Skydivers do not jump out of planes without personally checking that their harnesses have been properly rigged and that their chutes have been correctly packed. Skydivers have an intimate knowledge and responsibility for the equipment upon which their lives depend. We should take the same responsibility for our patients' safety by selecting high quality laryngoscopes and having rescue ventilation devices immediately accessible. Unlike the American Society of Anesthesiologists, which has equipment recommendations within its Practice Guidelines for the Difficult Airway, emergency medicine organizations have no standards or guidelines regarding availability of airway devices in emergency settings. As clinicians ultimately responsible for the patient, each of us should assume personal responsibility for the laryngoscopy and rescue ventilation equipment upon which our patients' lives depend.

Chapter 5

Mask Ventilation, Rescue Ventilation, and Rescue Intubation

Mask Ventilation

Mask ventilation is fundamental to patient safety in emergency airway management. For basic EMS providers, it may be the only means of airway management en route to the hospital. In advanced airway management, mask ventilation is used prior to intubation and it is often needed after RSI has been started but before the onset of muscular relaxation. If the initial laryngoscopy effort fails, it is used between repeat attempts. Finally, if laryngoscopy cannot succeed, mask ventilation is used to maintain oxygenation prior to rescue intubation.

Despite the necessity of mask ventilation in emergency settings, it can potentially increase the risk of regurgitation and aspiration. When rapid sequence induction was first conceived as an operating room technique to prevent aspiration in high-risk patients, ventilation after induction was considered contraindicated because of this risk.

In emergency airway situations, an immediate need for ventilation should always take priority over the potential threat of aspiration because critical hypoxia for more than a few minutes causes catastrophic brain injury and ultimately cardiac arrest. Even in short duration, critical hypoxia may precipitate bradycardia, brain injury, or myocardial injury. Depending upon the physiologic state of the patient and the underlying pathologic process, the onset of critical hypoxia occurs dramatically fast with the cessation of spontaneous ventilation. This is especially true when using RSI on patients whose original indication for intubation is hypoxia and respiratory distress. First pass laryngoscopy success becomes critical in these cases.

The best means of preventing critical hypoxia during RSI is the administration of 100% oxygen prior to the administration of RSI medications. A 100% non-rebreather facemask should be applied to all patients who are making adequate respiratory efforts for a period of at least four minutes. The facemask should be well fitting, the reservoir bag should be fully inflated, and the oxygen should be checked to ensure high flow (15 lpm). A 100% pulse oximetry reading may correlate with a PaO_2 on blood gas of 90-100. By administering 100% oxygen via a non-rebreather mask, the PaO_2 can potentially reach 600 or more depending on the patient. This difference, which is not apparent by pulse oximetry reading, provides an added margin of safety by delaying the onset of critical hypoxia. Elevating oxygen concentrations in the alveolus, the blood stream, and body tissues creates the longest possible safe apneic period, protecting the patient from hypoxia while awaiting muscle relaxants to work and during subsequent laryngoscopy efforts.

According to the alveolar gas equation, oxygen concentration in the alveolus is positively influenced by the concentration of inspired oxygen and negatively affected by the partial pressure of carbon dioxide in the alveolus. Maximizing oxygenation requires maximizing the inspired concentration of oxygen as well as the effective elimination of carbon dioxide from the alveolus. Patients who are not making adequate respiratory efforts require bag mask ventilation prior to RSI drug administration and while awaiting onset of muscle relaxation. This is always required with patients who are critically hypoxic on 100% oxygen prior to RSI.

Aspiration, Gastric Distention, and Mask Ventilation Technique

Patients in cardiac arrest and in RSI situations are at particular risk for regurgitation of stomach contents because of decreased lower esophageal sphincter tone and supine positioning. Increased gastric volume in such circumstances is particularly hazardous, whether resulting from air, gastrointestinal contents or blood. Gastric distention is usually a consequence of over aggressive mask ventilation, but can also be caused by underlying medical conditions.

Many emergency conditions can decrease gastric motility and potentially result in gastric distention. For patients who need emergent intubation, time may not permit stomach decompression with a nasogastric (NG) tube prior to intubation. In urgent, but non-emergent high-risk situations, such as mechanical bowel obstruction or upper GI bleeding, decompression with a NG tube is recommended. In the author's experience, it is best to remove the nasogastric tube prior to laryngoscopy and after the stomach has been evacuated. The NG tube can interfere with laryngoscope insertion and affect target visualization.

Numerous patient variables, as well as several subtle aspects of operator technique, affect the balance between effective oxygenation, gastric distention and aspiration risk in the unprotected airway during mask ventilation. To minimize the risk of aspiration, the overall strategy is to create a patent upper airway and to use lower mask volumes (6-7 cc/kg), delivered at low pressure (<20 mm), over a relatively long inflation time (1-2 seconds).

Patient Positioning

A patent upper airway is essential for effective ventilation with lower pressures and volumes. The creation of a patent airway is itself a three step process: 1) proper patient positioning; 2) insertion of an oral or nasal airway; and 3) lifting of the mandible and submandibular structures.

To appreciate the patient position that maximizes effective ventilation, it is helpful to observe how patients position themselves when faced with respiratory distress. While many clinicians focus on tilting the head backward, or atlanto-occipital extension, patients in respiratory distress do not use such positioning. Instead, they lean their heads and necks forward and sit upright. This position maximizes the dimensions of the upper airway, and unless contraindicated by cervical spine precautions, the ideal position for mask ventilation is to recreate this position, albeit with the patient supine. Exaggerated atlanto-occipital extension, or tilting the head backward, increases the difficulty of ventilation, because it pushes the tongue and soft tissues of the hypopharynx backward onto the posterior pharyngeal wall.

Positioning is also important when pre-oxygenating patients who are ventilating themselves, especially in morbid obesity. In a recent study addressing this issue, the safe apneic period (pulse oximetry falling from 100% to 92%) was more than three minutes in patients in a head elevated (reverse Trendelenberg) position compared to only two minutes if the patient was positioned lying flat. An additional minute without hypoxia may be clinically significant if repeat laryngoscopy is required.

The amount of head elevation necessary to optimize ventilation varies depending upon body habitus, although many reference texts suggest a uniform 8 to 10 centimeters of head elevation. It is the author's belief that the ideal ventilation position is not reliably created by a specific amount of head elevation, but instead depends upon the position of the patient's head relative to his or her chest. Such a position can be easily defined and is independent of body habitus, age, or total weight. The head and shoulders should be elevated until the ear canal is at the level of the sternal notch when viewed from a lateral perspective (Figure 5-1). For a thin person, a few inches of head elevation may achieve proper alignment, while a morbidly obese patient may need several feet of head elevation to create proper positioning. This relationship of ear canal to sternal notch is also independent of age. In infants and small children, the head is relatively larger than in adults and as a result, the ear canal and sternal notch line up without additional head elevation (Figure 5-2).

Proper positioning permits the maximal potential upper airway dimensions, but does not, in itself, ensure a patent airway because the tongue, epiglottis, and soft-tissues of the hypopharynx are soft and collapsible. In profound unconsciousness, cardiac arrest, and after muscle relaxation with RSI, the lack of muscular tone can cause the soft tissues of the upper airway to collapse. Without an oral or nasal airway, mask ventilation may not be possible.

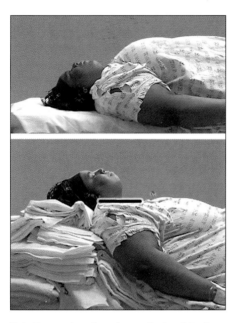

5-1 *Proper head to chest relationship for ventilation defined by a horizontal line connecting the external auditory meatus (ear) to the sternal notch.*

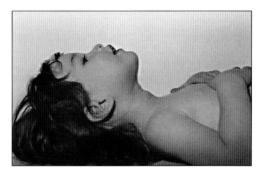

5-2 *Large occiput in child creates proper head to chest relationship (ear to sternal notch) without additional head elevation.*

Creating a Patent Airway Using Oral and Nasal Airways

Oral or nasal airways are often needed with mask ventilation in order to keep the tongue from lying against the posterior pharyngeal wall. The oral airway should fit around the curvature of the tongue. Under no circumstances should it push the base of the tongue downward. It is best inserted by rotating it down the curvature of the tongue, ideally with the use of a tongue blade or a laryngoscope blade. The historical practice of inserting the oral airway upside down and turning it over can cause trauma to the palate and does not ensure proper placement.

Mask Technique and Submandibular Lift

Oral and nasal airways help create patency of the upper airway but these devices do not prevent obstruction by the base of the tongue, epiglottis, and the soft tissues of the hypopharynx. Distracting the mandible and the submandibular tissue upward during mask ventilation prevents obstruction at this lower level. The top of the mask should be firmly pressed downward onto the bridge of the nose, but the lower portion of the mask should be held tightly to the face, avoiding downward pressure on the mandible. This is best achieved by using an "E-C" grip (Figure 5-3). The center of the mask fits within the "C" created by the thumb and first finger and the "E" represents the third, fourth, and fifth digits that hold the lower mask to the face. The fourth and fifth digits are at the same time used to lift the angle of the mandible upward. Additional lift at the level of the hyoid, where the base of the epiglottis attaches, is also important and can sometimes be provided by the fourth and fifth fingertips if they can reach beneath the mandible.

Proper mask technique overcomes problems with upper airway obstruction in almost all cases but there are special circumstances when mask ventilation may be especially challenging. Difficult mask ventilation is associated with beards, lack of teeth, older age, a history of sleep apnea, and known prior difficult laryngoscopy. One technique for overcoming the problem of a seal with beards is to apply a thin transparent adhesive film over the mouth and lower face, i.e., an Op-Site or equivalent plastic covering, and then to punch a hole through the center. The mask can then seal against the plastic. Another option is to use a surgical lubricant to compress the hair and permit a seal to the facemask. In the edentulous patient, leaving dentures in place is helpful for mask ventilation, but they should be removed prior to laryngoscopy.

When assistance is available for mask ventilation, extra hands should coordinate to improve the patency of the upper airway and not simply to squeeze the bag harder or push downward on the mask (Figure 5-4). Squeezing the bag too vigorously increases insufflation pressure and will lead to more gastric distention. Assistants can best help by providing a jaw thrust maneuver or by lifting up directly on the mandible and submandibular tissues (Figure 5-5). Extra hands can be used to create a better face seal, however, the lower part of the mask must never push the mandible downward.

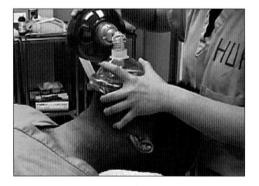

5-3 *"E-C" facemask ventilation hand position. "E" formed by 3rd, 4th, and 5th fingers, and "C" by 1st and 2nd digits.*

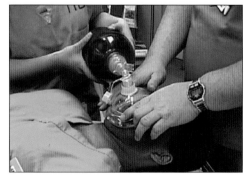

5-4 *Incorrect 2 person facemask technique pushing the mandible downward.*

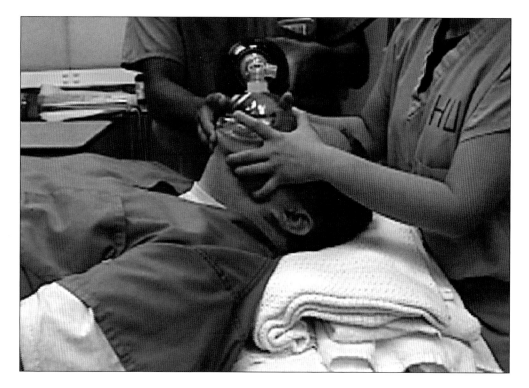

5-5 *Correct two person facemask technique with mask firmly applied to face but lifting mandible and submandibular tissues. Note the elevation of the head.*

Cricoid Pressure: Pros and Cons

Cricoid pressure is considered a standard of care when performing mask ventilation and RSI associated laryngoscopy. Cricoid pressure was first described by Sellick in 1961 to prevent aspiration, although its efficacy is largely unproven (Figure 5-6a–c).

In theory, application of downward pressure at the cricoid ring (with a recommended force of 20 Newtons) causes compression of the underlying esophagus and thereby prevents passive regurgitation of stomach contents. Unfortunately, it can have deleterious effects on both laryngoscopy and ventilation.

From a ventilation perspective, over aggressive cricoid pressure can cause tracheal compression and prevent ventilation or necessitate higher bag pressures. The vast majority of clinicians do not apply cricoid pressure correctly, either applying it at the wrong location or using excessive force. Even when cricoid pressure is correctly applied the esophagus is partially or completely lateral to the cricoid cartilage in approximately 50% of patients on CT examination. An excellent review of the literature on cricoid pressure and its effects on airway management is provided by Brimacombe (Brimacombe JR. Berry AM. Cricoid pressure. *Can J Anaesth*. 1997; 44:414-25.).

Cricoid pressure does not reliably protect against regurgitation in situations of poor mask ventilation technique and associated gastric distention. It is also frequently ineffective in high-risk

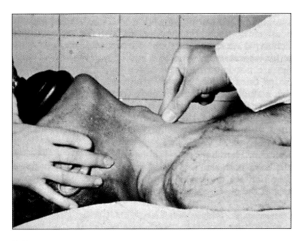

5-6a

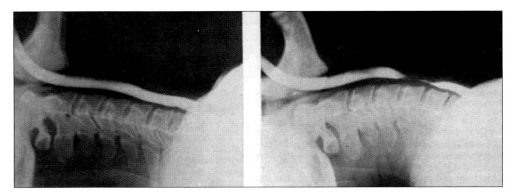

5-6b

5-6a *Original photograph of cricoid pressure from Sellick's 1961 article in the Lancet. Note lowered head position which Sellick recommended.*

5-6b *Radiographs of lateral neck with dye filled Penrose drain prior to application of cricoid pressure (left) and after application of cricoid pressure (right) showing indentation of dye column. (Reprinted from: Sellick BA. Cricoid pressure to control regurgitation of stomach contents during induction of anesthesia. Lancet 1961; ii: 404–6, with permission of Elsevier.)*

situations like complete bowel obstruction, in which nasogastric tube decompression should be done prior to RSI. In terms of patient safety, properly performed mask ventilation is the best way to prevent regurgitation, i.e., using low volumes delivered with low pressure and slow insufflation times.

It is the author's recommendation that RSI start with the application of cricoid pressure, but cricoid pressure should be released as needed to optimize laryngeal view and to allow for first pass intubation success. Cricoid pressure should also be lightened or released as needed to permit ventilation, assuming other aspects of ventilation have already been optimized (positioning, oral airway, mandible and submandibular elevation, etc.).

Decision Making About Repeat Laryngoscopy

Having addressed the technique of mask ventilation, we can turn our attention to decision making about the relationship of ventilation to repeat laryngoscopy. In the event of a failed laryngoscopy attempt, the decision about whether to temporarily suspend laryngoscopy efforts and bag the patient is dependent upon pulse oximetry readings and other clinical considerations. Individual laryngoscopy efforts should never exceed 15–30 seconds. Repeat laryngoscopy should never be initiated if the patient is hypoxic because if the subsequent attempt fails, a precipitous drop in saturation can trigger hemodynamic instability and catastrophe. The lag in pulse oximetry dictates that falling oxygen saturations need to be dealt with early. Even as ventilation is initiated, oxygen saturation on the monitor may transiently continue to fall, but this should improve within 60 seconds if ventilation is properly applied.

A proper dose of succinylcholine, i.e., 1.0–1.5 mg/kg IV, should permit at least three laryngoscopy attempts under good conditions. Beyond three of four attempts by an experienced intubator there is a declining likelihood of success and a greater risk of complications. A repeat dose of a neuromuscular blocker is rarely necessary and should be undertaken very cautiously. This decision should be based upon the patient's ventilation status and the perceived problem with the initial laryngoscopy attempts. Repeat succinylcholine dosing can cause profound bradycardia, although this is transient and responsive to atropine. Additional succinylcholine should not be considered unless the patient can be ventilated and well oxygenated. At that point, if laryngoscopy is to be reattempted, something significant should be changed that will likely result in laryngoscopy success. Most often this means changing the laryngoscopist.

Rescue Ventilation

The low rate of laryngoscopy failure, and the even lower rate of mask ventilation failure, means that rescue ventilation is rarely needed. Despite various predictive tests, however, unanticipated laryngoscopy failure can and does occur. Unfortunately, some of the patients predisposed to laryngoscopy failure will also have difficult ventilation. In operating room settings, combined inability to intubate and inability to ventilate leading to injury is estimated at fewer than 2 in 10,000 cases. This number predates widespread use and availability of the laryngeal mask airway, and so the actual incidence of "cannot intubate," "cannot rescue ventilate" is now significantly lower. Patient safety in RSI requires close attention to pulse oximetry coupled with proper mask ventilation techniques, and in rare instances, immediate availability of rescue ventilation devices.

In the author's experience, providers often underestimate how fast desaturation can occur during emergency airways and then fail to correctly provide mask ventilation in a timely manner. Assuming correct technique is applied, the rate of true failures of ventilation will be very low. Mask ventilation failure generally occurs due to faulty technique, not from abnormal pathology or patient characteristics that make mask ventilation impossible. In the exceedingly rare event of both laryngoscopy failure and true mask ventilation failure, the situation will be a crisis. Speed and simplicity are critical for any technique or device in these conditions. This is where the LMA and Combitube can be magical and life saving.

The LMA and Combitube overcome the problems associated with mask ventilation. Both devices can be inserted quickly, are relatively simple to operate with minimal prior experience, and transform the failed airway from a true emergency to an urgent but stabilized situation.

Laryngeal Mask Airway

The laryngeal mask airway provides a seal around the laryngeal inlet (Figure 5-7a, 5-7b), and is available in a variety of forms and sizes. One model is disposable (the LMA "Unique") (Figure 5-8), the standard model is reusable (LMA "Classic"), and a third model is specifically designed to allow for blind tracheal tube placement (the Intubating LMA, or "Fastrach"). There are three adult sizes of the device, and selection is based upon weight (30-50 kg = #3, 50–70 kg = #4, >70 kg = #5). A #4 LMA will be the proper size for most women and a #5 the proper size for most men.

To insert the standard or disposable LMA, the patient's neck should be flexed and the head extended, though less than would be done for laryngoscopy. Many different insertion techniques have been described. The recommended technique, however, is most likely to result in optimal positioning (Figure 5–9a–f). This technique involves completely deflating the device fully and pressing it against the hard and soft palate in a cephalad direction into the hypopharynx, until definite resistance is felt. Insertion can be from above the patient using the index and long finger of the dominant hand, or from alongside the patient using the thumb. Insertion is completed by using the non-dominant hand to continue cephalad pressure on the device, before the index finger or thumb is removed. Once advanced fully, the leading edge should be beneath the posterior cartilages in the upper esophagus. Inflate the mask without holding the tube; slight outward

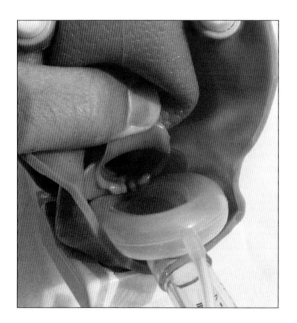

5-7a *Position of the LMA over the laryngeal inlet in an airway model.*

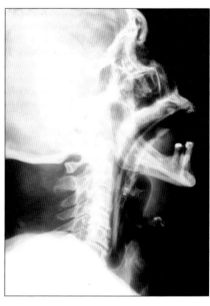

5-7b *Lateral neck radiograph showing LMA in position over laryngeal inlet.*

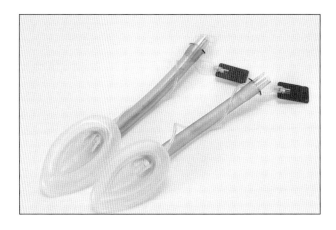

5-8 *LMA Unique sizes 5 and 4.*

movement is expected. Inflation of the mask varies from 20–40 cc, depending upon which of three adult sized masks (#3, #4, or #5), are used. Over-inflating the cuff is detrimental because it causes the LMA to slide upward out of proper position (no longer wedged into the upper esophagus). The best fit and seal pressures with the device actually occur with slight under-inflation of the cuff. In the anesthesia setting, the cuff is commonly inflated only until a seal is created, which can be verified by listening with stethoscope over the neck. Similar to a tracheal tube, the device is secured by tape to the patient's face and a bite block is inserted.

It is important that the leading edge of the LMA is not downfolded as it is placed. If this occurs, it may push the epiglottis downward and cause airway obstruction. This is prevented by correct deflation and positioning of the mask edge before insertion, and by directing the device posterior and downward (into the upper esophagus) throughout insertion. Lubricating the undersurface of the LMA mask enables it to glide easily down the posterior pharyngeal wall.

Two other simple techniques of LMA insertion include insertion with the device half inflated and using a malleable stylet. With the mask half inflated, the device can be inserted into the mouth upside down and then rotated around the tongue, similar to the original technique of placing an oral airway. Alternatively, a malleable stylet can be placed within the LMA (shaping it into a J shape like the rigid intubating LMA), so the device can be rotated down into position and the stylet removed. The stylet must not extend out of the distal portion of the LMA or it will injure the patient. The proximal section of the stylet should be bent to secure its position before inserting the stylet and the LMA into the mouth.

The LMA is easy to insert, even by non-skilled persons, and when used by novice airway managers it has much higher effective ventilation rates than a facemask or tracheal tube. Reluctance to use the LMA in emergency situations has centered around concerns over aspiration risk, as suggested by dye studies and pH probes in anesthetized patients. Other studies using similar methods have concluded that the LMA is protective. Proper LMA positioning is not critical for ventilation, but to prevent gastric insufflation and aspiration the device needs to overlie the laryngeal inlet and the distal tip must be wedged into the esophagus. Studies in cadavers have shown that a properly positioned LMA is an effective barrier at the upper esophageal sphincter. Additionally, a large clinical series in the operating room and a meta-analysis of 547 studies on the LMA have shown that the aspiration risk with the LMA in the OR is no different than with

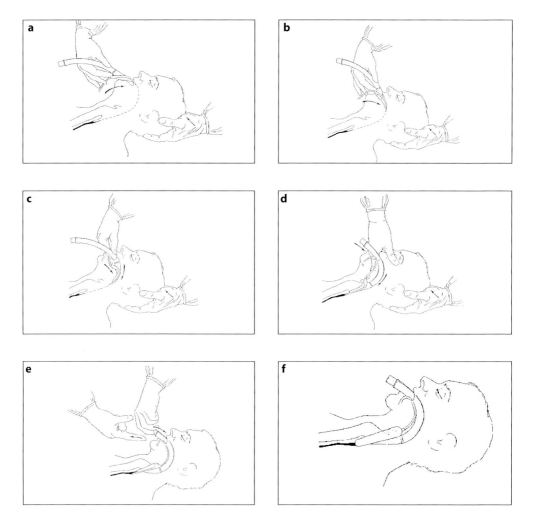

5-9a–f *Recommended LMA insertion technique. (Reprinted from: Brimacombe JR. The laryngeal mask airway: A review and practical guide, 1997, with permission of Elsevier.) See text for details.*

facemasks and tracheal tubes. Clinical studies have shown its efficacy as a rescue device for failed intubation and its utility in cardiac arrest. It is recommended for rescue ventilation in the American Society of Anesthesiology Difficult Airway Algorithm, along with the Combitube. In the ACLS guidelines, the LMA and Combitube are recommended for cardiac arrest above mask ventilation because of improved ventilation and less gastric distention, with less skill required to effectively ventilate.

When using the LMA in cardiac arrest and failed emergency intubation, it is important to understand the effects of cricoid pressure on LMA insertion and performance. Cricoid pressure causes compression of the upper esophagus and has been shown to prevent the LMA from fitting into the upper esophagus during insertion. This may negatively impact on ventilation and theoretically increases aspiration risk since the tip of the LMA may be superiorly displaced. The clinical significance of using cricoid pressure with the LMA in true "cannot intubate" conditions is unknown. It has already been noted that cricoid pressure can worsen laryngoscopy and if done with excessive force may prevent mask ventilation. Cricoid pressure has detrimental effects on LMA insertion and sealing the upper esophagus, and theoretically can worsen LMA ventilation.

Apart from the risk of aspiration, which as noted above appears to be low, rare complications reported with the LMA have included minor bleeding, hoarseness, sore throat, dysphagia, and case reports of injury to the recurrent, hypoglossal and lingual nerves.

Tracheal-Esophageal Combitube

The tracheal-esophageal Combitube has not one, but two inflatable balloons and two lumens (Figure 5-10a, Figure 5-10b). It is designed to seal the upper airway and isolate the tracheal and esophagus with one balloon in the esophagus and a second balloon in the pharynx (Figure 5-11). It is comparable to a tracheal tube in terms of gas exchange and oxygenation. The Combitube's combined ability to effectively ventilate and at the same time provide a full seal of the esophagus, thereby preventing aspiration, has made it useful in the management of failed airways and as a primary means of airway management in cardiac arrest.

Because the Combitube is designed for insertion into the esophagus, its use is contraindicated in hiatal hernia, esophageal pathology, caustic ingestion, and patients below four and a half feet tall. Patients must have no gag response to tolerate insertion. Rare instances of pneumomediastinum and esophageal rupture have been reported, and minor mucosal bleeding is not uncommon.

Early problems with the device have led to some significant changes from the original recommendations regarding its use. The first is that it now comes in two sizes: SA for small adult (size

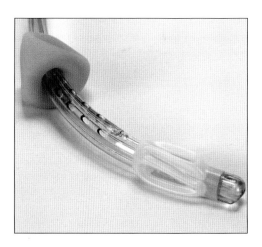

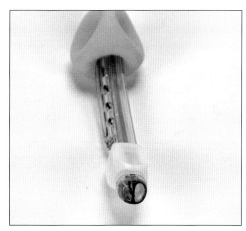

5-10a *View of Combitube ventilation holes (lumen #1) between esophageal balloon (white) and pharyngeal balloon (beige).*

5-10b *Close up view of Combitube tip showing lumen #1 (left side of tip, with ventilation holes between balloons) and lumen #2 (on right side).*

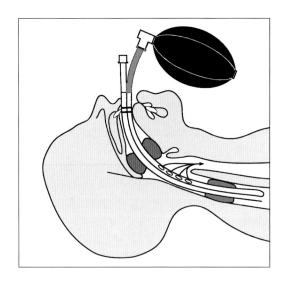

5-11 *Combitube in esophagus with ventilation of the trachea through lumen #1 (blue color).*

4.5–6 feet), and the original adult size, which the inventor now recommends only for patients taller than 6 feet. The smaller size (37 F vs. 41 F) increases the likelihood of successful first time placement. It is only slightly smaller in longitudinal dimension, but it is much more flexible (Figure 5-12). Several studies have used the smaller size in patients up to 6.5 feet and reported near universal success, unlike the original size, which had an insertion failure rate as high as 25%, even in the OR.

Although originally designed for blind placement in the mouth, a laryngoscope is useful for deliberately placing the device into the esophagus. Esophageal placement under direct vision with a laryngoscope, is also less likely to cause trauma to the posterior pharynx, hypopharynx, or larynx. It is important to appreciate that inadvertently placing the Combitube into the trachea (Figure 5-13) mandates that the clear tube (#2) must be used to ventilate the lungs or the patient will not be oxygenated. Unrecognized tracheal placement of the Combitube (and ventilating the wrong lumen) is equivalent to unrecognized esophageal placement of a tracheal tube. An esophageal intubation detector or end-tidal CO_2 detection device should always be used to verify ventilation of the trachea, i.e., Combitube location in esophagus with ventilation through lumen #1, in addition to the standard clinical signs.

To insert the Combitube: 1) each balloon should be checked and deflated, and the device well lubricated with water soluble jelly; 2) the SA size should be used for all patients less than 6.5 feet tall; 3) a laryngoscope or the non-dominant hand can be used to distract the jaw as the device is inserted until the heavy double line markings are at the dental line or alveolar ridge; 4) the two balloons and corresponding syringes are color coded blue and white, and well marked #1 and #2; the balloons are inflated sequentially with 85–100 cc, and 5–15 cc of air, respectively, depending on whether the SA or Adult size is used; 5) with inflation of the first balloon (oropharyngeal) the device may move slightly out of the mouth; 6) the distal balloon (esophageal) is then inflated; 7) ventilation is done through the first lumen (blue) and assessed with clinical signs and esophageal detection devices or CO_2 detection if available. The possibility of inadvertent tracheal intubation must be considered if ventilation through the first lumen is not successful. In this case, ventilation should be done through the second lumen (clear). If there is no leak from the pharynx (in which case add air to the pharyngeal balloon), and ventilation is not possible through either lumen, the device should be withdrawn 3 cm with the balloons deflated. The balloons should be re-inflated in order and ventilation attempted with

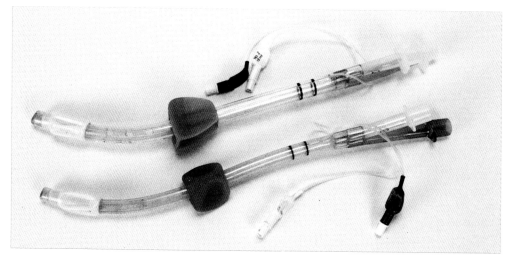

5-12 *41 F Adult size Combitube (above) and 37 F Small Adult size (below). Note color-coding of balloons and lumens and double line markings that line up with teeth or alveolar ridge when inserted.*

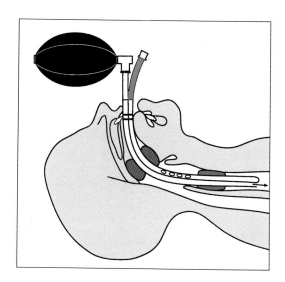

5-13 *Combitube in trachea with ventilation of trachea through lumen #2 (clear lumen).*

the blue (#1) lumen first. The oropharyngeal balloon may have caused the epiglottis to fold downward or may have been blocking the entrance into the trachea.

Compared to the LMA, the Combitube has several advantages and a couple of disadvantages. The advantages include isolation of the airway from the esophagus. Another advantage is that the stomach can be decompressed via the second lumen, assuming the device is inserted into the esophagus. The device comes packaged with a small nasogastric tube for this purpose. The Combitube has higher peak airway pressures and leak pressures compared to the LMA. The device stabilizes itself very well with the pharyngeal balloon, which is an important consideration in the pre-hospital setting. In terms of disadvantages, two lumens and two possible positions (esophagus or trachea) create the potential pitfall of ventilating the stomach. It is a more difficult task to convert the Combitube to a tracheal tube, unlike the LMA, that if properly positioned can serve as a conduit (often with a fiberscope) to the laryngeal inlet and larynx.

Trans-Tracheal Jet Ventilation

Trans-tracheal jet ventilation was once considered a standard option for ventilation in the failed laryngoscopy situation. It was listed among the acceptable approaches in the ASA Difficult Airway Guidelines in 1993 and for many years was routinely mentioned in ACLS texts. Trans-tracheal jet ventilation (TTJV) permits effective oxygenation and ventilation when used with a high-pressure oxygen source, passive exhalation through a non-obstructed upper airway, and appropriate I:E ratios. It provides no protection against aspiration, and definitive airway management requires intubation through conventional or surgical means.

For emergency rescue ventilation, TTJV is not now recommended because it has many potential drawbacks. Though inexpensive, it requires multiple pieces of specialized equipment, including specialized high-pressure tubing and a non-kinking catheter. The clinician must also have prior familiarity with its set-up and use. In upper airway obstruction, it can cause life-threatening barotrauma unless air egress is assured (it should always be used with oral and nasal airways). The combination of a thin lumen passing through the skin and the high-pressure jet coming from the end of the catheter makes TTJV inherently unstable. If the tip of the catheter is incorrectly placed outside the lumen of the trachea (in subcutaneous tissue or through the posterior tracheal wall), even one or two high-pressure ventilations may be lethal.

TTJV is established using a 14-gauge catheter that is placed through the cricothyroid membrane in a caudal direction. Air should be aspirated as the needle is inserted to verify the correct depth of placement. Although standard intravenous catheters can be used, such catheters can kink and make ventilation impossible. Catheters specifically designed for trans-tracheal ventilation are reinforced to prevent kinking, and have a gentle curve or a distal bent tip to facilitate insertion. Once inserted, the catheter must be manually stabilized throughout its use, otherwise dislodgment or subcutaneous inflation will occur.

Numerous different ventilation systems and equipment have been described for TTJV. The most efficacious of these systems are commercially pre-assembled systems comprised of high-pressure hoses, an in-line regulator, and a controllable valve switch. When a 14-gauge cannula is connected to wall oxygen at 50 psi, this type of system will have a 1 second tidal volume of 1600 ml. Accordingly, an inspiratory time of 0.5 seconds with an I:E ratio of 1:3 is recommended to prevent barotrauma and to allow for adequate exhalation.

Exhalation during trans-tracheal ventilation is a passive process through the mouth or nose. Oral or nasal airways are required to permit passive air egress. In cases of significant upper airway obstruction, trans-tracheal ventilation with a high-pressure oxygen source can quickly lead to lung distention, hemodynamic compromise, and barotrauma.

If specific equipment for trans-tracheal ventilation is not available, several different combinations of routine equipment have been described which can be connected through a 15 mm connector to a bag resuscitator. For example, a 5 cc syringe with a Luer lock can be attached to the 14-gauge catheter, and the tracheal tube connector from a size 8.0 mm ID tube can be fitted into the barrel of the syringe (with the plunger removed). This can then be attached to a bag resuscitator (in turn connected to 15 lpm oxygen tubing). This type of system permits oxygenation, but the slower inflation period limits time for exhalation and will not accomplish effective ventilation, and hypercarbia develops quickly. According to Benumof, in situations of complete airway obstruction, this type of lower pressure system may be advantageous for limiting barotrauma.

The efficacy of the LMA and TTJV in rescue situations was assessed in a study by Parmet involving more than twenty thousand OR cases. There were 25 cases of simultaneous difficulty with intubation and ventilation leading to saturation below 90%. The LMA successfully provided rescue ventilation in 16 out of the 17 instances in which it was used. The one LMA failure involved a large thrombus in the airway and ultimately required a surgical airway. The average oxygen saturation prior to the LMA was 80%. Subsequent to the LMA it was 100% in 15 of 16 cases, and 92% in the other. By comparison, even though TTJV was immediately available, it only worked in one of the three cases in which it was tried. The catheter kinked in one case and extra-tracheal insertion in the other case caused massive subcutaneous emphysema, bilateral pneumothoraces, and electrical mechanical dissociation with only one jet of air (delivered at 50 psi).

Transition to Rescue Intubation

Rescue ventilation allows the clinician to take a step backward and make a carefully considered judgment about how to proceed. In emergency airways, this most often means bringing in a different laryngoscopist or moving on to a rescue intubation technique. Because rescue intubation follows rescue ventilation, the transition to a tracheal tube is also a function of which rescue ventilation approach is being used to stabilize the situation.

In situations where mask ventilation is adequate but laryngoscopy cannot be accomplished, the full variety of approaches can be used for rescue intubation. Mask ventilation provides no aspiration protection, so proper ventilation technique must be adhered to in order to not distend the stomach and trigger regurgitation. As has been repeatedly mentioned, this includes small tidal volumes (6–7 cc/kg), delivered at slow speed, with use of oral and or nasal airways and lifting of the mandible and submandibular tissue to provide a patent airway.

The Combitube Following Failed Laryngoscopy

In the field situation, leaving the Combitube in place following failed laryngoscopy is an appropriate stopping point. Assuming oxygenation and ventilation have been achieved, aspiration is prevented by the esophageal balloon and the device is well stabilized for transport by the pharyngeal balloon. Within the time frame of almost any EMS system transport time, it may be best to leave well enough alone and let the emergency department place a tracheal tube in a more controlled setting with more resources. Depending upon the patient's mental status and muscular tone, the use of neuromuscular blockers may be required to prevent the patient from biting down or gagging.

The Combitube is also an appropriate stopping point in failed laryngoscopy and cardiac arrest, even in ED settings. If the patient is subsequently resuscitated, placement of a tracheal tube can be addressed once the situation has stabilized. In the interim, while the code is being run, the patient is receiving maximal therapeutic respiratory management. Prior studies with the Combitube have verified that oxygenation and ventilation in the cardiac arrest situation are equivalent to a tracheal tube. No studies have looked at the maximal length of time the Combitube can be left in place, but it should be considered a bridging device only, since the pharyngeal balloon can cause venous compression of the tongue.

In patients in whom the Combitube is placed and who then need placement of a tracheal tube, several options exist. Laryngoscopy after Combitube placement can be accomplished with the Combitube left in place and selective deflation of the pharyngeal balloon (Figure 5-14). This is recommended instead of withdrawing the device because of the risk of regurgitation. In the author's experience in cadavers, this is easier with a straight blade than with a curved blade. The smaller flange and smaller spatula of a straight blade is easier to insert with the Combitube in place. The straight blade also permits direct control of the epiglottis, which can be difficult to elevate indirectly with a curved blade while the Combitube is present. Laryngoscopy after Combitube placement is noticeably easier with the smaller version of the device, the 37 F SA size, compared to the 41 F Adult size.

While it may seem counterintuitive that laryngoscopy would be appropriate after initial failed laryngoscopy and subsequent Combitube placement, this situation may arise through a variety of scenarios. Initial failed laryngoscopy in the field could have been a function of difficult intubation conditions from numerous causes. With the patient in the ED, subsequent laryngoscopy efforts under better circumstances is usually warranted. This decision is also dependent upon how many prior attempts have been made and what type of blade was used, as well as on the experience of the pre-hospital provider.

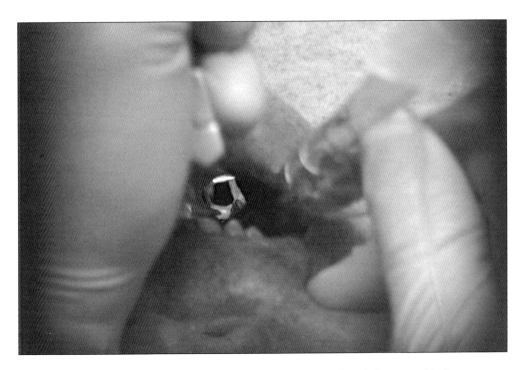

5-14 *Laryngoscopy using straight blade with Combitube inserted and pharyngeal balloon deflated.*

Other options for rescue intubation via the oral route around the Combitube involve the use of fiberoptic devices or a lighted stylet. After the patient has been well oxygenated, the pharyngeal balloon can be deflated and intubation attempted. In the author's experience, this is done most quickly and effectively with a rigid optical stylet. Assuming a Combitube can be inserted into the mouth, there is no particular reason to consider a nasal route for intubation. That said, it is probably easier to intubate with the flexible fiberscope via the nose than through the mouth because it is a less acute curvature. If flexible fiberoptic intubation via the mouth is attempted specialized oral airways for this purpose are very helpful. If efforts at oral intubation are unsuccessful, the balloon can be re-inflated and preparations made for a surgical or semi-surgical approach through the neck.

The Combitube can also provide continuous ventilation with both balloons up while a surgical airway is established. In practice this does not come up often. Surgical airways are most commonly needed in situations of the surgically inevitable airway, obstruction, and intrinsic laryngo-tracheal pathology. The Combitube, like any blindly inserted device, may worsen such situations, and it is not recommended in cases of distorted anatomy of the hypopharynx or larynx. Lastly, the Combitube can be used with a retrograde intubation approach, though wire retrieval from the mouth may be challenging around the tube and pharyngeal balloon.

Intubation Through the LMA

The LMA is unique as a ventilation device because of its ability to be used as a conduit for tracheal intubation. The intubating LMA (Fastrach) was specifically designed for this purpose, but the standard LMA can also be used for blind and fiberoptically guided intubation. When properly positioned overlying the laryngeal inlet, a tracheal tube can pass directly through the device into the larynx. The standard and disposable LMAs, however, have small aperture bars designed to prevent the epiglottis from falling backward into the lumen of the device. Because of these bars, and because of the relatively small lumen of the device, only a 6.0 tracheal tube can pass through a #3 or #4 LMA. Although the #5 LMA should accept a 7.0 mm tracheal tube, in the author's experience, this fits very tightly, particularly through the disposable LMA.

The technique for blind intubation through the LMA as recommended by Heath is as follows: 1) correctly position the LMA with mask inflated (slight under-inflation of the LMA, i.e., 10–15 ml may help); 2) position the patient in usual intubating position; 3) a well lubricated 30 cm long tracheal tube (previously checked for easy passage), is passed through the LMA lumen; 4) the tube is rotated 90 degrees counterclockwise as the tube passes into the glottis, and then allowed to rotate back to its normal position; and 5) the tracheal tube is inflated and the patient is ventilated. Rotation of the tracheal tube counterclockwise is beneficial because the bevel on a traditional tube is asymmetric (faces leftward as it is inserted). By rotating it counterclockwise, the bevel is directed downward, the leading edge is kept midline, and passage into the trachea is improved. Following intubation, the safest thing is to leave the LMA in place with the mask deflated. If it needs to be removed, a smaller or equal sized tracheal tube can be used as a pusher on the tracheal tube already in place to rotate out the LMA.

The length of the LMA and a standard tracheal tube also pose a problem for intubation. Only a few centimeters of tube will extend beyond the LMA because of the relatively long length of the proximal tube on the LMA. As has been pointed out by Osborne, with the disposable LMA, it is beneficial to shorten the length of the device so more of the tracheal tube can be passed through the distal part of the LMA and into the trachea.

The Intubating LMA, a.k.a. "Fastrach"

A modified version of the LMA, the intubating LMA or "Fastrach" (Figure 5-15), is specifically designed for blind placement of a tracheal tube through the device. Compared to the standard LMA, the device has a larger, rigid metal lumen with a sharper angle, and a metal handle that allows for more manipulation once placed. Instead of aperture bars over the lumen at the mask end of the device, there is an epiglottis elevating bar. This bar is pushed upward as a tracheal tube is passed, and it is designed to elevate the epiglottis away from the leading edge of the tracheal tube (Figure 5-16a–b). Because of its larger lumen it will accept up to a size 8.0 tracheal tube. The manufacturer supplies a custom-made straight silicone tracheal tube with a soft tip with the device. The rationale for this special tube is that blind insertion of a standard tube can cause trauma to the larynx. Additionally, standard curved tubes can exit out the lumen of the ILMA in the wrong manner and will not pass into the trachea (Figure 5-17a). This problem can be overcome by inserting a standard tube with the natural curvature upside down as it is placed into the ILMA, so that it exits in a straighter fashion out of the lumen of the ILMA (Figure 5-17b).

Like the standard LMA, the mask needs to be fully deflated before insertion. The device is rigid, so it must be rotated into position following its curvature. As with the traditional LMA, the goal is to keep the device along the hard and soft palate upon insertion so that the leading edge of the mask does not catch the epiglottis and cause downfolding. The handle can be used to keep the

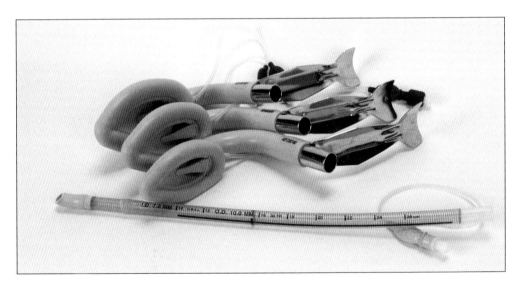

5-15 *Intubating LMA's (ILMA or "Fastrach"), sizes 3, 4 and 5 with specially designed Fastrach tube (7.0 mm ID wire-reinforced flexible tracheal tube with soft tip).*

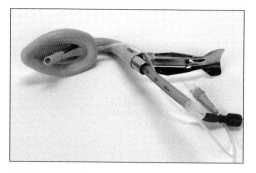

5-16a *ILMA showing lifting of epiglottis elevating bar as Fastrach tracheal tube advances.*

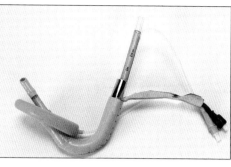

5-16b *Side view of specially designed Fastrach tracheal tube. Note tube tip exits straight out of device.*

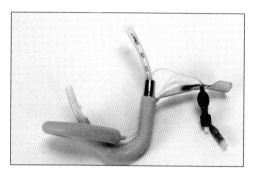

5-17a *Standard tracheal tube exits ILMA at wrong angle if inserted with curvature facing up.*

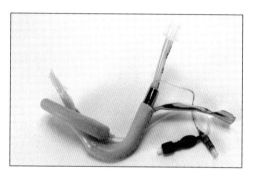

5-17b *Standard tracheal tube exiting ILMA at correct angle after tracheal tube was inserted with curvature facing downward.*

device midline and to finalize positioning. Once in place, the mask is inflated and ventilation assessed. After verifying ventilation, a very well lubricated tracheal tube is inserted directly down the lumen of the device to a depth of 26 cm. Ventilation through the tracheal tube should then be confirmed using end-tidal CO_2 detection and clinical signs of tracheal placement. To remove the ILMA, it is rotated out of the mouth while the tracheal tube is stabilized, with a special 20 cm long tube pusher. If the pusher is not available, a same size or smaller tracheal tube can be used for the same purpose.

If tracheal tube placement does not occur easily, the device can be readjusted and lifted by the metal handle. If this does not allow for easy tracheal tube placement, one of four problems may be present: 1) downfolded epiglottis; 2) ILMA too small; 3) ILMA too large, or 4) inadequate anesthesia or muscle relaxation. Repositioning with the handle, or partially withdrawing the device 6 cm and reinserting, may correct the downfolded epiglottis.

The ILMA's combined ability for emergency ventilation and immediate conversion to tracheal tube placement is unique among rescue airway devices. Early reports described near universal success of the device, but were from anesthesiologists who had pioneered the LMA and ILMA. Its utility in difficult airways has also been reported in the OR, and in case reports from the emergency department. Novice intubators have high rates of success using the ILMA on manikins and cadavers with minimum training. In an operating room study, however, although novices had high rates of successful ventilation, the ability to intubate was no better than with direct laryngoscopy. The ability to blindly intubate through the ILMA, as with through the regular LMA, is dependent upon proper positioning over the laryngeal inlet. In an ED study using the ILMA after nine failed laryngoscopies, blind intubation with the ILMA was possible in 2 cases, a retrograde wire technique was used in one case, and 5 of the other 6 required use of a flexible fiberscope.

The difference between reported OR and ED success with blind ILMA insertion could relate to capnography as well as to operator skill. If the ILMA is to be used for intubation, capnography provides feedback about the optimal location of the device prior to attempting tube passage. Among experienced ILMA users in the OR setting, the device has been shown to be comparable in efficacy to fiberoptic devices for intubation in a large multicenter trial of known difficult airways.

The ILMA, like the regular LMA, can be used with fiberoptic guidance, although in the author's experience, the sharp angle of the device can make it more difficult to use with a fiberscope than the regular LMA. If a fiberscope is used with the ILMA, the fiberscope should be used to check positioning of the mask over the tracheal inlet. It should not be used as a stent to place or remove the ILMA over the tracheal tube, as this may break the fiberoptic bundles. Other studies have also combined use of a flexible lighted stylet or bougie with the ILMA, but the primary issue with tube insertion into the trachea is proper position over the laryngeal inlet, not the use of additional adjuncts.

Although the use of the ILMA in unstable cervical fractures has been described, its safety remains to be defined. One cadaver study has suggested it causes significant pressure upon the cervical vertebrae.

Rescue Intubation Considerations

The choice of rescue intubation following failed RSI in emergency settings is dependent upon access to alternative devices, the skills of the care provider, and the availability of consultants, in addition to the characteristics of the patient and the cause of failed laryngoscopy. Whatever approach is used, it should be undertaken only after the immediate need for rescue ventilation has been addressed. Rescue intubation must be done expeditiously with continual monitoring of oxygenation. Specific devices and alternative means of intubation will be reviewed later, but some general comments about selection are included here.

There is no one device that can be expected to effectively deal with the myriad of potential airway problems common in emergency situations. For most patients, a few different rescue intubation options will be appropriate, and it is operator skill and experience, as well as device availability, that determine which should be selected. All clinicians who use RSI must have immediately available a few rescue intubation devices and the knowledge of how to use them.

Surgical airways are often appropriate in situations of failed laryngoscopy, especially in trauma patients or others who have a predictable long-term requirement for respiratory support. Surgical airways are most challenging in patients with short, fat necks, who cannot be optimally positioned. Unfortunately, this is also the subset of patients who desaturate the fastest, and in whom surgical airways take the longest time. Although the scalpel is inexpensive and widely available, technical competence is a requirement, as is the mental commitment to use it early. Few providers will obtain practice with the procedure on a non-embalmed cadaver, let alone actual patients. For providers uncomfortable with the open technique, the percutaneously placed cuffed Melker airway uses a Seldinger technique involving wire placement through the cricothyroid membrane, followed by passage of a dilator and a 5 mm cuffed airway. Retrograde intubation is appropriate for the patient in whom ventilation is feasible, but an open surgical airway is not a desired outcome. Although theoretically simple, a number of subtle maneuvers are necessary to make retrograde intubation successful.

Numerous rescue intubation options involve fiberoptic and video imaging. Fiberoptic and other imaging approaches are difficult to use when there is blood, secretions, or vomitus in the airway. In addition to cost and cleaning issues, such devices represent major commitments of educational training and routine use if they are expected to be successful in emergency cases when truly needed. It is impossible for any clinician to achieve competence with all available products. Flexible fiberoptic scopes are widely available and can be effectively used following LMA placement, but recognition of landmarks is sometimes challenging and often made more difficult by prior repeat laryngoscopy efforts. Tube passage through the ILMA is easier than through the standard LMA because of its wider bore, but it also has a sharper curvature that makes fiberoptic placement very difficult. In general, flexible fiberoptics often perform poorly following failed RSI laryngoscopy because of the challenges created by a supine patient with no muscular tone. In the study by Parmet involving failed laryngoscopy noted above, flexible fiberoptic intubation worked in only two of four cases in the OR. Interestingly, six cases of failed fiberoptic intubation in anesthetized patients were rescued using direct laryngoscopy. Compared to flexible scopes, rigid imaging devices have the potential for greater speed and ease of use in these situations.

In the author's opinion, the future of rescue ventilation and rescue intubation will involve even greater use of supraglottic ventilation devices that will serve as conduits for intubation. These disposable devices will be inexpensive and specifically tailored to tracheal tube passage. Some supraglottic ventilation devices will also have built-in fiberoptic imaging. Direct laryngoscopy using standard shaped blades will be augmented by fiberoptic imaging, either in the form of optical stylets, or as combined fiberoptic light and optical bundles attached to laryngoscopes. Such devices will be routinely incorporated into first pass laryngoscopy efforts and will seamlessly merge with current practice, minimizing even further the incidence of failed laryngoscopy. These novel solutions for oral intubation, however, will never completely eliminate the rare need for intubation through the nose or the emergent surgical airway.

Chapter 6

Laryngoscopy Overview

Educational Issues

Direct laryngoscopy for the purpose of intubation is a remarkably simple procedure to define: the tongue and epiglottis are distracted by a rigid blade to expose the larynx to direct vision.

Given its apparent simplicity, it is surprising that laryngoscopy is so difficult to learn and master. Novice intubators, whether in the operating room or less controlled settings, have a success rate in their first attempts below 50%. In a study of anesthesia trainees' skill acquisition, laryngoscopy skill did not plateau above a 90% success rate until 57 laryngoscopy attempts. The slow rate of skill acquisition has enormous public health implications for emergency medical systems given the need for a definitive airway in resuscitation. Most emergency care providers have little or no opportunity for operating room training. Practice on the newly deceased, though commonly done in the past, is now considered ethically unacceptable without specific family consent. The slow rate of skill acquisition, combined with limited training opportunities on actual patients, has contributed to the promotion of alternative airways for resuscitation, such as the laryngeal mask and tracheal-esophageal Combitube.

Ironically, the problem with direct laryngoscopy is not its overall success rate. Even in emergency settings, the failed laryngoscopy rate is well below 1%. Although the procedure can sometimes be difficult, and on rare occasions impossible, the real problem with laryngoscopy involves the rate of skill acquisition. Instead of examining the methods used for training and teaching, there has been an almost resigned acceptance that this situation is uncorrectable.

Problems with Manikin Training

For fifty years, practice on plastic manikins has been a ritualistic part of learning laryngoscopy. Equally ubiquitous in training settings and instructional texts is the two dimensional line drawing of the entire larynx. Each of these training tools has serious shortcomings and each, in its own way, effectively sabotages the novice laryngoscopist's understanding of the anatomy and the procedure.

Manikins present a single, idealized view of the critical laryngeal structures. There is a significant gap between what the trainee visualizes on a manikin and how the airway appears in a real patient. In a manikin, the tongue and epiglottis, molded and semi-rigid in structure, are distinctly separated from the posterior pharynx. The epiglottis is suspended anteriorly and superiorly away from the laryngeal inlet. Even before the laryngoscope is inserted, the tongue and epiglottis, the two structures central to laryngoscopy, do not behave as they do in a real person with no muscular tone. Distinguishing structures on a manikin is not a challenge. The manner is which they are molded keeps everything distinct. Laryngeal exposure on a manikin involves only finding the correct depth of insertion before lifting upward and forward. On a manikin there is simply no way to be lost in the "pink mush" of the upper airway.

In a person without any protective reflexes, the tongue and epiglottis are obviously not suspended upward and out of the way, but rather collapse backward, filling the hypopharynx and supraglottic space. The combination of saliva, compressible fleshy tissue, and the uniform erythematous hue of the upper airway mucosa all contribute in real patients to making the structures of the upper airway appear very similar under the bright light of a laryngoscope. The leap from manikin training to an actual patient is considerable. The novice has never seen the structures as they really appear, and has never had to separate critical structures.

The separation of structures with blade insertion and advancement is a significant step in actual laryngoscopy. The difficulties in discerning structures are compounded by the narrow area for visualization as the tongue flops around the laryngoscope blade. In actual laryngoscopy, these problems necessitate a methodical step-wise approach. As the laryngoscope is inserted, it should distract the tongue forward, lifting the base of the tongue so that the edge of the epiglottis is separated from the posterior pharynx. Only after the epiglottis has been identified should efforts to expose the larynx itself be initiated.

Comparatively, laryngoscopy on a manikin does not require a step-wise approach. Some instructors have even taught a laryngoscopy technique that uses full blind advancement of the laryngoscope and then retraction until the larynx drops backwards into place. This technique should never be performed on real patients. It works well in a molded plastic manikin where getting lost is not an issue and where there is no potential for injury to the posterior pharynx or esophagus. In humans, the blind insertion of a laryngoscope can cause a variety of upper airway injuries and often will not result in visualizion of the larynx.

Apart from the differences in the feel and structure of the tissues, manikins do not behave mechanically like real patients. The manikin does not bleed and the tissues do not get edematous as they are repeatedly manipulated. The soft tissue structures are not accurately attached and supported by the cartilaginous and bony structures. The shortcomings of manikins are especially evident when it comes to the epiglottis.

The most crucial aspect of curved blade laryngoscopy is indirect elevation of the epiglottis by pressure with the blade tip at the vallecula, causing the hyoepiglottic ligament to flip the epiglottis upward. On a manikin, this action is not realistic. In fact, the rubberized nature of the manikin's structures allows much more levering of the laryngoscope handle backward in order to elevate the epiglottis. When this maneuver is done on real patients, the blade tip falls out of the vallecula and the epiglottis falls downward into the line of sight. This difference in action using a curved blade may explain why novice intubators who have practiced on manikins commonly fail to use the correct force vector on the laryngoscope.

Limitations of Line Drawings

Idealized line drawings of laryngeal structures further exacerbate the problems of mastering laryngoscopy. The traditional view of the larynx supplied in most instructional texts is that of indirect laryngoscopy, looking down at the larynx from above (Figure 6-1). The laryngeal structures are superimposed upon one another and flattened out. This type of image provides no depth and provides no information about the relationship of the structures around the laryngeal inlet to the vocal cords and glottic opening. A cross-sectional view of the head and neck better shows the position and orientation of the epiglottis, but still does not adequately show the structures of the laryngeal inlet and the relationship to the vocal cords (Figure 6-2).

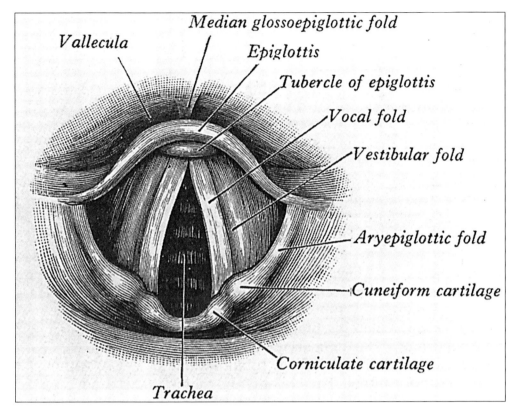

6-1 *View of indirect laryngoscopy from Henry Gray's Anatomy of the Human Body (1918). It is difficult to appreciate the three-dimensional nature of the structures about the laryngeal inlet or the distinction between true and false vocal cords. This view is also not representative of what is seen at direct laryngoscopy because this degree of full visualization almost never occurs.*

Drawings of idealized laryngeal views improperly suggest to the novice laryngoscopist that all of the structures shown will be visible. The tracheal rings, epiglottic tubercle, and the anterior commissure of the vocal cords, for example, are in fact rarely sighted during laryngoscopy.

Idealized drawings also contribute to an overall training emphasis on sighting of the vocal cords. The problem with this approach is that the vocal cords are often not well illuminated during direct laryngoscopy with curved laryngoscope blades. Shadowing of the vocal cords is caused by the position of the light source on the curved blade. When a curved blade is placed in the vallecula at the base of the tongue, the epiglottis is suspended between the light and the larynx. Depending upon how well the epiglottis is indirectly elevated, it can shadow the light directed at the inner larynx where the vocal cords are located.

Difficulties in Observation and Supervision

Apart from training tools, the slow learning curve of laryngoscopy is also related to the procedure itself. Even for those who have the opportunity to practice on actual patients, the educational experience from each individual case is limited by a number of factors.

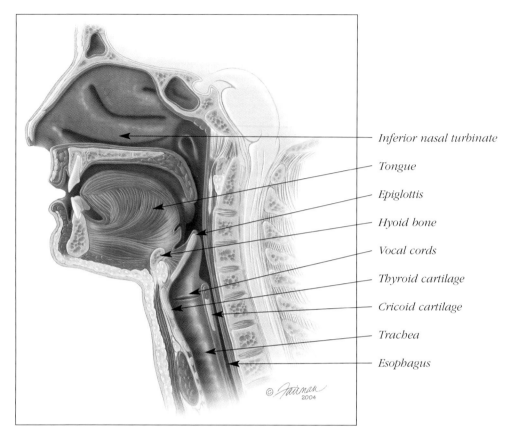

Inferior nasal turbinate

Tongue

Epiglottis

Hyoid bone

Vocal cords

Thyroid cartilage

Cricoid cartilage

Trachea

Esophagus

6-2 *Lateral cross-sectional view of head and neck showing vertical relationship of tongue, epiglottis, and vocal cords.*

Laryngoscopy, even in the elective OR setting, is a time dependent procedure. Patient safety demands that it be done quickly. This discourages repetitive laryngoscopy or manipulations simply for educational reasons. The actual sighting of critical structures during each laryngoscopy is usually less than 10 seconds. This type of brief visualization does not promote a detailed understanding of laryngeal anatomy.

The visual restrictions inherent to laryngoscopy make it impossible for two persons to simultaneously visualize the larynx. Observation of laryngoscopy is of little educational value to the trainee, unlike other major procedures in medicine that can be easily observed, since he or she cannot effectively see what is happening at the tip of the laryngoscope blade.

Visual restrictions also impact on the ability of a supervisor to provide feedback during the procedure. The lack of effective observation, and the subsequent inability to provide meaningful feedback or assistance, creates a difficult training environment for both supervisor and trainee. If the supervisor takes over the case, he or she is not able to effectively demonstrate the correct technique. Also, procedural errors made by a trainee are difficult for the supervisor to observe and correct.

The Lack of Imaging as a Contributing Factor to Poor Laryngoscopy Training

The final contributing factor to the slow learning curve of laryngoscopy relates to the lack of imaging from the operator's perspective. Although fiberoptic images of laryngeal anatomy have been commonly available for three decades, they are rarely used in intubation training materials and do not correlate with what is seen at laryngoscopy. The usual orientation of the larynx from the fiberscope is with the epiglottis at the bottom of the image and the posterior structures at the top. During laryngoscopy, this perspective is reversed; the epiglottis is at the top of the image and the posterior structures are at the bottom. Fiberoptic images of the larynx (Figure 6-3), like idealized line drawings, provide a more full view of laryngeal structures than laryngoscopy normally provides. For the novice intubator, fiberoptic images lack any familiar landmarks, such as the mouth, teeth, or tongue, and it is difficult to synthesize this view of the larynx with what is seen at laryngoscopy.

The Importance of the Laryngeal Inlet and Recognition of the Posterior Structures

Two aspects of laryngeal anatomy have been traditionally under-emphasized and yet are critical for mastering laryngoscopy. The first of these has to do with the concept of the laryngeal inlet. The second involves the interarytenoid notch, which is the dividing structure between the larynx and esophagus.

The larynx is a small cavity with the vocal cords and glottic opening positioned at its most inferior aspect. The structures that define the entrance of the larynx comprise the laryngeal inlet. These include the epiglottis, the aryepiglottic folds, the posterior cartilages, and the interarytenoid notch. The aryepiglottic folds and posterior cartilages are paired structures. The vocal cords and glottic opening are at the base of the laryngeal cavity. A drawing from the superior perspective (with the epiglottis retracted), using shadowing to denote depth, shows the vocal cords and glottic

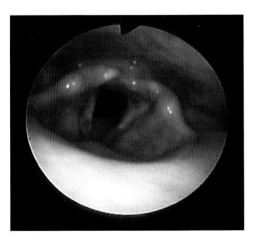 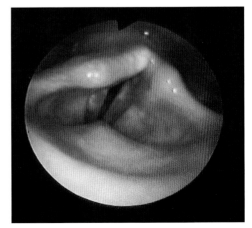

6-3 *Fiberoptic images of larynx obtained during nasoendoscopy. Epiglottis is at bottom of screen, posterior cartilages at top of screen. Vocal cords abducted during inspiration (left). Vocal cords adducted during phonation (right).*

opening visible at the base of the laryngeal cavity (Figure 6-4). This is more detailed than the line drawings that are typically shown, but even with shadowing, it is difficult to discern the laryngeal inlet as a distinct structure at a different level from the vocal cords.

From the posterior perspective, with dissection and reflection of the esophagus, the laryngeal inlet is easily appreciated (Figure 6-5). The vocal cords and glottic opening are not visible in this drawing since they are within the laryngeal cavity.

An oblique, posterior perspective with partial dissection permits the best appreciation of the laryngeal inlet and its positioning relative to the vocal cords (Figure 6-6a). From this perspective, the inlet can be seen as a ring of structures (inset Figure 6-6b) tilting downward and directed backward.

With the thyroid partially cut, it can also be appreciated that the vocal cords attach anteriorly at the thyroid cartilage. The cricoid ring is a complete circular structure, unlike the tracheal rings that are incomplete posteriorly. The relationship between the epiglottis and the hyoid bone is also visible in this drawing. The epiglottis is attached to the hyoid by the hyoepiglottic ligament. This structure is immediately below the vallecula, where the tongue and epiglottis meet. The vallecula is where the tip of the curved blade is placed in order to elevate the epiglottis indirectly. The relationship between the epiglottis and the hyoid bone, and the relationship between the thyroid cartilage and the vocal cords, will be reexamined later during the discussion on the use of the curved blade and external laryngeal manipulation.

The three dimensional nature of the laryngeal inlet can be well appreciated with the Glidescope video laryngoscope (Saturn Biomedical, Burnaby BC) (Figure 6-7). This device has a camera embedded into a plastic curved laryngoscope and effectively demonstrates the relative positioning of the structures about the laryngeal inlet and more deeply located vocal cords and glottic opening.

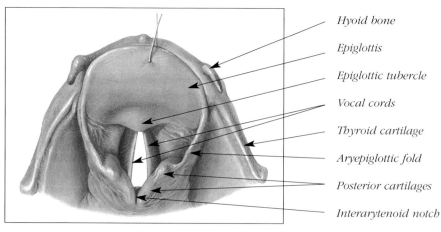

Hyoid bone

Epiglottis

Epiglottic tubercle

Vocal cords

Thyroid cartilage

Aryepiglottic fold

Posterior cartilages

Interarytenoid notch

6-4 *Drawing of larynx with epiglottis retracted. Hyoid bone and epiglottis are at top of image (anterior) and posterior cartilages and interarytenoid notch at the bottom of the image. Lateral are the laminae of the thyroid cartilage. (From LifeART, copyright 1998, Lippincott, Williams & Wilkins. All rights reserved.)*

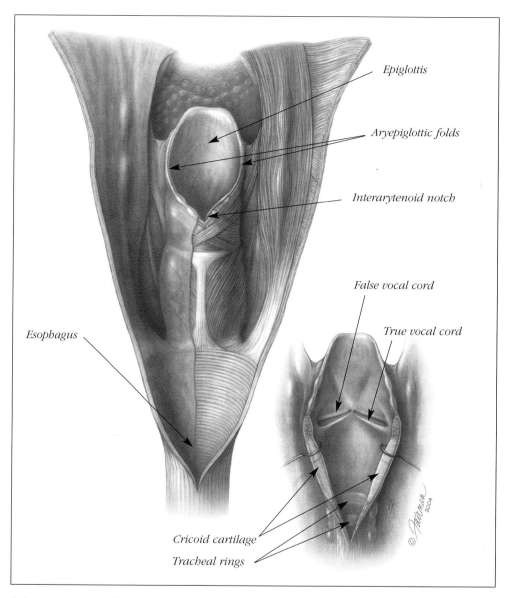

Epiglottis

Aryepiglottic folds

Interarytenoid notch

False vocal cord

True vocal cord

Esophagus

Cricoid cartilage

Tracheal rings

6-5 *Posterior view of laryngeal inlet and hypopharynx with retraction of cervical esophagus. Right side of image shows underlying musculature. Base of tongue can be seen behind epiglottis. Inset image below, right, shows inner larynx and vocal cords after cricoid cartilage has been bisected and retracted.*

Illumination and Visualization of the Vocal Cords During Laryngoscopy

The position of the vocal cords within the cavity of the larynx and their location inferior (caudal) to the structures of the laryngeal inlet explains in part why the true vocal cords may be shadowed and poorly visible during laryngoscopy. When a curved blade is used, the epiglottis is

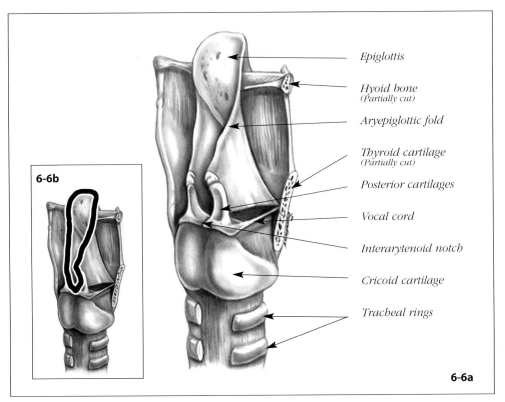

6-6a *Oblique perspective of larynx with partial removal of right side of thyroid and hyoid cartilages and view within inner larynx showing true vocal cords. The hyoepiglottic ligament connects the epiglottis to the hyoid. The large posterior aspect of the cricoid ring is immediately below the posterior cartilages. Beneath the cricoid are the incomplete tracheal rings.*
6-6b *Structures about laryngeal inlet marked by bold black line. These include epiglottis, aryepiglottic folds (bilaterally), posterior cartilages (bilaterally), and interarytenoid notch.*

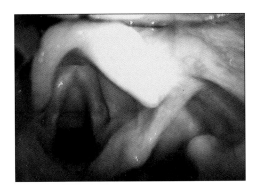 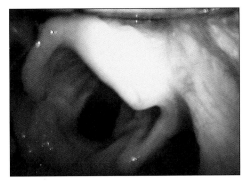

6-7 *Images of larynx and laryngeal inlet from Glidescope videolaryngoscope (Saturn Biomedical, Burnaby BC). The epiglottis forms a hood covering the deeper structures of the larynx. The vocal cords and glottic opening are the deepest structures within the larynx. The curvilinear structure lateral to epiglottis on right side of image is the pharyngoepiglottic fold. The tip of the Glidescope is in vallecula and at the top of image. Light from the blade is coming from above the epiglottis. The inner larynx is shadowed by the epiglottis.*

positioned between the light source and the larynx (Figures 6-7, 6-8). The degree of epiglottis elevation, the positioning of the light source on the laryngoscope blade, and the intensity of the light all contribute to how well the larynx is illuminated.

The true vocal cords are located inferior (caudal) to the false vocal cords that are sometimes labeled as the vestibular or ventricular folds. The distinction between the true and false vocal cords is clearly seen on stroboscopic images of the larynx (Figure 6-9). The true cords have a distinctive white appearance, whereas the false cords have the same appearance as the rest of the mucosa of the larynx. The false cords lie superior and lateral to the true cords. Beneath the false vocal cords, and between the false and true vocal cords, is a small recess, called the laryngeal vestibule or ventricle. The positioning of the true and false cords and their relationship to other laryngeal structures can be appreciated in a coronal cross-sectional perspective (Figure 6-10).

During direct laryngoscopy, the visibility of the true vocal cords is also affected by the muscular tone of the patient. The vocal cords adduct, or close, during phonation, and abduct, or open, during inspiration. Laryngoscopy is a strong gagging stimulus. Unless the patient has been given neuromuscular blocking agents for intubation or is deeply comatose or moribund, laryngoscope blade insertion and manipulation will cause vocal cord adduction. Another factor affecting the degree of vocal cord adduction is the upward lifting force from the laryngoscope tip, which also causes vocal cord adduction.

Stroboscopic, fiberoptic and videographic images of the larynx provide remarkably detailed and close-up images of laryngeal anatomy from within the mouth. By comparison, the view during direct laryngoscopy is visually analogous to looking down a small pipe, approximately 12 to 18 inches, at a target the size of your thumbnail. Recognition of laryngeal structures from this more challenging perspective is essential for mastering direct laryngoscopy.

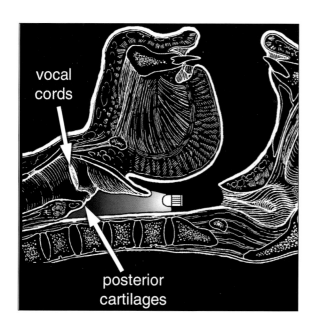

vocal cords

posterior cartilages

6-8 *The epiglottis is located between the light source on a curved blade and the larynx. This contributes to poor illumination of the inner larynx and true vocal cords. Conversely, the posterior cartilages and interarytenoid notch are almost always well illuminated during curved blade laryngoscopy even if the vocal cords cannot be seen. (Modified from LifeART, copyright 1998, Lippincott, Williams & Wilkins. All rights reserved.)*

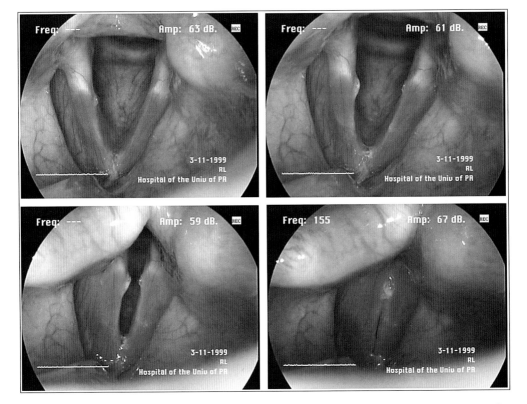

6-9 *Stroboscopic images of the larynx showing full abduction (top left) and full adduction with phonation (bottom right). The distinction between the true and false vocal cords is well delineated. The true cords are the vocal ligaments and change position during phonation. The false vocal cords are a mucosal fold lateral to the true vocal cords. The epiglottic tubercle is at the bottom of the image and the blurred curvilinear structure is the epiglottis edge. At the top of the image are the posterior cartilages and the interarytenoid notch. The cartilages come together with phonation and cause the notch (defined by the space between the posterior cartilages) to change appearance from a broad gap in the top left picture to a vertical slit in the bottom right.*

The Interarytenoid Notch

The significance of the interarytenoid notch is that this structure is the most posterior (and inferior), aspect of the laryngeal inlet (Figures 6-3, 6-5, 6-6a). At laryngoscopy, the interarytenoid notch is the dividing structure between the larynx and the esophagus. The larynx is anterior (above) the interarytenoid notch and the esophagus is posterior (below) the interarytenoid notch. During vocal cord and posterior cartilage adduction, the interarytenoid notch is a small vertical cleft created by the close approximation of the posterior cartilages. With full relaxation and vocal cord abduction, it is a broad, almost flat ridge, between the laterally displaced posterior cartilages located on either side.

The interarytenoid notch is a visual landmark that can be useful for determining the location of the glottic opening and vocal cords, even when these latter structures cannot be directly seen. This occurs commonly during curved blade laryngoscopy because of problems elevating the epiglottis. It also occurs frequently when head positioning cannot be optimized, such as in cervical

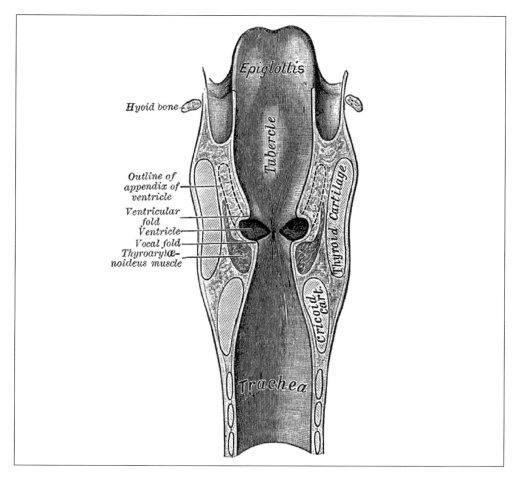

6-10 *Henry Gray's Anatomy of the Human Body (1918) drawing of laryngeal structures in coronal plane. Dark round structures at narrowest portion of larynx comprise the paired laryngeal ventricles created by the gap between the true vocal cords (vocal folds) and the false vocal cords (ventricular folds). Lateral to the epiglottis is the piriform recess on each side.*

spine immobilization. Recognizing the interarytenoid notch and directing the tip of the tracheal tube anterior to the notch, usually permits intubation even in instances of poor laryngeal view.

Historical Perspective

Laryngoscopy has changed little since Kirstein reported successful direct visualization of the larynx using his "autoscope" in 1895 (Figure 6-11). Awake diagnostic laryngoscopy, without the benefits of modern anesthetic agents, required meticulous attention to proper technique and positioning. The discoveries made by these early pioneers have relevance today for facilitating laryngeal exposure in difficult cases.

Fifty years before Kirstein's report, Czermak used external laryngeal manipulation to improve laryngeal exposure during indirect or mirror examination of the larynx. As noted above, the vocal cords attach anteriorly at the thyroid cartilage. Images of Czermak from the 1850s show the use of a two-handed technique, with one hand holding a small mirror inside the mouth and aimed at the larynx, and the other hand pushing the thyroid cartilage backward to bring the larynx into better view (Figure 6-12).

External Laryngeal Manipulation (Bimanual Laryngoscopy) and Direct Laryngoscopy

Shortly after the turn of the century, using ether anesthesia, patients were placed into a supine position for laryngeal surgery. Killian designed a laryngoscope that could permit suspension of the patient's head with the mouth open and the larynx exposed. This allowed the surgeon to have two free hands for operative procedures. In order to maximize laryngeal exposure, in 1911 Brunning invented a "counter-pressor attachment" that was connected to the laryngoscope and mechanically applied pressure to the thyroid cartilage (Figure 6-13). This device drove the larynx downward into the surgeon's line of sight. In the 1920s and 1930s, Chevalier Jackson, one of the pioneers of laryngoscopy in the United States, described two-handed laryngoscopy techniques for diagnostic purposes, as well as for the insertion of breathing tubes.

The utility of external manipulation of the larynx remains today. It is perhaps the single most useful technique for facilitating laryngeal exposure during intubation. Bimanual laryngoscopy, i.e., the laryngoscopist using his or her right hand to improve laryngeal view while the left holds the

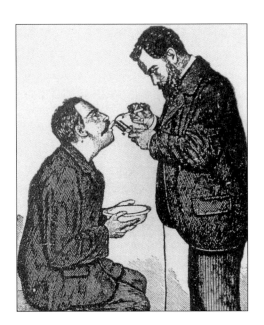

6-11 *Alfred Kirstein performing awake direct laryngoscopy with "autoscope" in 1895. Note the position of the patient's head and neck.*

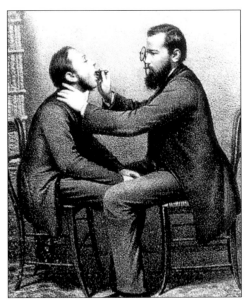

6-12 *Johann Czermak in 1865 using intraoral mirror for indirect laryngoscopy. Left hand is manipulating thyroid cartilage to improve laryngeal view.*

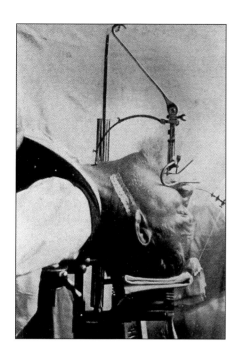

6-13 *Brunning's counter-pressor attachment with Killian's suspension laryngoscope, circa 1911. Killian did not appreciate that head elevation improves laryngeal view, an idea later advocated by Chevalier Jackson.*

laryngoscope, will be discussed in detail later in this text. Modern day laryngeal surgery also uses external manipulation, but with a rubber cushion to improve laryngeal exposure. The cushion is placed over the patient's thyroid cartilage and secured in place and pushed backward by cloth tape attached to the operating table.

In addition to external laryngeal manipulation, the pioneers of laryngoscopy focused on two other aspects of laryngoscopy that remain remarkably applicable to modern day emergency airway management. The first of these involved a slow methodical insertion of the laryngoscope using progressive visualization of landmarks. The second aspect of the procedure that received a great deal of attention was correct patient positioning.

Progressive Visualization of Landmarks

Progressive visualization of landmarks emphasizes the consistent relationship of critical structures, and it is the best means of ensuring first pass intubation success. Jackson described the technique of laryngoscopy as being comprised of three stages. The first was identifying the edge of the epiglottis, the second involved tilting the blade and advancing the tip under the epiglottis, and the third stage involved increased lifting to expose the larynx. Although Jackson used a straight tubular laryngoscope, the technique is essentially the same with modern-day straight blade designs. With a curved blade the tip of the blade is positioned into the vallecula, and the epiglottis is lifted indirectly by pressure on the hyoepiglottic ligament. Proper use of any blade, however, still depends upon knowledge of where the tip of the blade is located. Without progressive visualization, i.e., identifying the epiglottis first, it becomes very difficult to know where in the mucosal folds of the upper aerodigestive tract the blade are located, and accordingly, it is difficult to plan a response to poor laryngeal view.

Historical Origins of Laryngoscopy Positioning

The other area of focus for the early pioneers of laryngoscopy was proper positioning of the patient so as to maximize laryngeal exposure. For diagnostic purposes it was necessary to visualize the anterior commissure of the vocal cords, since many pathologic conditions occur at this location. The pictures of Kirstein and even those of Czermak show the patient sitting upright in what is now commonly referred to as "sniffing" position with the neck flexed and the head extended. Practitioners experimented with different head and neck positions as laryngoscopy changed to a procedure performed with the patient supine.

In 1909 Richard Johnston described supine laryngoscopy in five patients, keeping the head straight and the neck flexed on the chest and improving laryngeal view by the placement of a small pillow under the head. That same year Chevalier Jackson used radiographs of the chest and neck to illustrate the importance of raising the head, and keeping the cervical spine "strongly inclined forward," so that the axis of "peroral bronchoscopy" correlated with the axis of the trachea both in the neck and the thorax.

In his 1915 text on Peroral Endoscopy and Laryngeal Surgery, Jackson reiterated the significance of head elevation: "Whether the head is flexed or extended or kept midway, the fundamental principal of all positions is the anterior placement of the cervical spine." Jackson's classic textbook on Bronchoscopy, Esophagoscopy and Gastroscopy included drawings on proper positioning and specifically recommended the 10 centimeters of head elevation above the level of the table (Figure 6-14). In cases of poor laryngeal view Jackson commented, "the lifting motion and elevation of the head should be increased." In his discussion of difficulties with direct laryngoscopy he cited: "Over extension of the patient's head is a frequent cause of difficulty. If the head is held high enough extension is not necessary, and the less the extension the less muscular tension there is in the anterior cervical muscles."

Progressive visualization of landmarks, external laryngeal manipulation, and head elevated laryngoscopy position, each of which have their origins dating back more than a hundred years, are as valuable today as when they were first discovered. For the pioneers of the procedure, proper technique was critical for effective diagnostic laryngoscopy. Direct laryngoscopy is now done primarily for intubation, but these same techniques can help maximize first pass intubation success.

Ocularity and Mechanics of Laryngoscopy

A lack of appreciation of how the larynx is sighted and the impact of operator positioning and posture are additional issues facing the novice intubator. They have been essentially ignored in instructional guides, yet must be addressed by every laryngoscopist. It is appropriate that they be identified upon initial training.

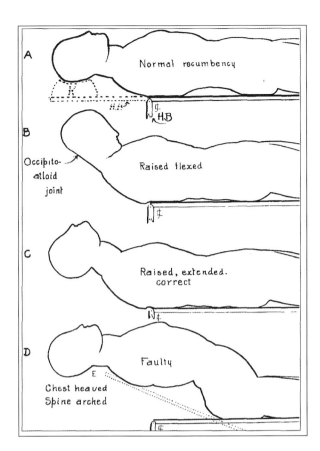

6-14 *Chevalier Jackson's comparison of various head and neck positions for direct laryngoscopy, circa 1915. Note the degree of head elevation in his "Raised, extended, correct position."*

Ocularity of Laryngoscopy

Target visualization at the level of the larynx is a monocular task. Textbooks routinely state that the left arm should be held straight out so that the head is held far enough back that a binocular view of the target is achieved. This does not happen, and in fact, the lack of attention to monocularity probably inhibits faster acquisition of the skill.

New trainees at intubation routinely rotate their heads from side to side when trying to perform laryngoscopy and sight the target. It becomes evident observing this that they are trying to figure out which eye to believe, since the view from the right and left eye are too dissimilar to be fused.

Normal stereoscopic sight involves the right and left eye having a slightly disparate view of a target. The minor difference between the images received by the left and right eye permits the brain to construct a 3-dimensional image of the target. With laryngoscopy, however, the procedure is analogous to looking down a pipe from a distance of 12–18 inches. The "pipe" is created not only by the laryngoscope blade, but also by the tongue and mouth that collectively create a narrow viewing area. The visual restrictions inherent to the procedure prevent simultaneous sighting of the target by both eyes. Without simultaneous sighting of the target the images from the left and right eye cannot be fused and stereoscopic sight cannot occur. Binocular suppression occurs subconsciously. The brain ignores the visual input from the non-dominant pupil even if both eyes are open. The same thing happens when you keep both eyes open and look through a peephole or shoot at a target.

The vast majority (>80%) of persons sight the larynx with their right eye. This is because laryngoscope blades have a left-sided flange, laryngeal view is mostly down the right paralingual space, and also because the vast majority of persons are right eye dominant (eyedness follows handedness in about 98% of people). Persons with left eye dominance tend to either be left-handed or wear glasses or have noticeably worse short range vision with the right eye. A very few individuals, far less than 1%, can equally use both eyes for short-range tasks. If you are not cognizant of which eye you use, it will become very apparent by sighting the larynx and, while keeping your head still, alternatively closing one eye and then the other. When you close your dominant eye, the view of the larynx disappears and instead, the view that is normally suppressed from the other eye appears.

This information is useful for novice intubators to appreciate upon initial instruction. Since most physicians are not routinely tested for visual performance at short-range, the impact of unrecognized poor short-range vision is not known. In the author's experience, many novices who wrestle with laryngoscopy initially, moving their heads about and assuming off center and tilted head positions, seem to have a longer learning curve for the procedure. Adjustments and alterations in head and body position seem to detract from being able to focus on manipulations about the tip of the blade. Experienced laryngoscopists know through practice, even if not through conscious awareness, how to sight and position themselves to focus on manipulations about the blade tip and other interventions that improve view.

Operator Positioning and Posture

Which eye is used for sighting and the manner in which the operator's head is positioned also affects how the operator positions himself or herself in relation to the patient. Ideally, the laryngoscopist should have his or her shoulders parallel to the patient's shoulders. The operator's head should be positioned relatively straight, facing forward, and not significantly tilted or rotated to one side or the other. Note that left eye dominant laryngoscopists tend to rotate their heads slightly to the right (the patient's right as well) (Figure 6-15), because this brings the dominant pupil closer to the target and widens the field of view, especially down the right side of the patient's mouth. Without making this compensation, the left-sided flange of the laryngoscope would somewhat restrict vision. Right-eyed laryngoscopists do not need to compensate for this, because standard left flanged laryngoscopes create a larger visual field down the right side, especially at the right corner of the mouth. Right-eyed laryngoscopists keep their heads straight relative to the patient (Figure 6-16).

The height of the patient relative to the laryngoscopist is also relevant. Traditional instruction is that the patient's stretcher should be elevated until it is at the level of the operator's xiphoid. While this approach eliminates the need for the laryngoscopist to bend over, it does not allow the clinician to elevate the head higher in case of poor laryngeal view. As will be addressed under laryngoscopy technique, increasing head elevation is an effective and easy to apply intervention that can significantly improve laryngeal view. If the patient is initially elevated to the level of the xiphoid, additional lifting in case of poor laryngeal view becomes difficult or impossible.

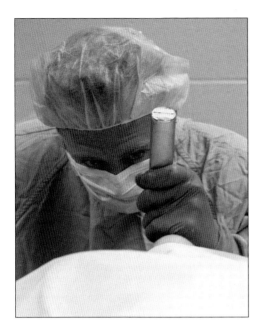

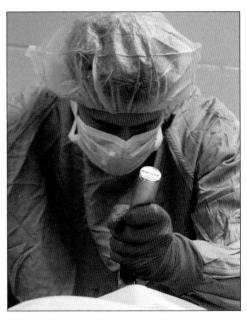

6-15 *Left eye dominant laryngoscopist. Note slight head rotation toward right side (nose pointed slightly to right) so that left eye is closer to target.*

6-16 *Right eye dominant laryngoscopist keeps head straight relative to target.*

Holding the Laryngoscope

Another commonly ignored aspect of laryngoscopy technique has to do with biomechanics, specifically, how the left hand grips the instrument. The handle should be gripped from the base so that the hypothenar eminence, i.e., the base of the palm on the ulnar aspect of the wrist, is at the base of the handle and proximal end of the flange (Figure 6-17). The handle is gripped by the second, third, and fourth fingers primarily. The thumb is less involved with gripping and does not fully wrap around the handle, but is directed more upward. Holding the handle higher up or completely wrapping the fingers and thumb around the handle does not provide the best leverage on the handle or the blade tip (Figure 6-18). The main force vector with laryngoscopy is directed longitudinally down the forearm using lift provided by the triceps and extension at the elbow. By gripping the handle low, the laryngoscope blade lines up better with the forearm.

While some texts have promoted the idea that the arm should be completely straight, this does not provide mechanical advantage and it places the laryngoscopist's eye very far from the target. As already noted, binocular view is a myth. Operating as far from the target as possible is not helpful, even if getting extremely close to the patient's mouth is not desired. A mid-range position with the elbow at approximately 90 degrees seems to be the most comfortable and effective. If the elbow is kept close to the body and the handle gripped as described, force can be increased along the blade simply by leaning inward, thus relieving much of the need for forearm and shoulder straining (Figure 6-19 and 6-20). Minor movements at the tip of the laryngoscope blade, both in terms of force and vector orientation, can cause marked changes in laryngeal exposure. Properly gripping the handle and holding the arm as described facilitate fine control of the blade tip.

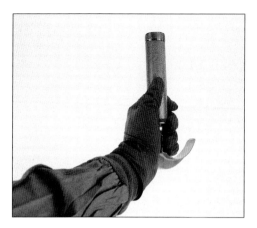

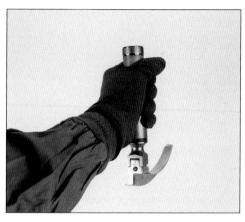

6-17 *Correct grip of laryngoscope low down on the handle, with thumb pointing upward.*

6-18 *Incorrect grip of laryngoscope high on the handle requires significantly more work to create same lifting force and pressure at the hyoepiglottic ligament.*

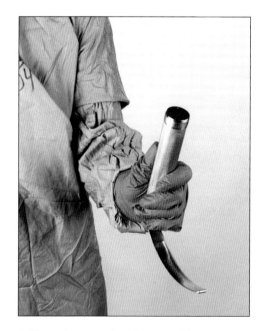

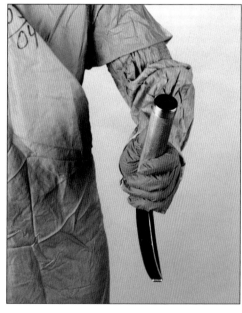

6-19 *With proper hand grip and keeping elbow close to torso, it is easy to transmit force along forearm and to blade tip, making effective use of instrument without straining.*

6-20 *Elbow out strains the arm and increases operator work.*

Direct Laryngoscopy Imaging: The Airway Cam™

Sophisticated imaging of laryngeal structures has been possible through fiberoptic and other imaging technologies for more than 30 years. In the 1980s, several different academic anesthesiologists reported attaching a fiberscope to a laryngoscope to observe how trainees placed the tip of the blade and to confirm intubation. While such a marriage of devices achieves this goal, it does not provide a view of what the laryngoscopist is seeing, and instead provides an intraoral view of laryngeal structures. Imaging from the perspective of the operator cannot provide the same diagnostic quality that a fiberscope or stroboscope can, and it does not add anything in terms of tracheal tube placement in challenging cases. For teaching and documenting laryngoscopy, however, capturing the perspective of the operator is very useful.

Imaging of direct laryngoscopy from the perspective of the operator requires placing a camera within the line of sight of the dominant pupil. The Airway Cam™ Direct Laryngoscopy Video System (Airway Cam Technologies, Inc., Wayne PA) uses a head-mounted miniature video camera that has been optically aligned with the dominant pupil. This alignment occurs through a beam-splitting penta-prism wedge assembly (Figure 6-21). Approximately 50% of the light passes straight through the prism to the operator's eye. The glass prism also serves as a targeting mechanism for the laryngoscopist. By consciously sighting through the prism, the operator can ensure that the camera will display what he is seeing. The other 50% of the light from the target is reflected through the penta-prism to a vertically mounted miniature video camera. Passing through two reflections and a 90 degree change in orientation before reaching the camera, the target image arrives at the camera right-left correct. The camera and prism assembly is mounted on a headset that allows adjustment for right and left-eyed laryngoscopists (Figure 6-22). The other components of the direct laryngoscopy video system are a camera cable and a camera control unit. The cable is wrapped in Kevlar for protection and durability. The control unit permits modification of aperture and white balance, allowing for variation in laryngoscope light.

The Airway Cam is easy for experienced intubators to use, but novices sometimes have problems because of the added burden of sighting through the prism during a procedure that is already stressful. Apart from practicing on manikins and reviewing the operator's ocular dominance, head position, and body posture beforehand, it is helpful to have the trainee go from landmark to landmark as a reminder to continuously sight through the prism. Typically this involves first sighting the patient's nose, then the uvula, the posterior pharynx, etc. and continuing until the glottic opening is exposed. If sighting is done incorrectly, the operator may have an adequate laryngeal view, but the supervisor will not see this on the video monitor.

Because of the requirements for fine positioning of the sighting mechanism, and because it does not add anything to actually placing the tracheal tube, the author has avoided use of the device by trainees in the emergency setting. It has worked well in the OR for about 90% of residents who have worn the device, and has permitted documentation of their airway experience. Supervisors have generally liked being able to see what the operator is seeing, but this has been a function of the resident's skill at properly sighting the target. The other effective use of the device is for video documentation of laryngeal view. This has been an essential aspect of the author's research on laryngoscopy techniques.

The most valuable educational contribution of the Airway Cam has been the imaging itself, not the use of the device per se. All residents in the author's institution watch Airway Cam

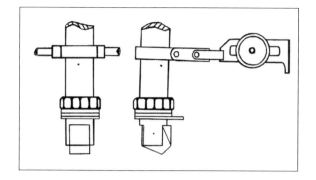

6-21 *Drawing of the Airway Cam™ Direct Laryngoscopy Video System (Airway Cam Technologies, Wayne PA) showing beam splitting penta-prism wedge assembly at end of vertically oriented camera tube.*

videotapes of laryngoscopy prior to their OR rotation, and this has markedly improved their comfort level with the procedure. The author has also shown that using video imaging as a teaching tool resulted in higher initial intubation success by paramedic students. There are currently four Airway Cam videotapes commercially available (www.airwaycam.com).

Sending the trainee to the OR having never effectively seen laryngoscopy (i.e., looking over a shoulder or using a manikin as a visual reference) has been the traditional approach to training and is a prescription for poor initial performance. This erodes the trainee's confidence and stresses the relationship with anesthesia supervisors. Video imaging of the procedure permits the trainee to instantly recognize critical structures and more effectively communicate this to supervisors. Instead of trial and failure (manikin and line drawing teaching), video imaging as an integral part of teaching is better for the patient, better for the supervisor, and better for the trainee.

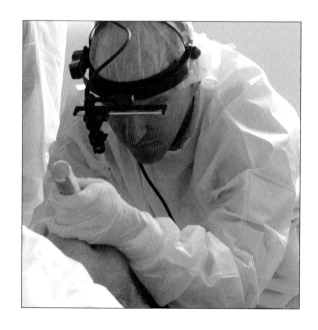

6-22 *Author using Airway Cam™ during laryngoscopy, sighting through glass prism with dominant pupil at the target.*

Laryngoscope Lighting

Standard laryngoscopes have a bulb located at the distal end of the blade and an electrical connection between the handle and the blade (Figure 6-23). When snapped into place, the circuit between the power source and light is completed, illuminating the bulb. Because the bulb is screwed into position at the end of the blade, it is possible for the bulb to become loose. This causes flickering or loss of light altogether, and for this reason, every time a standard bulb laryngoscope is used, the bulb should be checked to verify that it is secure. Bulbs also fail, so if the light is not working, the first step should be to secure the bulb, followed by changing or checking the batteries in the handle, and lastly, switching out the bulb.

Fiberoptically lit laryngoscopes, by comparison, do not have bulbs at the end of the blade. At the end of the blade is a fiberoptic element that carries light from a bulb located at the end of the handle (Figure 6-24). When snapped into position, a spring mechanism completes the circuit illuminating the bulb and the light is directed into the fiberoptic element at the base of the blade. The light is then carried by the fiberoptic element, exiting at the tip of the blade. The bulb at the end of the handle can become loose and the spring mechanism engaging the bulb can fail, either of which will cause illumination problems. Almost all laryngoscopes and blades fall into the categories above, however, there are blades that use a standard connection where, instead of locating the bulb at the tip, the bulb is located at the base of the blade. The light is then transmitted via a fiberoptic bundle down the length of the blade. This type of blade is compatible with standard handles, as it has an electrical connection at the base of the blade.

The author prefers fiberoptically illuminated laryngoscope blades, however, the quality of illumination is very dependent on the particular manufacturer and design. Comparative studies between fiberoptic and standard blades have shown either no difference or improved illumination with standard blades. This may be due to several reasons. With time and repetitive sterilization, fiberoptic bundles can become cloudy or opacified, decreasing light transmission. Also, the size of the light bundle on the fiberoptic blade determines how much light can possibly be transmitted. Many fiberoptic blades use relatively small fiberoptic elements (Figure 6-25).

A final variable in laryngoscope illumination is the power source. Some fiberoptic devices have rechargeable 3.5 volt handles, while standard batteries provide 2.5 volts. Variation in the state of charging, the memory pattern of the battery, and the age of the rechargeable battery can all impact on how well rechargeable batteries perform. Having the ability to switch batteries instantly is valuable in emergency settings, and the author now prefers to use standard batteries, keeping an extra set on hand, rather than using the rechargeable handles exclusively. NiCad batteries, especially over time, have a habit of dying precipitously and without warning.

It is important to note that standard and fiberoptic handles, as well as standard and fiberoptic blades, are not interchangeable. In the Unites States, all fiberoptic handles and blades are marked with a green circle at the base of the blade or green ring at the top of the handle. There are also some proprietary handle and disposable plastic blade configurations that use custom fittings and therefore are not interchangeable with any other blades or handles.

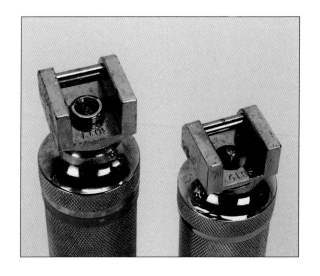

6-23 *Close up view of fiberoptic handle (left, green line around handle) with bulb in top of handle compared to electrical connection at top of handle in standard laryngoscope.*

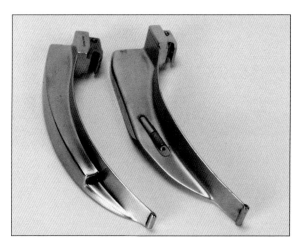

6-24 *Fiberoptic blade (left) showing flat distal end of light conducting bundle, compared to bulb of standard blade. Notice different flange shapes and distances from tip of blade to light source.*

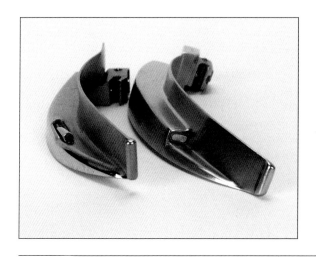

6-25 *Two fiberoptic curved blades showing differences in overall size and shape of light conducting bundle. Larger bundle on right transmits significantly more light.*

Chapter 6

Grading of Laryngeal View

Although direct laryngoscopy is the primary means of tracheal intubation in all settings objective research has been limited by several factors. One limiting factor in laryngoscopy research is its low failure rate. The low failure rate makes successful intubation an inadequate outcome measure in research studies. In order to demonstrate differences in blade design or intubation techniques, tens of thousands of patients would be required if the only outcome measure were tracheal tube placement.

Historically, the quality of laryngeal view has been used as a surrogate marker of ease of intubation. The standard means of describing laryngeal view was described by Cormack and Lehane in 1984.

Cormack and Lehane Grading

The CL grading system uses identification of landmarks to grade laryngeal view (Figure 6-26). Visualization of the vocal cords is a CL grade 1, a partial view of the glottic opening is a grade 2, an epiglottis-only view is a grade 3, and inability to sight the epiglottis is a grade 4. CL grading has been used as the standard means of assessing laryngeal view in most laryngoscopy studies, even without validation, and despite conflicting definitions and ambiguity of the different grades. While the definition of a grade 3 view, i.e., epiglottis-only, is relatively explicit (though this has been subdivided to whether the epiglottis can be lifted off the posterior pharyngeal wall, grade 3a, versus when it cannot be lifted, grade 3b), more than 99% of laryngeal views in most studies are either grade 1 or 2. The distinction between grade 1 and 2 is particularly ambiguous. In the original paper of CL grades, a grade 1 view was "all or most" of the glottis (with visualization of the vocal cords), whereas a grade 2 view is "the posterior extremity of the glottis." Benumof has pointed out that a grade 1 view may range from visualization of 1% to 100% of the vocal cords. In many studies and diagrams a grade 2 view has been represented as visualization of any portion of the glottis less than full visualization. Therefore, there are a wide range of views within grades 1 and 2, as well as ambiguity between these two grades which apply to 99% of all patients.

Direct laryngoscopy imaging permits for more detailed assessment of laryngeal view and it was apparent that among many imaged cases CL grading could not permit any distinction even though some views had far better laryngeal exposure than others. Aware of prior work that sought to quantify how much of the glottis is actually seen, and seeking to overcome the shortcomings of the CL grading scale, the author developed a new means of grading laryngeal view based upon how much of the glottic opening is visible. The method takes CL grades 1 and 2 and replaces them with a percentage of glottic opening: the POGO scale.

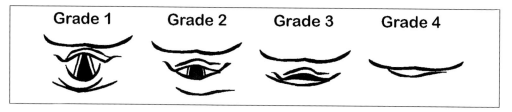

6-26 *Cormack-Lehane grading system. (From Cormack RS, Lehane J. Difficult tracheal intubation in obstetrics. Anaesth. 1984; 39: 1105–11. Used with permission.) See text for details.*

The Percentage of Glottic Opening (POGO) Score

A POGO score of 100% denotes visualization of the entire glottic opening in linear fashion from the anterior commissure to the posterior cartilages (Figure 6-27). If none of the glottic opening is seen, the POGO score is 0%. This scale has been shown to have excellent intra and inter-rater reliability when assessed by emergency physicians and anesthesiologists, and it has better reliability than the CL grading scale.

The POGO score has several distinct advantages over CL grading, especially for research purposes. The POGO score, unlike CL grading, does not depend on visualization of the vocal cords per se. It is a measure of how much of the glottic opening is seen, regardless of whether the true cords are identifiable. During laryngoscopy, the dark glottic opening is frequently well delineated, even though the vocal cords are not explicitly seen. This is because of the bulb position on a curved blade and shadowing created by the epiglottis (Figure 6-8). POGO scoring also has the advantage of being a continuous numerical scale that allows for much finer distinction between different laryngeal views. In terms of statistical analysis and the ability to distinguish differences in techniques or equipment, a continuous numerical scale is easier to use and more likely to demonstrate statistical significance.

Unlike CL grading, however, the POGO score does not provide a differentiation between epiglottis visualization and visualization of the tongue only. In each case the POGO score would be zero. Epiglottis-only views (using external manipulation) represent approximately one in 100 cases, and CL grade 4 (tongue only) is reported to have an incidence between one in 300 to one in 1,000.

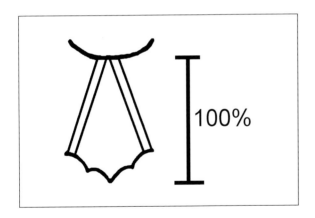

6-27 *The Percentage of Glottic Opening (POGO) score. See text for details.*

Intubation Difficulty Scale

The ultimate issue with any means of laryngeal view grading is what relevance does it really have to clinical outcome, and, secondarily, does a poor laryngeal view necessarily correlate with a difficult intubation? As was mentioned in the chapter on difficult airway prediction, almost all patients labeled in studies with a difficult airway are, in fact, readily intubated with a laryngoscope, or occasionally with the supplemental use of a bougie or tube introducer. Introducers and stylets can permit successful intubation when laryngeal view is very poor, or even when only the epiglottis is seen. If intubation occurs on first pass, does this count as a difficult airway?

Adnet devised a means of characterizing intubation difficulty that is more comprehensive and reflects the practical aspect of passing the tube, not simply the quality of laryngeal view. In Adnet's Intubation Difficulty Scale (IDS) (Figure 6-28), glottic exposure (CL grade minus 1) is just one of many components including the number of operators >1, the number of attempts >1, the number of alternative techniques, use of external laryngeal manipulation (0 or 1), the degree of lifting force (0 or 1), and the position of the vocal cords (0 or 1). Moderate to major intubation difficulty in this scale is characterized by scores greater than 5. When compared to a visual analog score of difficulty, the IDS had excellent correlation. In a subsequent prospective study, an IDS of 5 was found to occur in 8% of elective anesthesia cases but that minor difficulty occurred in as many as 37% of cases. Despite the high rate of minor difficulty, 89% of cases were successful on first attempt, and simple changes in technique almost always permitted laryngoscopy success. These included the use of external laryngeal manipulation, increasing the lifting force, addition of a stylet, repositioning the patient, and changing the operator or the blade.

Intubation Difficulty Scale

Parameter	Score
Number of Attempts >1	N_1
Number of Operators >1	N_2
Number of Alternative Techniques	N_3
Cormack Grade - 1	N_4
Lifting Force Required	
Normal	$N_5 = 0$
Increased	$N_5 = 1$
Laryngeal Pressure	
Not applied	$N_6 = 0$
Applied	$N_6 = 1$
Vocal Cord Mobility	
Abduction	$N_7 = 0$
Adduction	$N_7 = 1$
TOTAL: IDS = SUM OF SCORES	N_1-N_7

IDS Score	Degree of Difficulty
0	Easy
0 < IDS ≤5	Slight Difficulty
5 < IDS	Moderate to Major Difficulty
IDS = ∞	Impossible intubation

Rules for Calculating IDS Score:

N_1	Every additional attempt adds 1 pt.
N_2	Each additional operator adds 1 pt.
N_3	Each alternative technique adds 1 point: Repositioning of the patient, change of materials (blade, ET tube, addition of a stylette), change in approache (nasotracheal/orotracheal) or use of another technique (fibroscopy, intubation through a laryngeal mask).
N_4	Apply Cormack grade for 1st oral attempt. For successful blind intubation $N_4 = 0$.
N_6	Sellick's maneuver adds no points.
Impossible intubation:	IDS takes the value attained before abandonment of intubation attempts.

Cormack Grade[1]

I   II   III   IV

[1] Cormack RS, Lehane J. Difficult tracheal intubation in obstetrics. Anaesthesia 1984;39:1105-1111.

6-28 *Adnet's Intubation Difficulty Scale. (From Adnet F, Borron SW, Racine SX et al. The intubation difficulty scale (IDS): Proposal and evaluation of a new score characterizing the complexity of endotracheal intubation. Anesthesiology. 1997; 87: 1290–97. Used with permission.) See text for details.*

Preparation for Laryngoscopy

A useful acronym for remembering the equipment and preparation for intubation is SOAPME, which stands for Suction, Oxygen, Airways, Positioning and Preoxygenation, Monitoring and Medications, and End-tidal CO_2 and Esophageal intubation detection devices.

Suction. A Yankauer suction catheter should be on the right side of the patient's head, so it will be within reach of the operator's right hand during laryngoscopy. A convenient location to put the catheter just prior to the procedure is under the patient's right shoulder, or under the top right corner of the spine board. The suction should be checked immediately before the procedure. When properly connected the suction is audible and palpable when the tip of the catheter is touched against the hand.

Oxygen. A bag valve mask resuscitator should be connected to an oxygen source at 15 liters per minute. There are many different types of reservoir systems and valves on these units and the provider must be familiar with the design and operation of the device beforehand. The flow of oxygen should be audible and high enough to fill the reservoir bag or tubing. A hand should be held against the mask and the bag squeezed to verify the unit is functional.

Airways. Oral and nasal airways must be immediately accessible for bag mask ventilation, along with rescue ventilation devices, such as the LMA (#4, 5) and Small Adult Combitube. The cuff of the tracheal tube should be checked and fully deflated. If the cuff is not fully deflated it may block target visualization during tube placement. High-volume, low-pressure cuffs have a significant amount of plastic material, even when the cuff is deflated, that is best pulled toward the proximal end of the tube to keep it from bunching up near the tip. Some tracheal tubes have cuffs designed to have a slimmer profile when deflated (Mallinkrodt Lo-Pro, Nellcor, Pleasanton CA). The tracheal tube should be styletted with a straight-to-cuff shape.

Positioning. Optimal positioning for laryngoscopy is identical for optimal positioning for ventilation. The head is elevated and the neck is flexed relative to the chest. When viewed from a lateral perspective, a horizontal line can be drawn from the external auditory meatus (the ear) to the sternal notch. The degree of head and shoulder elevation is a function of the patient's body habitus and can be substantial in obese patients (Figures 5-1, 6-29, 6-30).

Successful laryngoscopy in morbidly obese patients mandates optimal positioning, while positioning is generally less important in non-obese persons. Morbidly obese patients have historically been considered to have "difficult airways," but this may not be true if positioning is optimized. In a recent study in which the author was involved, 60 morbidly obese patients undergoing bariatric surgery were randomly positioned either with 7 centimeters head elevation or positioned using the ear to sternal notch line. Laryngeal view was significantly better in the ear to sternal notch group (Collins JS, Lemmens HJM, Brodsky JB, Brock-Utne JG, Levitan RM. Laryngoscopy and morbid obesity: a comparison of the "sniff" and "ramped" positions. Publication submitted).

Patients who are being intubated with C-spine precautions cannot have their head and neck position optimized, and instead should undergo laryngoscopy using in-line stabilization. It is essential when performing laryngoscopy in this group of patients that the front of the cervical collar is taken off. An assistant, at the head of the bed but to the left of the laryngoscopist, stabilizes the patient's head (Figure 6-31). If the collar is not removed mouth opening and jaw distraction will be severely limited; this will certainly make the procedure more difficult, if not impossible.

Pre-oxygenation. As described in Chapter 3, pre-oxygenation should be done for four minutes on all patients who are effectively ventilating themselves. Patients with inadequate spontaneous ventilation require bag mask ventilation.

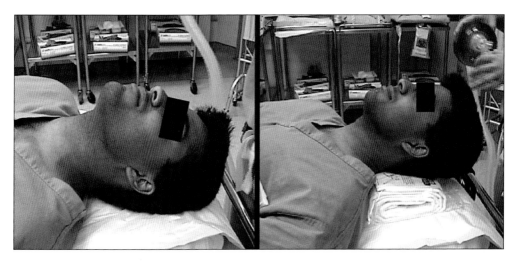

6-29 *Ear to sternal notch positioning for laryngoscopy in a thin person. Note the small amount of material needed for proper head elevation.*

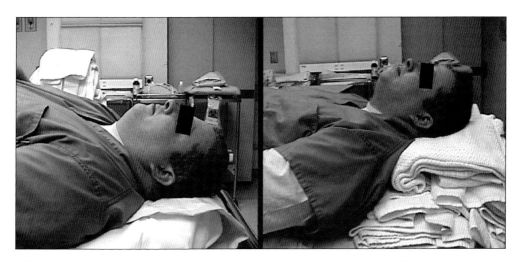

6-30 *Ear to sternal notch positioning for laryngoscopy in an obese person. Blankets have been placed underneath upper thorax, shoulders, and head. Head will need to be slightly extended during laryngoscopy, so care must be taken to avoid putting too much material under the occiput that could limit this movement.*

Monitoring. In patients without a pulse, laryngoscopy will occur as monitoring is being established. With RSI, the patient should have continuous pulse oximetry and cardiac monitoring, and pre-procedure and post-procedure blood pressure monitoring.

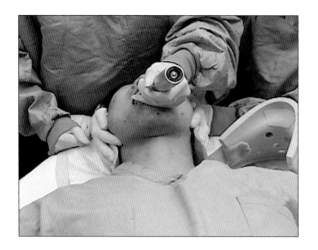

6-31 *Laryngoscopy with in-line stabilization of the cervical spine by an assistant. The front of the collar has been removed so that it will not limit mouth opening or jaw distraction.*

Medications. All medications should be drawn and labeled. The laryngoscopist should explicitly communicate with all members of the care team regarding the sequence and timing of medications. Timing of medication delivery must be clear to everybody, including the person holding in-line cervical stabilization, the person applying cricoid pressure, and the person administering the medications. The front of the cervical collar is taken down first and cricoid pressure is applied upon induction.

End-tidal CO2 monitor, esophageal intubation detector. To verify tracheal placement after the tube has been placed, all patients with a pulse should have end-tidal CO2 testing, either by capnography, capnometry, or colormetric testing. An esophageal intubation detector is useful for verifying tube location in cardiac arrest.

Chapter 7

Curved Blade Laryngoscopy

Laryngoscopy and intubation can be broken down into several steps that are useful not only for presentation purposes but also for ensuring success. These include: 1) opening of the mouth; 2) identifying the epiglottis; 3) controlling the tongue; 4) laryngeal exposure and landmark identification; and 5) tube placement.

Opening the Mouth / Identifying the Epiglottis / Controlling the Tongue

The easiest way to open the mouth is by using the first and third fingers of the right hand between the upper and lower right-sided incisors of the patient (Figure 7-1). The first and third fingers provide more strength for scissor opening than the first and second. The fingers used to open the mouth should be removed as soon as the tip of the blade has been introduced. Many novice laryngoscopists immediately focus on tongue control as the blade is inserted, instead of careful, progressive exposure of landmarks. The author believes that as the blade is being inserted the priority should be epiglottis identification, not tongue control. Finding the epiglottis, and then properly controlling it by placing the blade tip correctly into the middle of the vallecula, takes precedence over tongue control at this stage. Inserting the blade down the right side in an effort to immediately control the tongue can cause the tip of the blade to be laterally positioned relative to the vallecula and larynx. Should this occur, epiglottis control will be compromised. Additionally, blade insertion down the right is awkward mechanically, since the operator's right hand is opening the mouth on the right. Advancing down the right side of the mouth makes it harder to determine landmarks at the tip of the blade as it is advanced.

A hundred years ago, Chevalier Jackson recommended a strict midline approach in order not to misinterpret critical landmarks, specifically noting that unless the blade was kept midline, the right aryepiglottic fold could be mistaken for the epiglottis. In Jackson's day, all laryngoscopes were

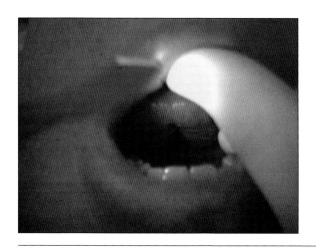

7-1 *Scissor technique of opening the mouth using the first and third fingers.*

tubular, whereas current laryngoscopes have a spatula design with a left-sided flange to permit sweeping of the tongue and tracheal tube insertion from the right. Nonetheless, the value of an initial midline approach for finding the epiglottis remains. The author recommends midline blade insertion until the edge of the epiglottis comes into view.

To find the epiglottis, the laryngoscope force (and handle) is initially directed downward (toward the patient's feet), to lift the epiglottis off of the posterior pharyngeal wall (Figure 7-2a–b). Separating the epiglottis off the posterior hypopharynx is necessary because the epiglottis does not have a distinctive mucosal appearance. It is phenomenal how easily the epiglottis can be camouflaged against the mucosa of the posterior hypopharynx, especially with secretions or blood. Gentle lifting with downward distraction of the tongue allows the edge of the epiglottis to become visible as the light from the blade creates a shadow against the posterior pharynx. The force used to distract the tongue downward and expose the edge of the epiglottis at this stage in the procedure is much less than the force subsequently used for laryngeal exposure (Figure 7-2c).

Once the epiglottis edge is seen, the handle and proximal blade can be gently shifted slightly toward the right side so that the mass of the tongue can fall to the left of the blade (Figure 7-3). The tongue actually does fall to the left, since the blade is under the tongue and the flange of the blade is oriented leftward. Only slight effort is needed to reposition the blade in this manner, assuming the upward force remains gentle. If the blade is lifted too early with too much force, the edge of the blade's spatula catches the tongue, and a section of tongue will be caught to the right of the blade.

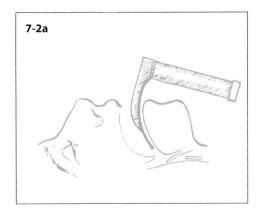
7-2a

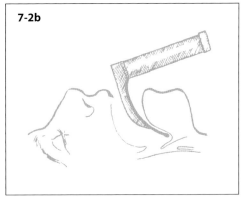
7-2b

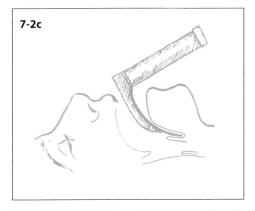
7-2c

7-2a At initial insertion the laryngoscope is tilted to facilitate insertion along tongue. The initial force vector of laryngoscopy is downward to distract the tongue and lift the epiglottis off of the posterior pharyngeal wall.
7-2b Blade tip is advanced into the vallecula.
7-2c After tip placement into the vallecula is maximized, the angle of the laryngoscope changes to expose the larynx. Handle approaches 40 degree position by the end of the procedure.

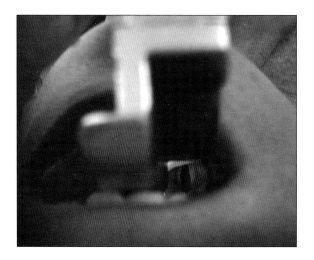

7-3 *Proper tongue control with the large flange of the curved blade. Excellent view of laryngeal structures with effective elevation of epiglottis.*

In practice, blade insertion, epiglottis identification, and control of the tongue happen within seconds. Once the proximal aspect of the blade has been gently repositioned to the right side of the mouth, and it is seen that no section of tongue is to the right of the blade, the force vector on the blade is changed, and the degree of force can be increased in order to expose the larynx. At this point, the laryngoscopist's viewing angle also changes. Initially, the viewing angle is relatively vertical as the blade is introduced and the operator is looking from above down into the mouth. After the epiglottis is found and seated into the vallecula, however, the angle drops backward concurrent with the change in the force vector on the laryngoscope. Originally the direction of force is oriented to direct the tongue and jaw downward, while after blade insertion, it changes to lift the tongue and jaw upward (Figures 7-2a–b). The handle, which had initially been oriented nearly parallel to the patient, changes orientation to approximately 40 degrees (Figure 7-2c).

Laryngoscopy as a Predictable Sequence of Exposed Structures Beginning with Epiglottoscopy

Success at laryngoscopy hinges entirely on successful epiglottoscopy. The epiglottis is consistently located at the base of the tongue. Slow and careful incremental advancement of the tip of the blade down the tongue helps locate the epiglottis. Novice laryngoscopists commonly advance the blade too aggressively, succumb to epiglottis camouflage, and become lost in the pink mucosa of the esophagus with no idea of what they are looking at or how to fix the problem. Practice on manikins fails to emphasize the importance of slowly advancing the blade. Progressive visualization of landmarks is the key to determining where the tip of the blade is located and what is being seen. In situations of distorted anatomy from trauma, edema, infection, bleeding, or emesis, a thorough knowledge of the sequence of different landmarks, both underneath the blade and visible down the lumen, is essential.

One way of conceptualizing the progressive visualization of landmarks is to consider the sequence of structures that the line of sight traverses as the blade is inserted and advanced. If the lumen of the airway is used as the dividing line, these structures can be divided into those that are above this line (the tongue and epiglottis), and those that are below the line (the palate, uvula, posterior pharyngeal wall, and posterior portion of the larynx) (Figure 7-4). The posterior aspect of the larynx is the first portion visible as the line of sight traverses from the epiglottis to the larynx (Figure 7-5). If the blade is inserted too deeply and enters the upper esophagus, the posterior laryngeal structures will not be seen.

There is no continuous direct visual connection that can be followed from the palate, uvula and posterior pharyngeal wall to the larynx. This is the reason epiglottis identification is so important. It is reliably located at the base of the tongue and it comprises the superior aspect of the laryngeal inlet. It is the only structure that bridges the gap between the tongue, from where the procedure starts, to the larynx.

Apart from the fact that an epiglottis first approach reliably guides the laryngoscopist from the tongue to the larynx, it has two other benefits. If the larynx cannot be seen but the epiglottis edge is visualized, the operator then knows exactly where the larynx should be. If a blind approach is needed, such as with a styletted tube or an introducer, the epiglottis serves as the signpost to follow as the tube or introducer is placed under the epiglottis edge.

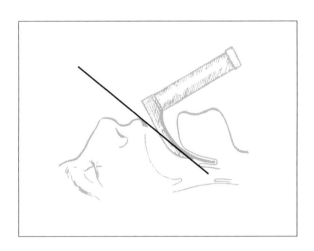

7-4 *Dividing line of visible structures within the airway during laryngoscopy. Above the line are the tongue and epiglottis. Below the line are the palate, uvula, posterior pharyngeal wall, and the posterior structures of the larynx.*

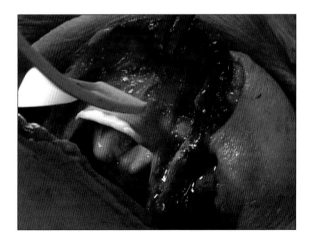

7-5 *Block neck dissection at the level of the hyoid bone. The tip of the curved laryngoscope blade is located at the vallecula. The pharyngoepiglottic folds can be seen coming down from each side of the epiglottis. The rounded prominences of the posterior cartilages and the narrow cleft of the interarytenoid notch are located beneath the epiglottis.*

The second benefit of an epiglottis first approach is the avoidance of mistaking the esophagus for the trachea. When the epiglottis is missed upon blade insertion, the tip of the blade will enter the esophagus. With enough of an upward force, a round hole will be seen that may erroneously appear to be the target. The author believes this is a common error in emergency settings when the operator is rushed and visualization is often sub-optimal. Even if quickly recognized, incorrectly intubating the esophagus is dangerous in many respects. It delays the time to ventilation and exposes the patient to hypoxia. Second, if the stomach is ventilated, it causes gastric distention and a high probability of regurgitation with repeat laryngoscopy. If esophageal intubation is not quickly recognized, the patient will be neurologically devastated or die from prolonged hypoxia.

Laryngeal Exposure and Landmark Identification

Landmark identification refers specifically to identification of structures about the larynx that will permit correct placement of the tracheal tube. The epiglottis defines the superior aspect of the laryngeal inlet, but in order to ensure that the tracheal tube is in fact entering the larynx and not just passing beneath the epiglottis into the esophagus below, it is necessary to have a landmark that the tube must pass above. This important landmark is the interarytenoid notch and adjacent posterior cartilages.

The operator's line of sight, at first almost vertical looking downward into the mouth, pivots backward (more parallel to the patient), after the blade has been inserted. Sighting the larynx occurs when the operator's visual axis converges with the plane of the laryngeal inlet, subsequently passing beneath the epiglottis and revealing the posterior laryngeal structures (Figure 7-5, 7-6a–f).

The true cords are not necessary for correct placement of the tracheal tube, and as explained earlier they are often not visible due to shadowing by the epiglottis. Visualization of the interarytenoid notch is a required minimum to ensure correct placement, because if the tube tip is directed above this landmark, it will enter the trachea.

Landmark recognition and effective epiglottis control are directly related since the epiglottis is the final visual obstruction to sighting the larynx. The best means of effectively elevating the epiglottis with the curved blade is by fully directing the blade tip into the vallecula. Under the mucosa of the vallecula, where the tongue and epiglottis meet, is the hyoepiglottic ligament. Pressure at this location causes indirect lifting of the epiglottis. Correctly holding the laryngoscope at the base of the handle, with the hypothenar eminence against the proximal end of the blade, allows the operator to effectively transmit force longitudinally down the forearm, through the blade and into the vallecula (Figures 6-17, 6-19, 6-20).

In practice, the author has found that the correct force vector and ideal blade tip position can be simultaneously and most efficiently achieved by bimanual laryngoscopy, also called external laryngeal manipulation (ELM). Another means of improving laryngeal view if ELM is not sufficient is to lift the head and increase flexion of the head on the chest, also known as head elevated laryngoscopy position (HELP). Each of these techniques is addressed below.

7-6. Progressive Visualization and Landmark Identification During Curved Blade Laryngoscopy

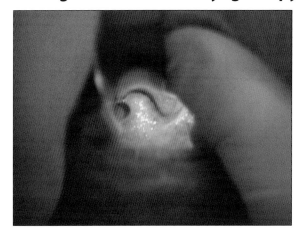

7-6a *Uvula.*

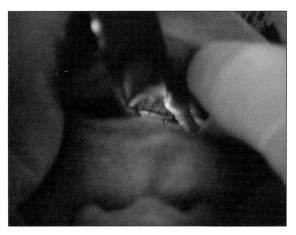

7-6b *Epiglottis edge.*

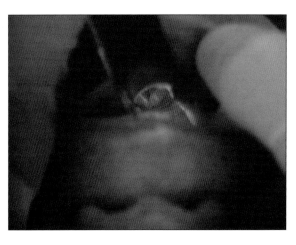

7-6c *The posterior cartilages and the thin vertical cleft of the interarytenoid notch are barely visible.*

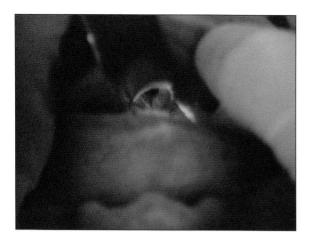

7-6d *Additional lift exposes a small portion of the glottic opening.*

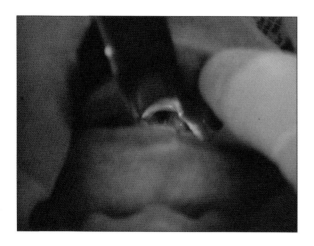

7-6e *More of the glottis becomes exposed but the vocal cords are still not seen.*

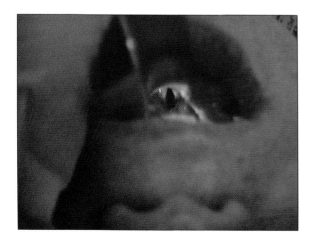

7-6f *The true vocal cords (white) are well seen with a nearly completely visible glottic opening, spanning from anterior commissure to interarytenoid notch.*

Improving Laryngeal View by External Laryngeal Manipulation: Bimanual Laryngoscopy

ELM transforms laryngoscopy from a one handed technique to a bimanual technique. With the laryngoscope held in the left hand, the laryngoscopist's right hand is placed on the thyroid cartilage, manipulating it backward, upward, or side to side while observing the effect on laryngeal exposure (Figure 7-7). After ELM is used to optimize view, an assistant can take over laryngeal manipulation at that same location, thereby allowing the laryngoscopist to place the tracheal tube (Figure 7-8).

ELM improves laryngeal view by three possible mechanisms: 1) it improves alignment of the larynx with the line of sight; 2) it more effectively elevates the epiglottis; and 3) it decreases the anterior tilt of the larynx.

The vocal cords attach anteriorly to the thyroid cartilage. By directing the thyroid cartilage backward, ELM brings the larynx, particularly the anterior larynx, into better alignment with the laryngoscopist's line of sight (Figure 7-9a–c).

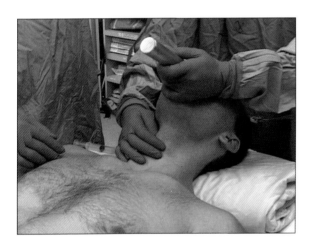

7-7 External laryngeal manipulation (ELM) by the laryngoscopist—bimanual laryngoscopy. Operator's right hand presses on anterior neck, most commonly at thyroid cartilage, while directly observing the effect on laryngeal view.

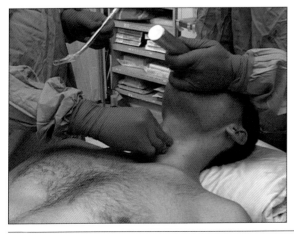

7-8 Once the view has been optimized by the laryngoscopist, an assistant takes over maintaining external laryngeal manipulation at the optimal spot, freeing the operator's right hand to place the tracheal tube.

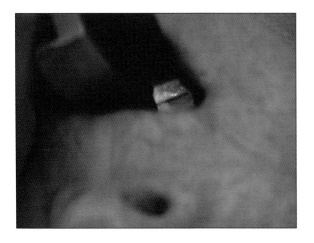

7-9a *The epiglottis edge.*

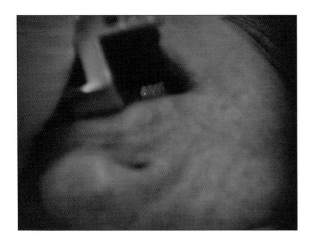

7-9b *The interarytenoid notch and posterior cartilages.*

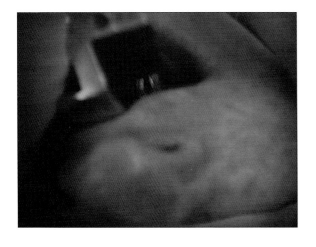

7-9c *With bimanual laryngoscopy excellent laryngeal exposure is obtained, although a small portion of the tongue is poorly controlled to the right of the spatula. The operator's right hand can be seen in the upper right hand corner of the image (compare to 7-9b).*

The second mechanism by which ELM facilitates laryngeal exposure is through more effective elevation of the epiglottis. The Macintosh blade fits the natural curvature of the tongue, has a natural stopping point at the vallecula, and the large flange provides for easier tongue control when compared to the smaller flange of the Miller or other straight blades. Laryngeal exposure with a curved blade however, is completely dependent upon proper pressure at the vallecula and the hyoepiglottic ligament. If the tip is loosely applied at the vallecula, or incorrectly directed, the epiglottis hangs downward and blocks exposure of the larynx (Figure 7-10a). Application of ELM drives the tip of the blade fully into the vallecula, into the ideal position for maximally elevating the epiglottis (Figure 7-10b).

The third mechanism by which ELM may improve laryngeal view is by changing the anterior tilt of the larynx. Several studies by Roberts have shown that the more pronounced the external anterior angle of the larynx (as measured by an inclinometer placed directly on the thyroid cartilage), the more difficult it is to achieve laryngeal exposure. ELM at the thyroid cartilage lessens this angle by directing the superior portion of the thyroid cartilage downward.

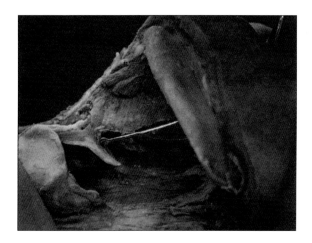

7-10a *Cross-sectional cadaver demonstration of epiglottis hanging down, blocking line of sight to larynx.*

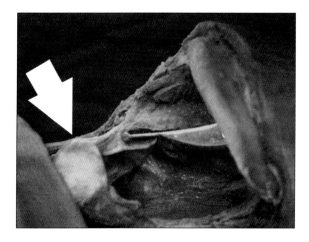

7-10b *Driving the tip of the curved blade into the vallecula causes the epiglottis to lift upward. ELM helps drive tip of curved blade fully into vallecula and it also drives larynx posteriorly into operator's line of sight (large arrow). (Images modified from Gorback MS. Emergency airway management. BC Decker, Philadelphia 1990. Used with permission.)*

ELM vs. Cricoid Pressure vs. Backward Upward Rightward Pressure

ELM is distinct from cricoid pressure. It is also not backward, upward, rightward pressure (BURP). Cricoid pressure and BURP, as originally described, are both performed by an assistant without feedback from the laryngoscopist.

According to a study by Benumof, cricoid pressure provided maximal improvement in laryngeal view in only 11% of cases, versus 88% of cases when the view was maximized by thyroid manipulation. Prior work by Roberts suggested that cricoid pressure worsens laryngeal view by increasing the anterior tilt of the larynx. Cricoid pressure can clearly worsen laryngoscopy and also impede the ability to pass a tracheal tube, even when the tube tip has passed into the larynx. It can impede laryngoscopy by affecting how the curved blade tip interacts with the hyoepiglottic ligament, and it negatively affects tube passage by increasing downward pressure of the anterior tracheal rings onto the tube tip or in some instances, by actually collapsing the trachea. This phenomenon can also prevent effective ventilation. The author and his colleagues have witnessed numerous instances in which intubation was impossible with cricoid pressure and easily achieved when it was lightened or replaced by ELM.

While BURP involves manipulation of the thyroid cartilage and is specifically designed to improve view, it is not physically done by the laryngoscopist nor directly coordinated with the laryngoscopist's view. ELM can involve movements similar to BURP, i.e., backward and rightward pressure, but it can also involve any manipulation that improves view. In many instances, for example, ELM maximizes laryngeal view with only backward pressure.

Minor changes in the positioning of the laryngoscope and pressure on the thyroid cartilage can have marked effects on laryngeal view. ELM coordinates the operator's right hand with what is being simultaneously visualized, immediately permitting direct fine tuning of the manipulation to maximize laryngeal exposure. The author's experience, as well as preliminary studies comparing ELM, cricoid, and BURP, show a clear advantage to operator-directed ELM for optimizing laryngeal view. In a large trial done in the author's cadaver based airway courses during the past year and involving more than a thousand total laryngoscopies, ELM is dramatically better than BURP or cricoid pressure in terms of laryngeal view (publication submitted at time of press). This is intuitive, since pressure on the neck by someone other than the laryngoscopist can either positively or negatively impact the view. ELM permits optimal laryngeal view as determined by the operator, then uses the assistant's hand to maintain this position.

ELM, BURP, and cricoid pressure have different historical origins in addition to differences in their application and intended goals. The pioneers of indirect laryngoscopy in the 1850s, as well the pioneers of direct laryngoscopy in the early 1900s, both used the term "external manipulation" or "external pressure" on the thyroid cartilage in describing techniques for improving laryngeal exposure. External laryngeal manipulation precedes BURP or cricoid pressure by a century. Although some authors have suggested that BURP can be done by the laryngoscopist, this confuses the key differences between BURP and ELM. BURP involves specific movements of the thyroid cartilage dorsally 0.5 cm, 2 cm cephalad, and 0.5–2.0 cm laterally to the right. These measured movements and directions were defined for an assistant, who cannot observe what the laryngoscopist is seeing. When done by the operator, however, it is counterintuitive that the laryngoscopist must apply specific measured movements if the end point is improvement of view upon direct observation.

Benumof coined the term "optimal external laryngeal manipulation" (OELM), emphasizing that the laryngoscopist should attempt manipulation at multiple points if needed (thyroid, cricoid, or hyoid) to create the optimal improvement in laryngeal view. As noted by Benumof "optimal external laryngeal manipulation is not cricoid pressure (the cricoid cartilage is 2–3 cm caudad to the larynx), it may be backward and upward and to the right pressure on the thyroid cartilage, but the best way to determine the exact area on the neck and the amount of pressure for optimal external laryngeal pressure is for the laryngoscopist to determine this empirically with his/her own free right hand." (Benumof JL. Difficult laryngoscopy: obtaining the best view [editorial]. *Can J Anaesth* 1994; 41: 361–5.)

Benumof demonstrated the effectiveness of ELM in a study which operator-directed ELM on 181 patients was found to improve laryngeal view in all instances of partial visualization. Although ELM done by the laryngoscopist is probably superior to BURP (done by an assistant), Takahata found that BURP allowed for laryngeal visualization in all 273 cases studied, including 12 cases in which only the epiglottis was initially seen. Using videographic imaging, the author showed that ELM improved laryngeal view in 72 cases where the initial laryngeal view was poor (percentage of glottic opening score <50%), including 32 cases in which only the epiglottis was seen. It has been estimated that routine use of external laryngeal manipulation may reduce the incidence of epiglottis-only views from 9% to as low as 1.3%.

Improving Laryngeal View by Head Elevated Laryngoscopy Positioning (HELP)

Chevalier Jackson recognized the significance of head elevation on laryngeal view and in cases of poor visualization recommended that "the lifting motion and elevation of the head should be increased."

Four studies have investigated how changing head and neck position in the same patient affects the quality of laryngeal view.

Adnet et al. compared laryngeal exposure in the "sniffing" position (defined as 7 cm occiput elevation), versus simple head extension (head flat), with a curved laryngoscope blade. They found no significant advantage to the "sniffing" position over simple head extension in routine practice. Their study used Cormack and Lehane (CL) grading, no objective recording of laryngeal views, and seven different laryngoscopists performing the intubations. The most significant limitation of the Adnet study, though, was that they performed laryngoscopy with a Macintosh curved laryngoscope blade. Curved blades are significantly dependent upon minor changes in the force applied to the hyoepiglottic ligament and tip placement in the vallecula. Collectively, these variables may have obscured the impact of changes in head positioning.

Hochman et. al. studied the effects of straight laryngoscope blade size as well as head and neck positioning on the force required for optimal laryngeal exposure. They concluded that increasing head elevation and neck flexion increased the incidence of full laryngeal exposure with less required force. Hochman characterized the position that optimized laryngeal exposure as "flexion-flexion," referring to both atlanto-occipital flexion and cervico-thoracic vertebrae flexion. An analysis of their photographs, however, suggests that the atlanto-occipital joint is not truly flexed, i.e., the laryngoscopy angle is not > 90 degrees. For this reason, and also because "head elevated" is a simpler term to describe the primary movement, it is the author's belief that "head elevated laryngoscopy position" (HELP) is a better term for this type of positioning than is "flexion-flexion."

A third study recently investigated increasing head elevation in 21 patients in whom only the epiglottis was initially visualized. Schmitt et al. found that laryngeal view was improved in 19 out of 21 cases by elevating the head beyond sniffing position, which permitted at least some of the glottic opening to be visible. An assistant provided head elevation as well as external manipulation and the two techniques were found to be synergistic in improving laryngeal view.

The author recently studied the effect of head elevated laryngoscopy positioning using seven fresh cadavers and recording POGO scores while measuring the angle of laryngoscopy (Figure 7-11). In all seven cadavers, POGO scores (determined from video recordings with the Airway Cam) markedly increased with increasing head elevation and increasing the degree of flexion of the head on the chest.

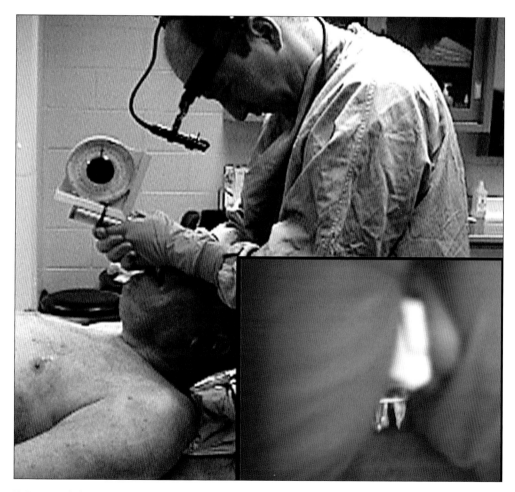

7-11 *Head elevated laryngoscopy study using matched videography of angle finder on laryngoscope and Airway Cam imaging of laryngeal view (inset right).*

Sequential Imaging of Curved Blade Laryngoscopy

7-12. Curved blade laryngoscopy using a McCoy blade

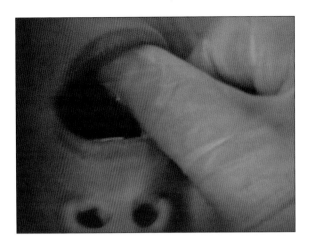

7-12a *A scissor technique is used to open the mouth.*

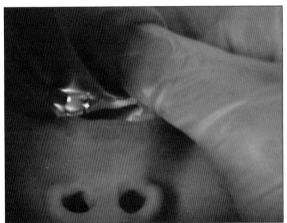

7-12b *Initial blade insertion along the curvature of the tongue.*

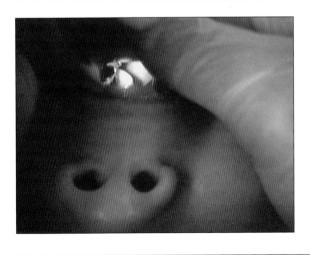

7-12c *The uvula is visible against the posterior pharyngeal wall.*

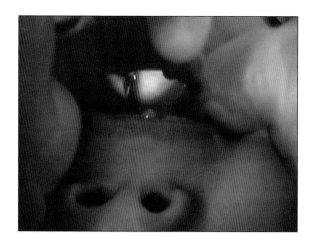

7-12d *Moving farther down the tongue and looking for the epiglottis. The posterior pharynx is seen through the lumen of the blade.*

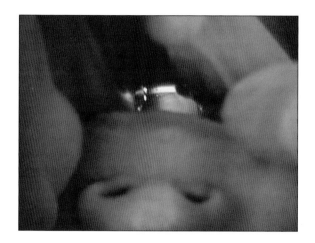

7-12e *The epiglottis edge is brightly lit beneath the tip of the blade.*

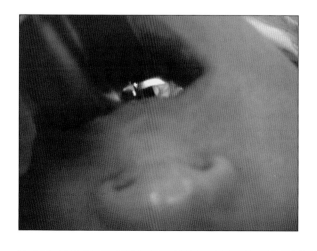

7-12f *With further insertion into the vallecula and lifting upward the glottic opening can be seen with a small section of the vocal cords.*

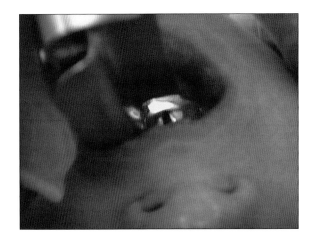

7-12g *Bimanual laryngoscopy exposes more of the anterior vocal cords.*

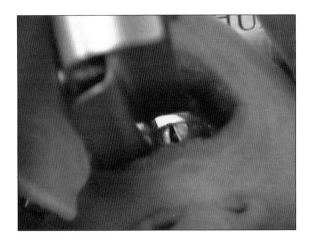

7-12h *As the tip of the blade is fully positioned into the vallecula and the larynx displaced downward, epiglottis elevation improves laryngeal exposure.*

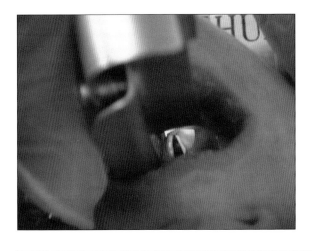

7-12i *Full elevation of the epiglottis exposes the epiglottic tubercle. The epiglottis itself is no longer visible.*

7-13. Curved blade laryngoscopy with a Macintosh blade

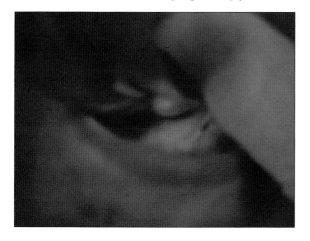

7-13a *Advancing the blade down the tongue after a scissor technique is used to open the mouth.*

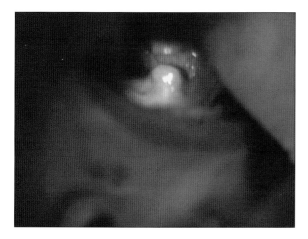

7-13b *Uvula.*

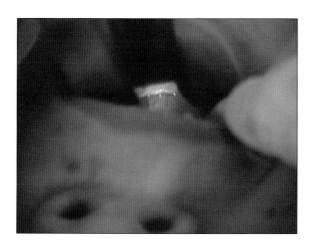

7-13c *The edge of the epiglottis.*

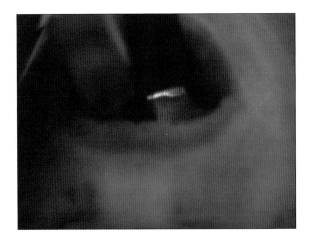

7-13d *The edge of the epiglottis is better defined. Beneath the epiglottis is seen the smooth mucosa of the posterior pharynx.*

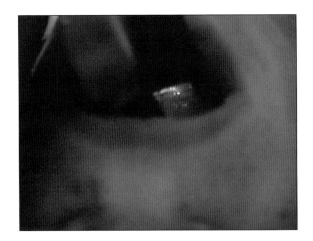

7-13e *A slight rounded prominence begins to appear beneath the epiglottis edge.*

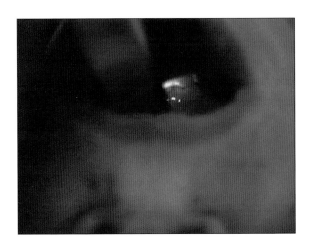

7-13f *The left posterior cartilage can be seen.*

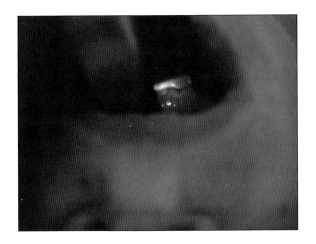

7-13g *The interarytenoid notch and left posterior cartilage are now visible.*

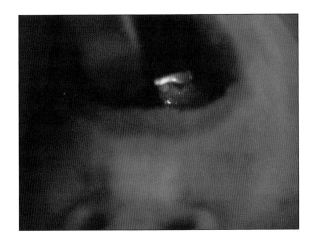

7-13h *The posterior cartilages can be seen with a small glottic opening.*

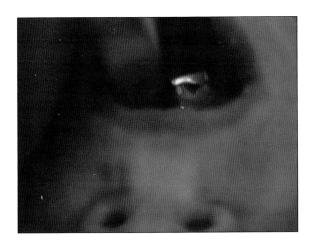

7-13i *More of the glottic opening becomes visible along with a better view of both posterior cartilages and the interarytenoid notch.*

7-14. Curved blade laryngoscopy with a Macintosh blade

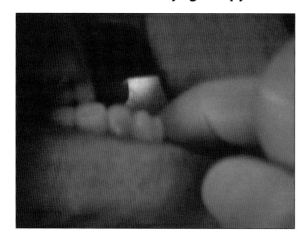

7-14a *Initial blade insertion trying to avoid injury to prominent upper dentition.*

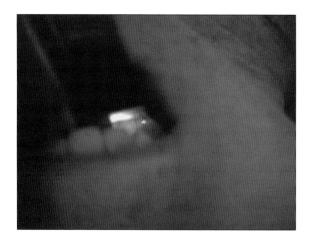

7-14b *The epiglottis edge is discernible against the posterior pharynx.*

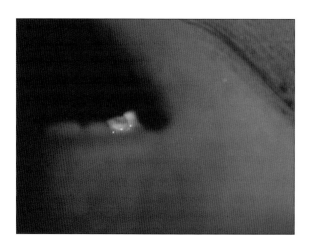

7-14c *The posterior aspect of the larynx.*

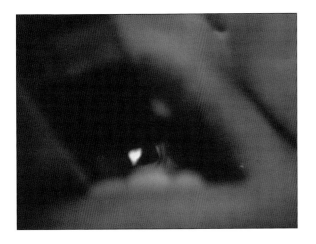

7-14d *The glottic opening can be well seen with a small section of the right vocal cord and right posterior cartilages. Under the left side of the spatula and immediately in front of the light on the blade is the tip of the epiglottis.*

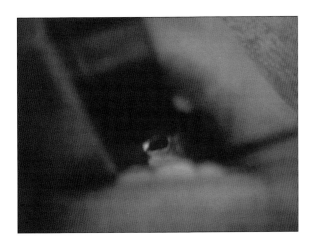

7-14e *The tracheal tube has been inserted and the tip is posteriorly displaced just prior to insertion through the glottic opening.*

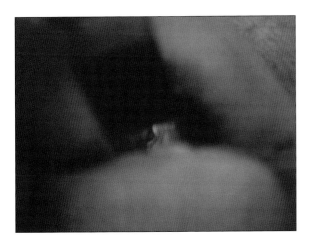

7-14f *The right vocal cord and the posterior cartilages can be partially seen laterally adjacent to the tracheal tube after it has been placed.*

7-15. Curved blade laryngoscopy using a McCoy blade

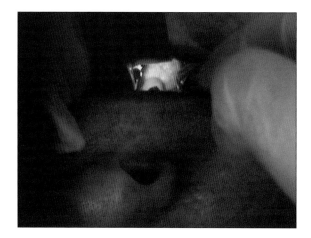

7-15a *Uvula.*

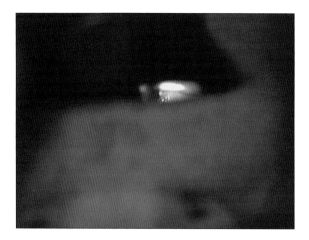

7-15b *The tip of the epiglottis.*

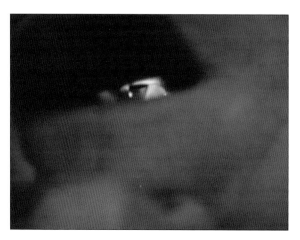

7-15c *The vertical cleft of the interarytenoid notch and a small portion of the glottic opening can be seen beneath the epiglottis.*

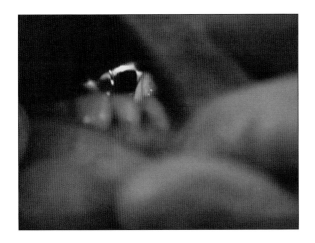

7-15d *A large section of the glottic opening is visible although the true vocal cords are not well seen. Note the rounded prominences of the posterior cartilages on the right.*

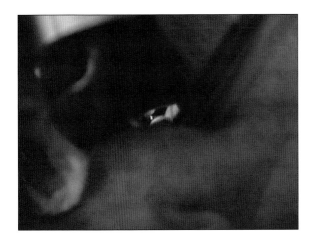

7-15e *The tracheal tube is inserted and the distal tip can be seen coming upward toward the glottic opening. This is a result of straight-to-cuff stylet shaping.*

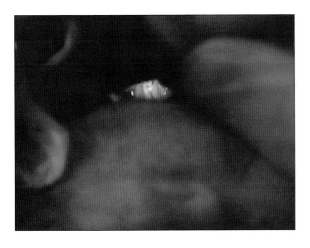

7-15f *After insertion the posterior cartilages on the right side are recognizable immediately adjacent to the tracheal tube.*

7-16. Curved blade laryngoscopy with a McCoy blade

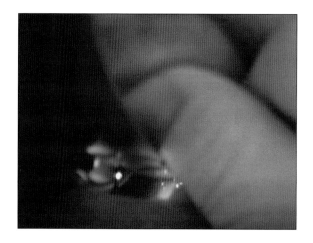

7-16a *Initial blade insertion. A scissor technique is used to open the mouth.*

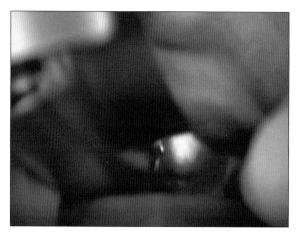

7-16b *The uvula and posterior pharynx.*

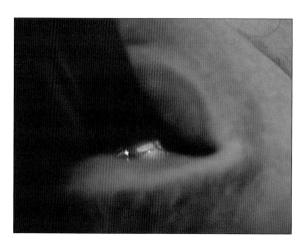

7-16c *The tip of the epiglottis.*

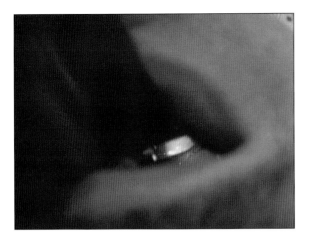

7-16d *A better view of the epiglottis.*

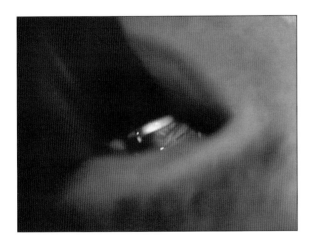

7-16e *Beneath the right edge of the epiglottis is the rounded edge of the right posterior cartilages.*

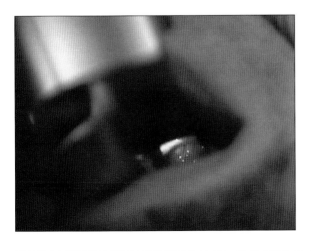

7-16f *With bimanual laryngoscopy the interarytenoid notch and the posterior cartilages become visible.*

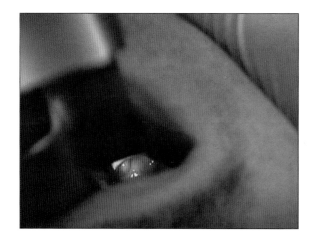

7-16g *As the epiglottis is lifted a little bit more the interarytenoid notch and posterior cartilages are slightly better seen.*

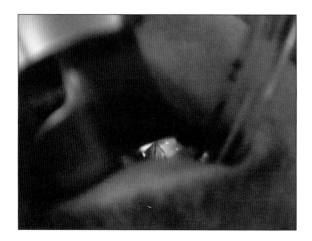

7-16h *Initial tracheal tube insertion into larynx shows the tube passing immediately adjacent to the right posterior cartilages and underneath the epiglottis.*

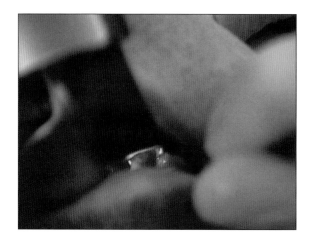

7-16i *With further tube advancement, the location of the tube beneath the epiglottis and alongside the posterior cartilages is evident. Even when the laryngeal view is poor, as occurred in this case, recognizing the posterior structures coupled with careful tube tip placement can result in successful intubation.*

7-17. Curved blade laryngoscopy with a Macintosh blade

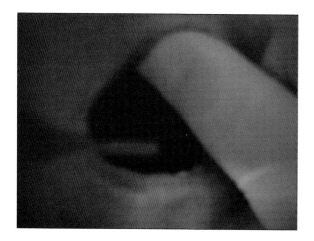

7-17a *Scissor technique opening the mouth.*

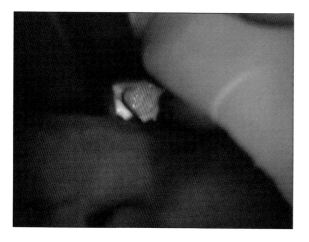

7-17b *The blade is advanced along the tongue and the uvula is seen just medial to the flange of the blade.*

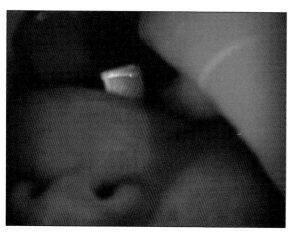

7-17c *The epiglottis edge is faintly visible against the mucosa of the posterior pharynx.*

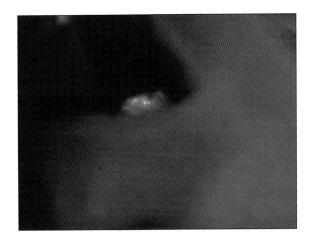

7-17d *Having found the proper location for the blade tip (in the vallecula), the jaw and tongue are lifted upward, revealing the posterior cartilages and the posterior aspect of the glottic opening.*

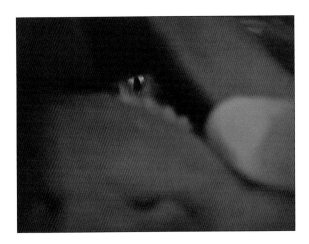

7-17e *With bimanual laryngoscopy and lip retraction the vocal cords and the glottic opening are exposed.*

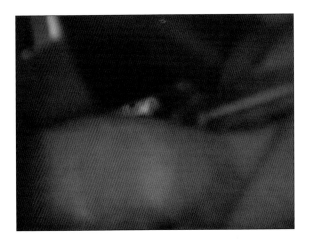

7-17f *The tracheal tube is inserted from the right side avoiding the line of sight. The posterior cartilages, the interarytenoid notch, and a small portion of the glottic opening are visible.*

Chapter 7

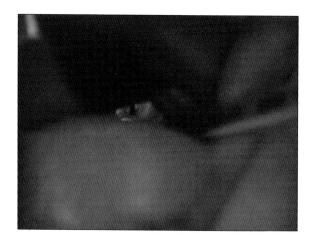

7-17g *Posterior displacement of the tracheal tube keeps the main section of the tube out of the line of sight.*

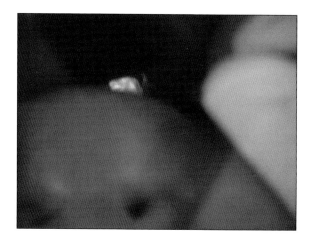

7-17h *Visualization of the target is compromised as the tracheal tube is advanced. This is the reason it is critical to observe the tube tip upon initial placement into the glottis.*

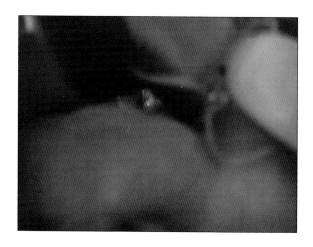

7-17i *After the cuff passes the right posterior cartilage, the right vocal cord can be seen next to the tracheal tube.*

7-18. Curved blade laryngoscopy using a McCoy blade

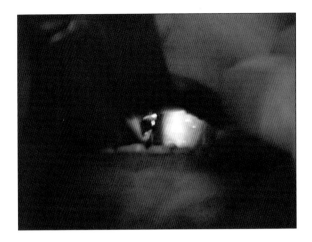

7-18a *Initial blade insertion advancing along the tongue.*

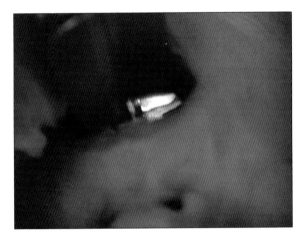

7-18b *The epiglottis tip.*

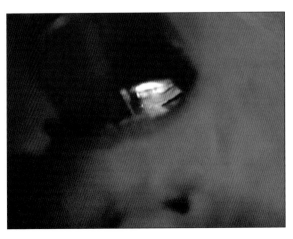

7-18c *The interarytenoid notch and the posterior cartilages start to appear beneath the epiglottis. To the right is a dark curvilinear line beneath which is the esophagus.*

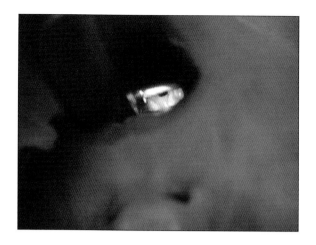

7-18d *The glottic opening is barely seen between the posterior cartilages and above the interarytenoid notch.*

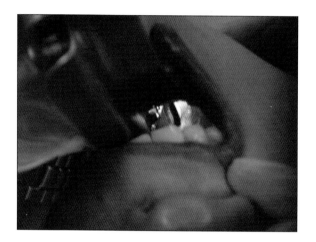

7-18e *With bimanual laryngoscopy the view is dramatically improved. The true and false vocal cords and almost the entire glottic opening are visible.*

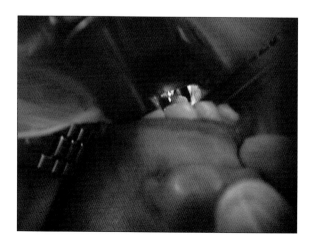

7-18f *Tracheal tube insertion with the tube tip about to enter the larynx.*

7-19. Curved blade laryngoscopy using a McCoy blade

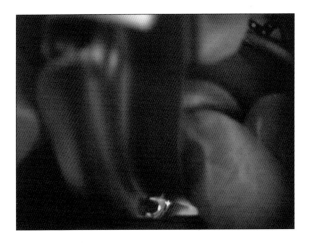

7-19a *Initial blade insertion.*

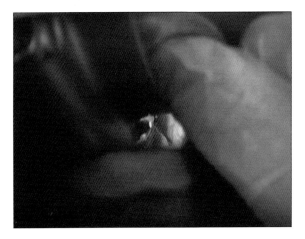

7-19b *The uvula and posterior pharynx.*

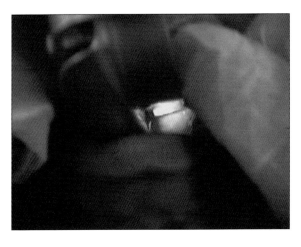

7-19c *The epiglottis tip.*

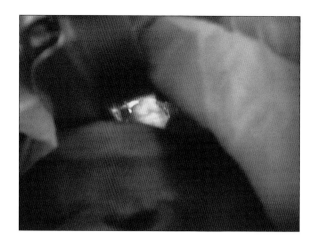

7-19f *With the blade fully positioned into the vallecula there is improved epiglottis elevation and the posterior structures begin to come into view.*

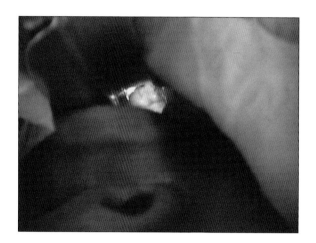

7-19g *The vertical cleft of the interarytenoid notch is well seen along with the left posterior cartilages.*

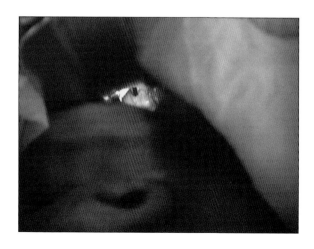

7-19f *The glottic opening starts to become visible.*

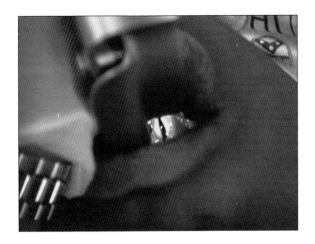

7-19g *This image shows an excellent view of the bright white true vocal cords.*

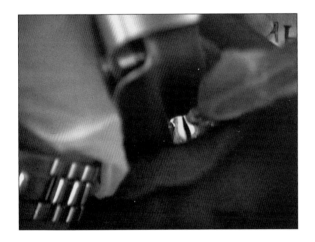

7-19h *Tube insertion using the right corner of the mouth.*

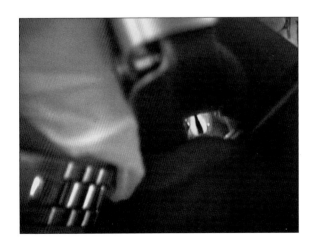

7-19i *The tracheal tube is advanced inside the mouth but the tip is kept beneath the line of sight so as not to obscure the target.*

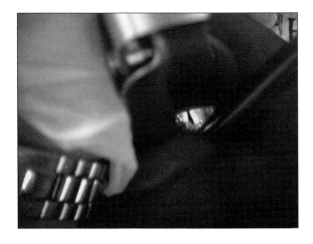

7-19j *Just prior to tube passage into the larynx.*

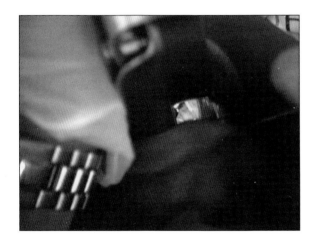

7-19k *The tracheal tube cuff is seen passing between the vocal cords.*

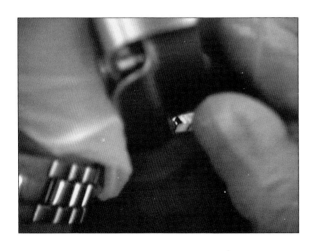

7-19l *With further advancement the tracheal tube can be seen adjacent to the vocal cords.*

7-20. Curved blade laryngoscopy using a Macintosh improved vision blade

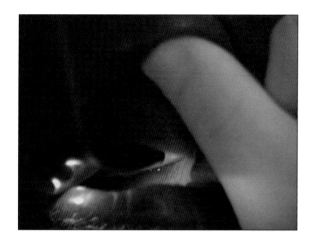

7-20a *The first and third fingers are used in a scissor technique to open the mouth.*

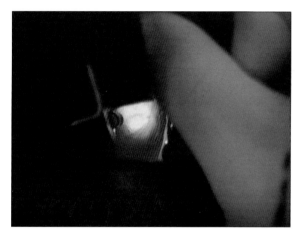

7-20b *With movement of the blade along the curvature of the tongue the uvula and posterior pharynx are illuminated.*

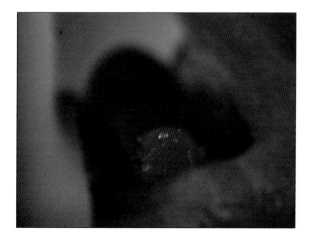

7-20c *Beneath the tubular shaped spatula of the Macintosh improved vision blade is seen the smooth mucosa of the posterior pharynx with no laryngeal landmarks visible.*

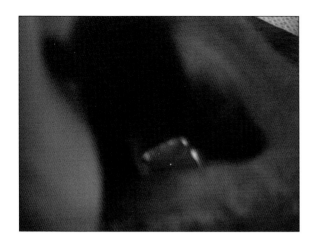

7-20d *The posterior structures of the larynx become visible, including the posterior cartilages and the interarytenoid notch.*

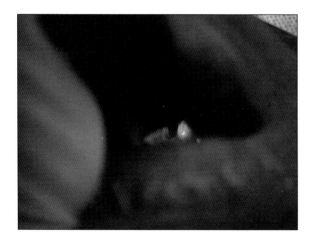

7-20e *With additional lifting the posterior aspect of the glottic opening is seen.*

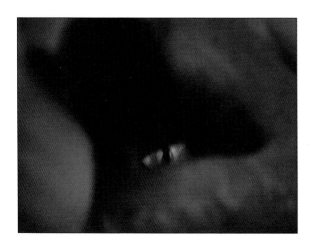

7-20f *After bimanual laryngoscopy a small portion of the vocal cords can be seen. It would be helpful to have an assistant retract the upper right lip.*

7-21. Curved blade laryngoscopy using a McCoy blade

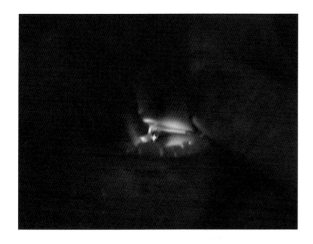

7-21a *Initial blade insertion.*

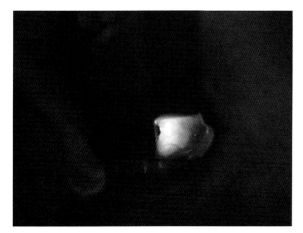

7-21b *The blade is advanced along the tongue.*

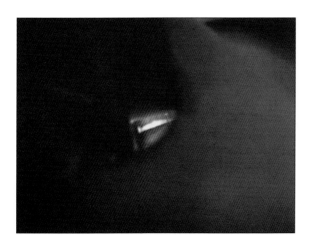

7-21c *The epiglottis tip.*

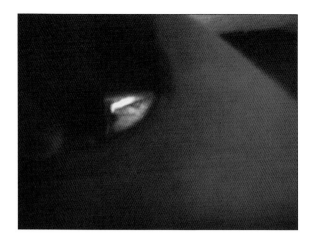

7-21d *The interarytenoid notch and posterior cartilages.*

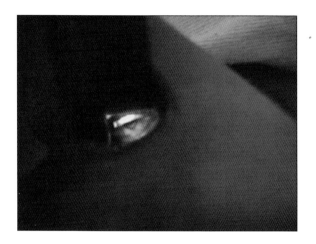

7-21e *A better view of the interarytenoid notch and adjacent cartilages.*

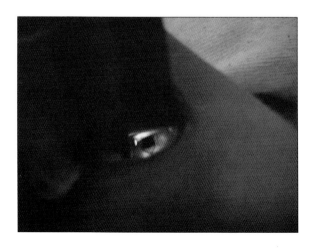

7-21f *Minor changes in blade force and direction, as well as the blade's location within the vallecula, cause the epiglottis to lift slightly higher and the view of the glottic opening improves.*

7-22. Curved blade laryngoscopy using a Macintosh blade

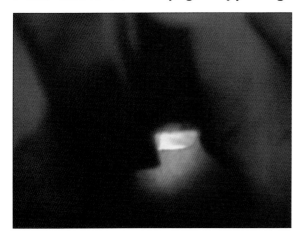

7-22a *The epiglottis edge is well seen against the smooth appearance of the posterior pharynx.*

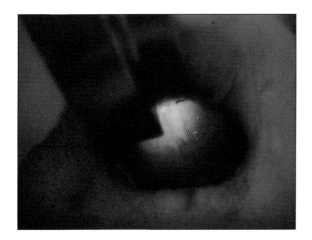

7-22b *The uvula and posterior pharynx.*

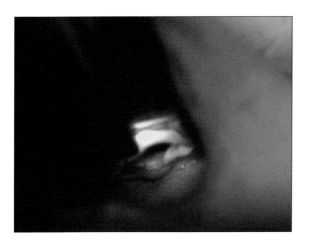

7-22c *The epiglottis edge and the posterior larynx can be seen, including the interarytenoid notch and the posterior cartilages.*

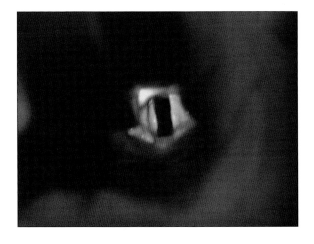

7-22d *Almost complete laryngeal exposure with excellent illumination of the inner laryngeal structures. Note how well the epiglottis is controlled and that the tongue is fully to the left side of the blade. Between the posterior structures of the larynx and the posterior pharyngeal wall is a dark space that narrows into the cervical esophagus.*

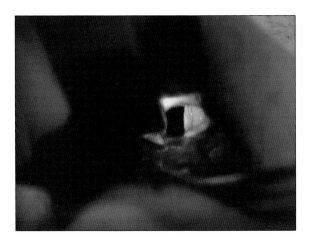

7-22e *The tracheal tube has been introduced and is positioned beneath the line of sight to the target. The tube tip is right at the interarytenoid notch.*

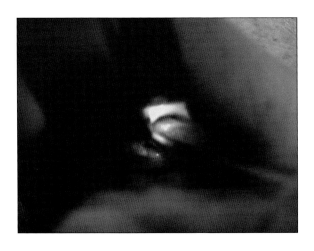

7-22f *Following insertion the tube is adjacent to the posterior cartilages and immediately beneath the epiglottis edge.*

7-23. Curved blade laryngoscopy with a Macintosh blade

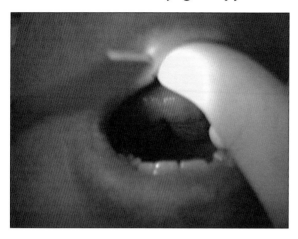

7-23a *The view of the tongue and mouth just prior to blade insertion.*

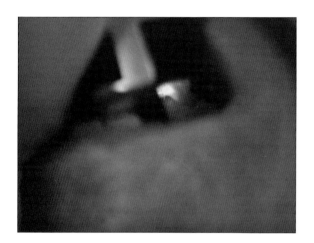

7-23b *The epiglottis tip is brightly lit beneath the dark spatula of the laryngoscope blade.*

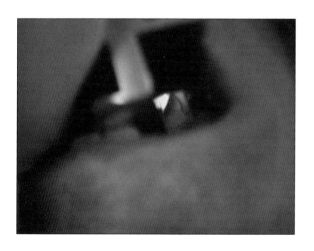

7-23c *The epiglottis in this patient is somewhat long and floppy and in this image has an inverted V shape.*

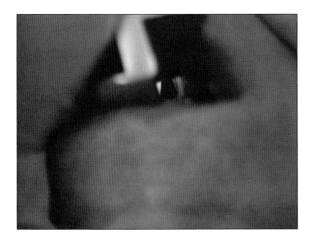

7-23d *The epiglottis in this image obscures the vocal cords, although the dark glottic opening is recognizable.*

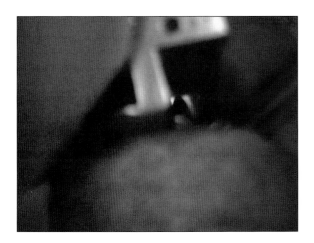

7-23e *Passing the tracheal tube under the epiglottis the tube tip must be carefully observed to be entering the larynx, which in this case is shadowed by the epiglottis. Ideally, the tube tip should always be seen to pass anterior to the interarytenoid notch.*

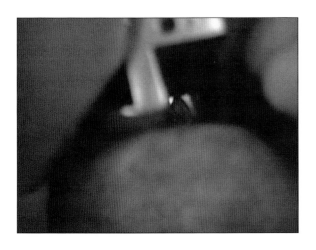

7-23f *With advancement the tube can be seen passing under the epiglottis.*

7-24. Curved blade laryngoscopy with a Macintosh blade

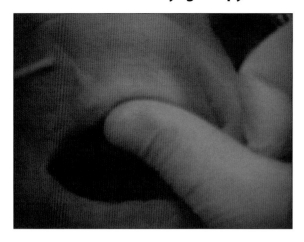

7-24a *Opening the mouth.*

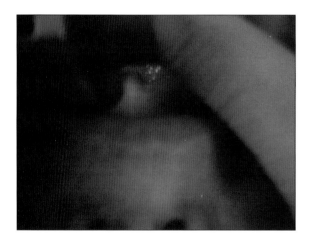

7-24b *Uvula.*

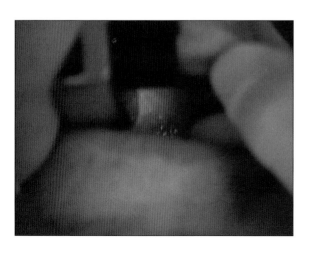

7-24c *The posterior pharynx.*

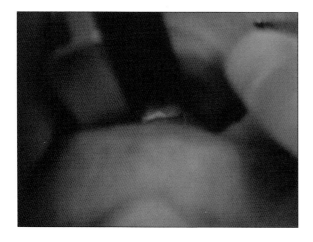

7-24d *The tip of the epiglottis.*

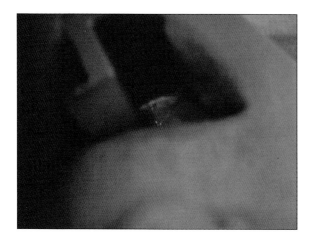

7-24e *The left posterior cartilages begin to be seen under the tip of the epiglottis.*

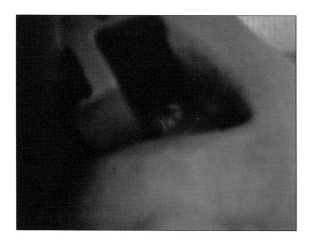

7-24f *A small portion of the glottic opening is now visible along with a good view of the vertical cleft of the interarytenoid notch and the posterior cartilages on the left side.*

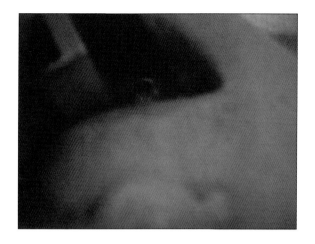

7-24g *A slightly larger view of the glottic opening.*

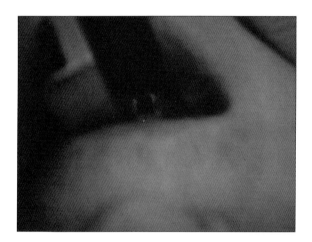

7-24h *With bimanual laryngoscopy the vocal cords, located deep within the larynx, can now be seen.*

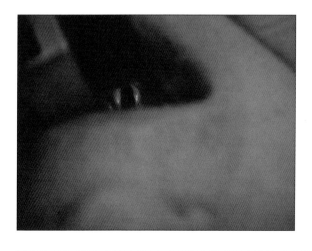

7-24i *A fuller view of the vocal cords.*

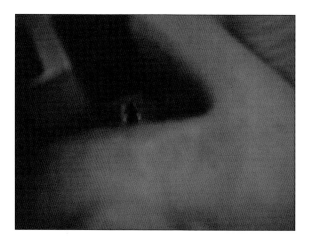

7-24j *More of the anterior aspect of the glottis is seen with additional manipulation, including the epiglottic tubercle.*

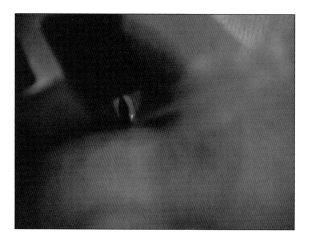

7-24k *The tracheal tube is inserted using the right side.*

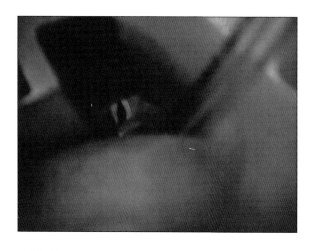

7-24l *As the tube is advanced toward the larynx it is positioned below the line of sight.*

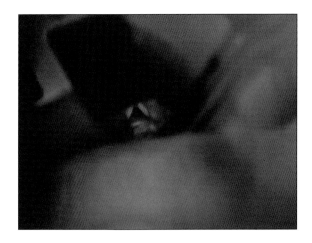

7-24m *The tube cuff can be seen passing adjacent to the vocal cords.*

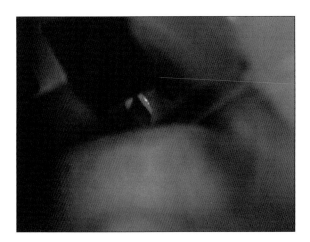

7-24n *The cuff has passed beyond the vocal cords and is no longer seen. The vocal cords can be seen alongside the tracheal tube.*

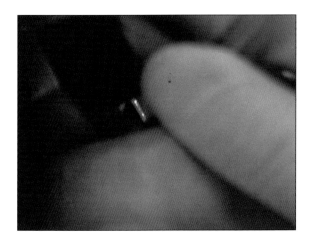

7-24o *The tube has been advanced until the markings of the tube at the teeth is at 21centimeters. The depth of insertion in men is 23 centimeters at the teeth.*

Chapter 8

Passing the Tracheal Tube

Stylet Shaping

Malleable metal stylets are widely recommended for emergency airway management, but optimal shaping and the rationale for their use has not been well explained. Stylets and other introducers have also been devised specifically for the "difficult airway," ranging from simple low-tech approaches such as the bougie, to technically complex approaches such as optical stylets.

In the author's opinion, mis-shaping of malleable stylets is a frequent cause of intubation difficulty and failure, even when the larynx is adequately exposed. The goal of the stylet is to improve placement of the tracheal tube. This involves two separate factors, target visualization and maneuverability. Stylet shape affects each of these. Simply inserting a stylet confers no advantages per se, and it may make intubation more difficult. Stylets stiffen tracheal tubes and can cause more resistance to placement if the tip of the tube catches on the tracheal rings. Stylets are frequently cited as causes of iatrogenic perforation of the pharynx, trachea, or esophagus. For these reasons, the stylet should stop at least 2 centimeters from the distal tip of the tube to avoid iatrogenic injury and to allow the tube tip some flexibility.

Regardless of the laryngeal view (epiglottis-only or 100% POGO score), there are two relative constants regarding laryngeal sighting and placement of a styletted tracheal tube. First, there is direct (straight) line of sight or axis from the operator's eye to the target (the laryngoscopy view axis), and second there is a separate axis defined by the orientation of the trachea. The tracheal axis with the patient lying in a supine position during laryngoscopy is generally of a shallower angle than the line of sight of the laryngoscopist, although there is great variability depending upon the amount of head elevation (neck flexion), atlanto-occipital extension, and other factors. On occasion, during easy laryngoscopy cases and optimal positioning, the axes converge and the anterior tracheal rings can be clearly seen. In cases of difficult laryngoscopy and epiglottis-only views, however, these axes tend to become more separated. In cases when the patient cannot be optimally positioned for laryngoscopy, such as with cervical spine precautions, morbid obesity, short neck and other situations, the axis of laryngeal view may be significantly different from the axis of the trachea. Commonly, only the posterior structures of the laryngeal inlet are seen.

The ideally shaped tracheal tube and stylet should mimic the line of sight axis in the main section of the tube (occupying as little space as possible when viewed down the long axis), and approximate or accommodate the tracheal axis in the distal section of the tube. This is the reason for a straight-to-cuff shape, with the main body of the tube being perfectly straight in all cases, and the section of the tube beginning just behind the cuff having the ability to be shaped as needed, in most instances angling slightly upward, i.e., about 35 degrees from the main section (Figure 8-1). The take-off point for the bend between these axes should be just behind the cuff, since insertion of the cuff past the cords is the stopping point of tube insertion.

Standard tracheal tubes have a pre-formed gentle arcuate shape and many manufacturers pre-package stylets in this shape purportedly for emergency situations. An arcuate shape is easiest for packaging tube and stylet combinations, and it seems intuitive that such a shape would best fit the curving contour of the tongue and curved laryngoscope blade during laryngoscopy. When viewed down the long axis of the tube from base to tip, however, this manner of shaping creates a relatively wide dimension from the base (or tip), to the middle section of the tube (Figure 8-2). It is difficult to manipulate this shape through the narrow confines of the mouth and hypopharynx and to aim it at a small target. Theoretically, such a shape lends itself to being rotated down the curvature of the tongue and laryngoscope blade, but this is awkward to accomplish, especially given the difficulties of depth perception and limited field of view inherent to the procedure. Moreover, even if rotation is used, visualization of the target is still obstructed by the mid-section of the tube as the tube is moved down into position.

Videographic and radiographic images on cadavers have shown that a gentle arcuate shape causes the mid-section of the tracheal tube to obscure the line of sight to the target (Figure 8-3). With the straight-to-cuff shape, and the tube bent 35 degrees just behind the cuff, the mid-section of the tube is out of the line of sight after placement within the pharynx (Figure 8-4). The distal tip of the tube appears to angle itself upward at the laryngeal inlet, and because the mid-section is out of view, the tip can easily be seen. It is especially valuable that the tip is angling itself upward toward the target. The dividing line between the esophagus and the trachea is the interarytenoid notch and the posterior cartilages. With the tip of the tube angling upward, it is easy to direct the tip above these structures.

A straight-to-cuff shape to the stylet also aids maneuverability. By having a small long axis dimension and with the bend point as noted, the tube can be easily tilted backward and forward, and the tip advanced toward the target or adjusted up or down. The pivot point of movement is at the teeth and the opening of the mouth, and the small shape permits a wide span of tip movement with only minor variation about the pivot point. The most valuable feature of the straight-to-cuff shape becomes evident in instances of poor laryngeal view, when the epiglottis is obstructing the view of the glottic opening. In these instances, the upward angle of the distal tip can be placed directly under the epiglottis and into the laryngeal inlet. For this technique to work, the tip of the tube must be kept upright, midline, and immediately beneath the epiglottis as it is advanced.

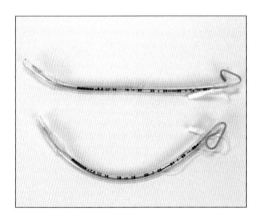

8-1 *Straight-to-cuff tube/stylet shape (above) and arcuate shaped tube/stylet (below). Note that the end of the stylet stops 1-2 centimeters before the tip of the tracheal tube.*

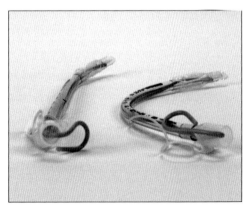

8-2 *The narrower long axis dimension of the straight-to-cuff shape (left) vs. the arcuate shape (right).*

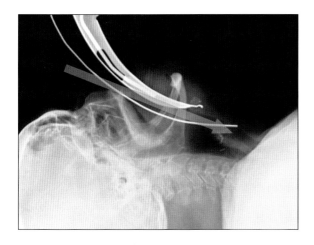

8-3 *Radiographic image of laryngoscopy with arcuate-shaped stylet demonstrates that mid-section of stylet is in the line of sight of the laryngoscopist.*

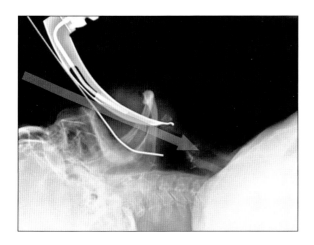

8-4a *Radiographic image of laryngoscopy with straight-to-cuff stylet demonstrates that mid-section and tip of stylet is below line of sight after insertion. Narrow long axis has improved maneuverability within hypopharynx vs. arcuate shape.*

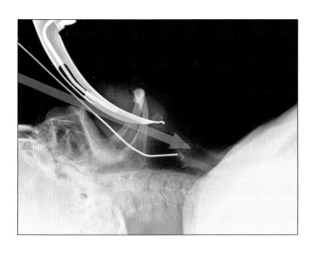

8-4b *As stylet tip advances toward larynx with straight-to-cuff shape it is angled correctly toward target and visible to laryngoscopist coming up from below line of sight.*

Conversely, when the tracheal tube and stylet is given a gentle arcuate shape, the larger long axis dimension takes up more space within the pharynx and hypopharynx. Trying to elevate the distal tube when the proximal end of the arcuate shape is contacting the upper palate and dentition causes bending of the stylet and tube over the teeth. The curved shape thus limits up/down maneuverability and forward and backward movements.

Advancement of the tracheal tube stylet combination is sometimes a problem when the tip of the tracheal tube catches on the anterior tracheal rings. When this occurs even when the larynx has been well visualized the tube and stylet cannot be advanced into the trachea. Conventional tubes have an asymmetric beveled tip that is rather firm and unyielding, especially when a stylet is used (Figure 8-5). Hanging up on the tracheal rings can occur with either an arcuate shape or a straight-to-cuff shape. This problem results from the tube and stylet not matching the shape of the trachea. When using a straight-to-cuff shape, the bend angle should not be overdone for this reason. Angles greater than approximately 35 degrees will predictably cause this problem to occur.

One response to catching the anterior tracheal rings is to rotate the tube and stylet. This will rotate the tube tip past the tracheal rings to the smooth posterior aspect of the trachea. If rotation of the tube is done, it should be done gently and with little force. A second means of handling this situation is to keep the tube tip at the same position and to have an assistant carefully withdraw the stylet. This permits more flexibility of the tube tip and advancement into the trachea over the tracheal rings.

As an aside, a new tracheal tube tip design (Parker Medical, Englewood CO, Flex-Tip), overcomes these issues by design (Figure 8-6). It has a patented ski-tip shaped end that has some built-in flexibility and can glide over the tracheal rings more easily than conventional beveled tubes. This tube may also be better for nasal intubation because of its ability to more easily glide over structures without impingement. Tube tip shape is also important in other situations when a

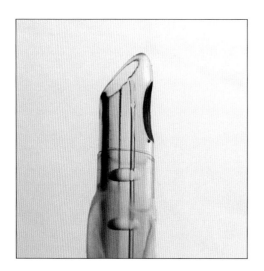

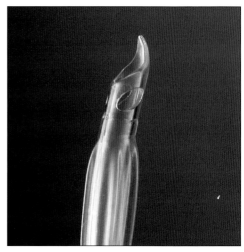

8-5 *Close up of beveled tracheal tube tip, with bevel facing leftward and curvature of tube perpendicular to the page.*

8-6 *The ski-tip shape of the Parker Medical Flex-tip tracheal tube. The curvature of the tube is directed to the right side in the same orientation of the page.*

tracheal tube is being slid off guides or introducers, such as with retrograde intubation, or with flexible fiberoptic intubation. In the author's experience, the Parker tube performs better than standard tubes in retrograde intubation, and one study has demonstrated easier tube passage with fiberoptic intubation.

A final issue with malleable stylets has to do with withdrawal of the stylet after placement, and is specifically related to the straight-to-cuff shape. Excessive angling of the tip will make withdrawal of the stylet very difficult. This does not occur with the gentle arcuate shape. If the bend angle is limited and deliberately not made too abrupt, this is easily managed. Lubricating the stylet with a water soluble jelly also helps. It is recommended that one stabilize the tracheal tube before pulling out the stylet to prevent unintentional withdrawal of the tracheal tube in the process.

Tracheal Tube Introducers: Eschmann Stylet, "Bougie"and Frova Introducer

The Eschmann Stylet (Portex, Kent UK), commonly called the gum elastic bougie, is a long, flexible, non-malleable introducer with a pre-formed upturned distal tip (Figure 8-7). The total length is 60 centimeters, and the distal bend occurs 3.5 centimeters from the tip with an angle of 40 degrees. Curiously, it is neither made of gum nor elastic, and it is not a true "bougie," which technically refers to a device that is used for dilation. The Eschmann is made of a resin covered, braided polyester, and is intended to be cold-sterilized and reused (the manufacturer suggests no more than 5 uses).

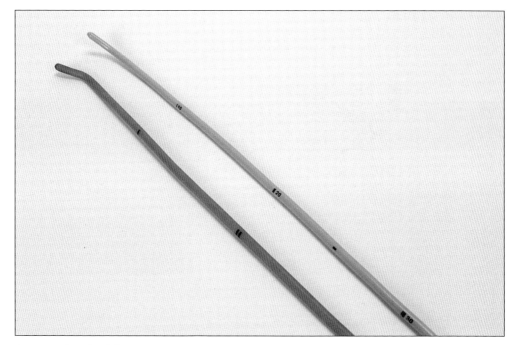

8-7 *Distal ends of the Portex Eschmann stylet (beige, left) and the disposable Sun-Med bougie. Markings on devices every 10 cm are useful for gauging depth of insertion during use.*

The Eschmann stylet and other bougies have a smaller outer diameter (5 mm) than the outer diameter of a tracheal tube (8.5–11 mm). This makes them easier to place and visualize within the narrow working space created during laryngoscopy. After the bougie is passed into the trachea, a tracheal tube is railroaded over the device. The outer diameter of the Eschmann and other bougies are not that dissimilar from the inner diameter of an adult tracheal tube, which generally makes it easy to slide the tube down the bougie and into the larynx (Figure 8-8). When passing a tracheal tube over a bronchoscope or a retrograde intubation wire, however, the gap between the devices may be significant. The asymmetric tip of a traditional tracheal tube can hang up at the laryngeal inlet, due to the size gap between the two devices (Figure 8-9). If resistance is encountered, regardless of what device is being used, a counterclockwise rotation of the tracheal tube will help. By rotating the tube counterclockwise, the bevel enters the laryngeal inlet under the epiglottis, symmetrically, instead of catching on the right aryepiglottic fold (Figure 8-9). In the UK, where a bougie is commonly used instead of a stylet, it is standard practice that laryngoscope is held in place after insertion of the bougie, and an assistant passes the tube down the bougie. This technique, along with counterclockwise tube rotation, prevents problems with tube passage into the larynx.

When properly placed into the trachea, the tip of the bougie can be felt to bounce over the tracheal rings as it is advanced in 65–90% of cases. Occasionally, the tip will impinge on a tracheal ring and stop; slight clockwise rotation rotates the tip off of the tracheal ring permitting insertion. The bougie will stop advancing between 24 and 40 centimeters when it is in the trachea because of the decreasing caliber of the airways. This resistance does not occur when it is placed into the esophagus. The device has markings to permit the clinician to readily identify depth of placement.

It is essential that the clinician note the location of the markings and the orientation of the upturned tip as a bougie is inserted. Minor rotational changes at the proximal end of the bougie can cause a significant change in the orientation and location of the tip (Figure 8-10a–c). For successful placement in cases of epiglottis-only views, the upturned distal tip must be kept midline and immediately underneath the epiglottis. The markings help identify which way the tip is

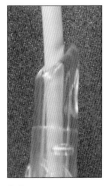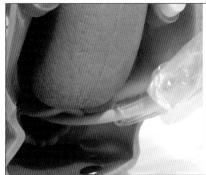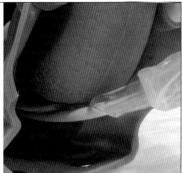

8-8   8-9

8-8 *Tracheal tube with bougie showing minimal gap between inner diameter of tracheal tube and 5mm outer diameter of bougie.*

8-9 *Effect of counter-clockwise rotation of tracheal tube and bevel orientation as tube slides over bougie. Counterclockwise rotation helps the tube pass into the larynx instead of catching the right aryepiglottic fold.*

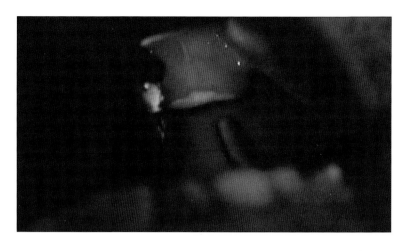

8-10a

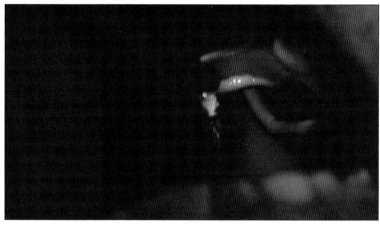

8-10b

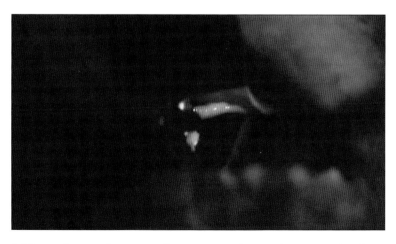

8-10c

8-10a–c *Correct placement of bougie in epiglottis-only view involves keeping tip midline, non-rotated, and immediately below epiglottis edge (8-10a–b). Minor rotation of bougie can cause angled tip to rotate significantly and miss laryngeal inlet (8-10c).*

directed, since they are printed on the same side that the tip is angled. Several studies have shown a benefit to shaping the bougie in a curved manner, especially in the epiglottis-only situation. The device works well in simulated epiglottis-only views when the epiglottis edge is not laying on the posterior pharyngeal wall (CL grade 3a), but there is less successful placement when the epiglottis cannot be elevated off the posterior pharyngeal wall (CL grade 3b).

Some studies have found the bougie more effective than the stylet for managing cases of epiglottis-only views, and it is used widely in Europe. It has recently achieved more attention in the ED in the United States, particularly since the marketing of single use, disposable plastic devices. The original version costs approximately $75, whereas the disposable variety ranges from $6–$10. Recent studies originating in the United Kingdom have questioned whether the performance of some of the disposable is inferior to the original version, but the reusable device has been acknowledged to be a potential vector for prion transfer between patients if improperly sterilized. The difference in performance may be due to differences in spring and shape retention, as the dimensions and tip design of the disposable and original devices are nearly identical.

The most sophisticated tube introducer available is the Frova Introducer (Cook Critical Care, Bloomington IN). It has a 3mm hollow lumen running its entire length, which permits it it to function as a ventilating aid after insertion. It is made of molded plastic, 65 centimeters long, and has an outer dimension and upturned tip similar to the bougie. After placement, the device can be fitted with a 15mm plastic adapter allowing ventilation with a resuscitator bag. Because there is no cuff, however, it is unclear how effective ventilation would be in a given patient, especially in situations of high airway resistance, like asthma, COPD, and CHF.

Lighted Stylets as a Laryngoscopy Adjunct

Lighted stylets come in a variety of designs and can act as a laryngoscopy adjunct similar to a standard stylet. A lighted stylet can also be used as an independent intubation device without a laryngoscope. Simple versions designed for single patient use have a single piece of malleable metal and a non-removable handle that contains the battery. Much more sophisticated and expensive is the Trachlight (Laerdal Medical, Wappinger Falls NY), which has a removable metal stiffener and reusable handle. The Trachlight stylets come in both reusable and disposable versions.

The potential advantage of a lighted stylet over a standard stylet or is that when the tip is placed beneath the epiglottis, trans-illumination through the cricothyroid membrane and trachea may verify tracheal placement. When used in this manner, it is recommended that the same straight-to-cuff shape be used. A more exaggerated bend, 70–90 degrees, is used when the lighted stylet is employed as an independent intubation device. The stiffness of the device can sometimes cause problems with advancing the tracheal tube and impaction on the tracheal rings, whether used either as a laryngoscopy adjunct or as an independent device. Rotating the device clockwise (to get past the tracheal rings) often overcomes this issue.

One study has addressed the use of the Laerdal Trachlight as a laryngoscopy adjunct. Agro, a world authority on the device, reported its use in 350 anesthetized patients with simulated epiglottis-only views. The overall success rate was 100%. Seventy-eight percent of patients were successfully intubated on first attempt with a median intubation time of 11 seconds. Difficulty with advancement happened in 6% of cases. The limitation of the lighted stylet is that trans-illumination tends to work poorly in the subset of patients who are most difficult for laryngoscopy, namely large patients with short necks. In this set of patients, especially those with dark skin, trans-illumination is often difficult to achieve.

Direct Laryngoscopy with Fiberoptic Augmentation

The ultimate means of augmenting direct laryngoscopy and tube insertion is by the addition of fiberoptic visualization. Combining laryngoscopy with a flexible scope has been described but this technique is slow and requires two persons. Intubation over a flexible scope is also more challenging in patients who are supine and flaccid because the tongue and soft tissues collapse downward, making the lumen of the airway harder to navigate. Techniques for overcoming poor visualization include a jaw thrust maneuver, retraction of the tongue with a gauze pad, or use of a laryngoscope to help lift the tongue upward. The other problem with flexible scopes is that the leading edge of the scope is exposed as it is placed. Any secretions or blood can obscure the small optical element of the tip.

Optical stylets that can be used by the laryngoscopist are much easier to use as laryngoscopy adjuncts compared to flexible scopes. An excellent review of these devices is by Liem (Liem EB, Bjoraker DG, Gravenstein D. New options for airway management: Intubating fibreoptic stylets. *Br J Anaesth*. 2003; 91: 408–418.).

Three optical stylets are commercially available in the United States (June 2004). The Storz Bonfils Intubating Stylet (Storz Endoscopy, Culver City CA) has a working length of 40 centimeters and a gently upturned distal tip with a deflection of 40 degrees. It uses a 12,000 pixel fiber and has a fixed shape (non-bendable). It comes with a handle battery or a light guide attachment, and one model has a working channel for suction or oxygen. Successful oral intubation (with and without a laryngoscope) has been described with extreme examples of micrognathia, macroglossia and spinal pathology. The Macintosh blade can be used to identify the epiglottis and the device is then placed beneath the epiglottis with subsequent reliance on the fiberoptic image to guide the device and the pre-loaded tube into the trachea.

The author has extensive experience using the Shikani Seeing Optical Stylet (Clarus Medical, Minneapolis MN) as a laryngoscopy adjunct (Figure 8-11). It has a long malleable stainless steel stylet coupled to a removable eyepiece. The stylet incorporates a high-resolution 30,000 pixel fiberoptic viewing element with a 70 degree viewing angle and a separate light conducting bundle. At the proximal end of the stylet, coming off at a right angle, is a light guide attachment. This can be connected to an external light source with a light guide cable, but other lighting options include a specially designed 6 volt battery handle, or an adapter to attach a standard fiberoptic laryngoscope handle (Figure 8-12). At the proximal end of the device is a tube-stop that engages the 15 millimeter connection of the tracheal tube, stabilizing the tube on the stylet. A small plastic connector that fits into the tube stop permits supplemental oxygen attachment. This helps to keep the tip of the scope secretion free as oxygen is blown down the inner aspect of the tracheal tube and out the distal end. The main body of the stylet can be shaped as desired using an overlying tracheal tube. Breaking the fiberoptic element is possible with extreme force and acute angulation, and that is the rationale for always bending the device with an overlying tracheal tube. Like any fiberoptic viewing device, it cannot be heat sterilized, but since it does not have a working channel, cleaning is a relatively simple matter and can be done with a Steris system, glutaraldehyde, or other cold sterilization solutions.

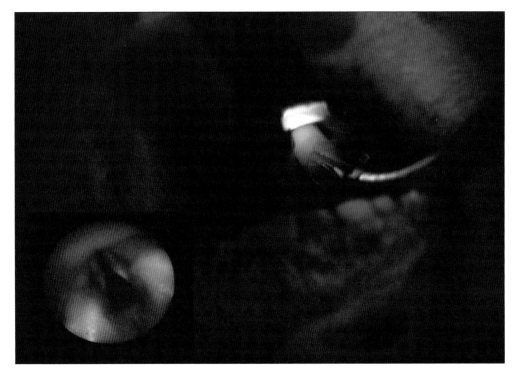

8-11 *Shikani optical stylet (Clarus Medical, Minneapolis MN) used as laryngoscopy adjunct, showing laryngoscopist's perspective of device placed under epiglottis. Inset shows corresponding endoscopic view from eyepiece. When using the device as a laryngoscopy adjunct it is essential to place the tip of the scope (and tube) under the epiglottis under direct vision, staying off of the mucosa, before the eyepiece is used to check the endoscopic view.*

In a study by the author performed on 40 non-embalmed cadavers with simulated epiglottis-only views, all tracheas were successfully intubated using the Shikani with a straight-to-cuff shape, with excellent laryngeal visualization in a mean time of 9 seconds. Although blood and secretions are significant in fresh cadavers, the recessed placement of the stylet tip within the tracheal tube prevented this from being a problem.

The Parker TrachView (Parker Medical, Englewood CO) is a flexible endoscope that is designed to be partnered with a malleable stylet to permit fiberoptic visualization from the tube tip. The device comes with an integrated endoscopic camera, color video monitor, and light source. Like the Shikani or Bonfils scope, the end of the scope is slightly recessed within the tip of the tracheal tube. A plastic connector that interfaces with the 15 millimeter hub on the tracheal tube holds the scope and malleable steel stylet in proper position. Compared to standard flexible scopes, the Parker scope is slightly larger in diameter and more durable because of its heavy-duty protective sleeve and lack of articulating tip. The integrated light source comes with a built-in spare bulb.

When using the Bonfils, Shikani, or Parker TrachView the tip of the tracheal tube extends beyond the tip of the optical element so design of the tube tip may affect the field of view looking through the scope. Many tracheal tubes have a rounded or shrouded tip in order to make the tip less traumatic (Figure 8-5). When viewed from the end of an optical stylet, however, this shrouded tip design can obscure a significant part of the visual field. Although this can be minimized by fine-

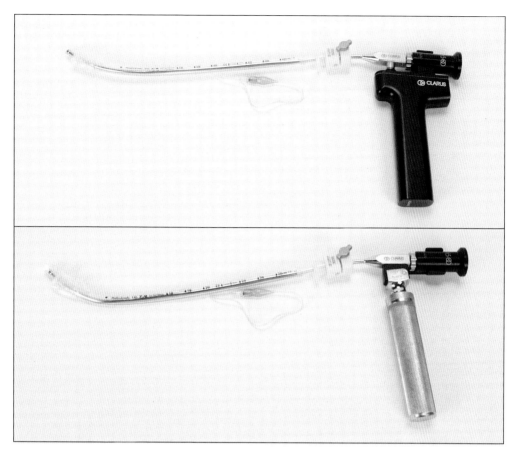

8-12 *Shikani optical stylet shaped as laryngoscopy adjunct and connected to 6 volt battery handle (top) and connected with an adapter to a fiberoptic laryngoscope handle (bottom).*

tuning the position of the tube on the tube stop, the best option is to use a tracheal tube that does not have a shrouded tip. An ideal tube for use with optical stylets is the 7.0 mm ID Mallinckrodt Lo-Pro tracheal tube (Nellcor Inc., Pleasanton CA).

Another flexible endoscope designed specifically for laryngoscopy use (but not yet available in the US), is the Intubationstylet (Acutronic Medical, Baar, Switzerland). It has an outer diameter of 3.9 centimeters and an overall length of two meters. Like the Parker TrachView, it works only with an attached video camera. The last 40 centimeters of the stylet incorporates a thin malleable wire. Unlike the Bonfils, Shikani, or Parker TrachView, however, the Intubationstylet is placed like the bougie in advance of the tracheal tube. Several studies have been done in Europe using a similar device called the Video Optical Intubating Stylet (VOIS).

Optical stylets are significantly simpler and faster to use than a flexible scope. Unlike other rigid fiberoptic or imaging devices (Bullard, Wu-Scope, Glidescope, etc.) that require direct or indirect elevation of the epiglottis to obtain visualization of the larynx, optical stylets can be independently inserted under the epiglottis, making them potentially useful in a broad array of difficult laryngoscopy situations. If the epiglottis cannot be seen directly down the laryngoscope lumen, the end of the stylet can be advanced along the curvature of the laryngoscope until the epiglottis edge comes into endoscopic view. The most important aspect of properly using an optical stylet is to keep the tip of the scope off of the mucosa. When placed directly on the mucosa, the entire view disappears. When dealing with the epiglottis-only situation, it is helpful to insert the device under direct vision, keeping the scope tip off of the mucosa and well away from the epiglottis, before viewing through the scope.

For ED practitioners, who are likely to be infrequent users of any fiberoptic device, the advantage of an optical stylet is its similarity to a standard malleable stylet. Optical stylets can fit easily within standard emergency airway practice. They can be used during first pass laryngoscopy efforts without switching from the laryngoscope to another device or requiring an intervening episode of ventilating the patient. A major hurdle to using fiberoptic devices is skill acquisition and familiarity with landmark recognition from a fiberoptic perspective. In order to be successful in problem cases, these devices must be used routinely so that the provider is thoroughly familiar with fiberoptic landmarks and comfortable handling the device.

The length of the Bonfils or Shikani is problematic for shorter persons because of the distance away from the patient and the arm stretch needed to hold the instrument out to length with initial insertion. A shorter version of the Shikani stylet, specifically designed for use with a laryngoscope, should be available in the near future.

Manipulating an optical scope while simultaneously doing laryngoscopy requires a significant degree of hand-eye coordination, especially when using an eyepiece on the stylet as opposed to a video monitor. The Parker TrachView and Acutronic devices can be handled almost exactly like a standard stylet, although each require an external light source and video monitor. The Bonfils and Shikani can be used with integrated batteries and self-contained light sources that do not require attachments, so they are not tethered to any one location or to an equipment cart. An endoscopic camera and external video monitor can also be attached to these devices if preferred, and this set-up is easier than working through the eyepiece, especially for an initial user. A potential pitfall in the ED setting with any fiberoptic device involves fogging, secretions, or blood obscuring the lens element, but this is less of a risk with the models in which the optical element is recessed within the tube tip. Supplemental oxygen flowing over the tip of the device also helps.

With the exception of the optical variety, stylets and bougies are very inexpensive and easy to use laryngoscopy adjuncts that can salvage poor laryngeal view. Assuming a standard malleable metal stylet is correctly shaped however, very few cases will require any other tube placement adjunct. It is the author's opinion that good laryngoscopy technique, coupled with properly shaped stylets and the rare use a bougie, can solve the vast majority of difficult airways in emergency settings. The departmental decision to acquire a fiberoptic device to augment laryngoscopy is dependent upon resources, the logistical ability to have it cleaned and restocked, and the providers' commitment for routine use. It is expected that disposable, single-use endoscopic sheaths will be available for optical stylets in the near future. Disposable sheaths will eliminate the need for cold sterilization or sending the device out of the department for cleaning, issues that have prevented some emergency departments from acquiring fiberoptic instruments.

Despite logistical hurdles and the fact that optical devices are rarely a necessity for intubation success, they have the potential to significantly enhance patient safety. Their use can transform tracheal tube confirmation from a delayed technique (end-tidal CO_2 confirmation) to immediate visual verification. In rare instances of unanticipated laryngoscopy difficulty they can be used on first pass, potentially eliminating the need for repeat laryngoscopy and rescue ventilation. In educational settings, when coupled to endoscopic cameras, optical stylets enhance supervision of the laryngoscopist as well as provide an educational experience for other observers. As the cost of these devices fall, and disposable endoscopic sheaths become available, the author believes optical stylets (specifically designed as laryngoscopy adjuncts) will become commonplace in emergency settings, especially in teaching hospitals.

Chapter 9

Straight Blade Laryngoscopy: Paraglossal Technique

Mechanics of Straight Blade Laryngoscopy and Direct Elevation of the Epiglottis

Straight laryngoscopes are used to directly lift the epiglottis, whereas curved blades do this indirectly with pressure at the vallecula. Proper epiglottis identification, tongue control, and tube passage, all of which are important with curved blades, are even more critical with straight blades. Compared to curved blades, most straight blades have a significantly smaller flange. The smaller flange means there is less blade to control the tongue, less of a window to look down at the larynx, and less space to place the tube without blocking the line of sight to the target.

The benefit of the smaller flange on most straight blades is a reduced overall displacement volume, i.e., the volume the blade takes up when placed within the mouth and pharynx. The smaller displacement volume translates into less tongue that needs to be moved out of the way, and it is accordingly easier to pass the blade down to the larynx. In patients with a small displacement space, such as small children and adults with a very short thyromental distance, the smaller displacement volume of a narrow lumen straight blade facilitates laryngeal visualization. This smaller lumen is not an issue when passing a non-cuffed tracheal tube, because the lumen of the blade is so large relative to the very small dimension of the tube. In adults with cuffed tubes however, the tracheal tube is significantly larger and tube passage becomes more difficult. Most adult Miller blades will not accept tracheal tubes larger than a 5.5 or 6.0 mm ID. In the design of any straight blade there is an inherent paradoxical balance between a smaller lumen, which facilitates ease of reaching the larynx, and a larger lumen, which broadens visualization and makes tube passage easier.

Direct control of the epiglottis also puts the tip of a straight blade within the laryngeal inlet, providing better and brighter illumination of the true vocal cords and glottic opening.

Mechanically, laryngeal exposure with straight blades does not depend upon pressure at the hyoepiglottic ligament, and they can overcome many causes of difficult laryngeal exposure stemming from problems at the vallecula and the base of the tongue (Figure 9-1a–c). Straight blade laryngoscopy has permitted intubation in cases of lingual tonsillar hyperplasia and other instances of failed curved blade laryngoscopy.

Another potential advantage of straight blades involves dentition problems. When there are dental gaps, the large proximal flange of a Macintosh blade may catch in this space, limiting the maneuverability of the blade and restricting the area for tube passage. Smaller flanged straight blades fit more easily and have fewer mechanical problems interacting with the teeth. They also need a smaller area for tube passage, assuming the extreme right hand corner of the mouth is used for tube introduction.

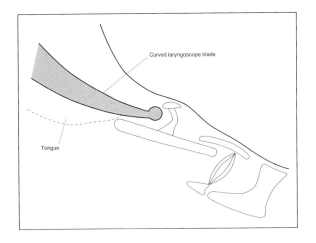

9-1a *In easy curved blade laryngoscopy, the tip of blade sits in vallecula and effectively elevates epiglottis by pressure at hyoepiglottic ligament.*

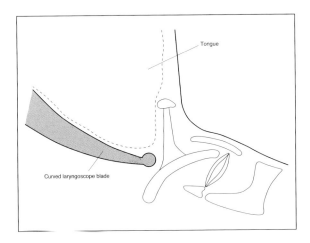

9-1b *When the tip of curved blade cannot be fully positioned into vallecula, the curved blade will not effectively elevate epiglottis.*

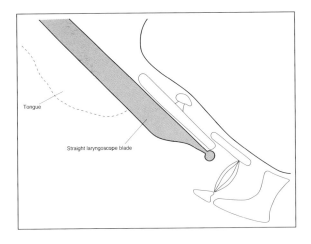

9-1c *Straight blade bypasses the mechanical issues of indirect epiglottis elevation and picks up the epiglottis directly.*

(Drawings courtesy of John Henderson, MD)

Finding the Epiglottis First and Paraglossal Placement

Finding the epiglottis first, before any effort is made to expose the larynx, is crucial to straight blade success. A slow methodical approach, advancing the spatula of the blade down the tongue is even more important with straight blades than with curved blades. Straight blades do not have a natural stopping point the way that curved blades fit in the vallecula. Their smaller spatula (the flat portion on the superior aspect of the blade that contacts the tongue) also makes it is easier to overlook the epiglottis. While the ultimate goal with a straight blade is to place the blade completely to the right side of the patient's mouth, the initial challenge is to locate the epiglottis edge. This is often easiest from a midline, straight down the tongue approach. As with the curved blade it is critical to distract the jaw in a caudal direction (toward the patient's feet) so that the epiglottis lifts off the posterior pharyngeal wall.

Once the epiglottis edge is identified, the blade can be adjusted and repositioned, and worked completely to the right of the tongue. The large flange on curved blades permits sweeping of the tongue, but this should not be done with straight blades. The goal with a straight blade is to achieve paraglossal right-sided placement. If the blade is not fully placed to the right side of the tongue, the tongue will flop over the small flange of most straight blades.

As the blade is being directed rightward, the epiglottis edge is lifted directly by the tip of the blade and the tip is advanced into the laryngeal inlet. This occurs by slightly changing the angle of the blade (tilting the top of the laryngoscope handle more toward the patient's feet) and advancing the blade a centimeter or two so that the tip has advanced beneath the epiglottis edge. Subsequent upward force will then expose the structures of the larynx, beginning from posterior to anterior. The first structure seen is the interarytenoid notch, followed by the posterior cartilages, and then the vocal cords and glottic opening.

It is important to note that great care must be taken with advancing straight blades beneath the epiglottis. At this point in the procedure the tip of the blade will be pointing directly at the posterior hypopharyngeal wall. This area is particularly prone to puncture and perforation if an over aggressive approach is taken. The tip of the straight blade should never be blindly advanced into the esophagus and then withdrawn. While such a technique works reliably in a training manikin, in real patients it carries a significant risk of trauma to the hypopharynx, upper esophagus, and larynx. It is also likely to result in failure to identify any landmarks. Without knowing exactly where the blade tip is positioned, it is difficult to apply specific strategies for improving laryngeal view.

Improving Laryngeal View with Straight Blades: ELM and Head Elevation

External laryngeal manipulation (ELM) and increasing head elevation are both effective means of improving laryngeal exposure once the epiglottis is identified and the tip of the straight blade has been inserted into the laryngeal inlet. ELM works with straight blades by pushing the larynx down into the line of sight of the laryngoscopist. An assistant can take over once the view is optimized. Increasing head elevation and neck flexion is particularly advantageous with straight blades because such positioning decreases the tension on the anterior neck muscles. It becomes easier to move the jaw and tongue forward if the head is not over extended, but rather lifted higher with the neck more flexed relative to the chest. In addition to requiring less force to distract the jaw and tongue forward, neck flexion also shortens the distance from the mouth opening to the larynx.

Tube Placement and Stylet Shaping with Straight Blades

The final step to successful intubation with the straight blade is placement of the tracheal tube. The narrow flange height (particularly of the Miller blade) makes passage of the tracheal tube through the lumen impossible with adult-sized tracheal tubes. As already noted, placing the tube via the lumen of a straight blade is possible with a small uncuffed tracheal tube on infants and children because of the relatively large size of the pediatric laryngoscope blade lumen compared to the small external diameter of the tracheal tube. Whether with adults or children, however, the best continuous visualization of the target is achieved by deliberately not placing the tracheal tube down the lumen of the blade.

With the blade located all the way to the right side of the mouth, the styletted tube should be inserted into the extreme right corner of the mouth. The tip of the tracheal tube is advanced toward the target from a position below the lumen of the blade so that visualization of the target is not obstructed. A straight-to-cuff stylet shape is especially useful, given the limited working area along the right paraglossal space. Using the extreme right corner of the mouth is essential. By swinging the tube into this area the base of the tube and stylet can be pivoted down, allowing the tube tip to come upward to the larynx. This space for tube manipulation exists because of the curvature of the upper dentition. If the styletted tube is manipulated from a midline position there is no space to move the tube backward over the central incisors, and bringing the tube tip upward cannot happen.

Sequential Imaging of Straight Blade Laryngoscopy

9-2. Straight blade laryngoscopy with a Wisconsin blade

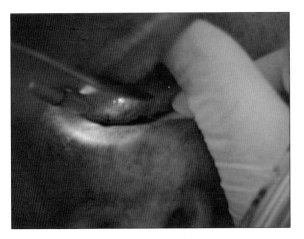

9-2a *Scissor technique opening of the mouth.*

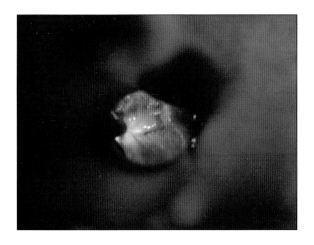

9-2b *Epiglottis edge camouflaged against posterior pharyngeal wall. Note the C-shaped flange of the Wisconsin blade.*

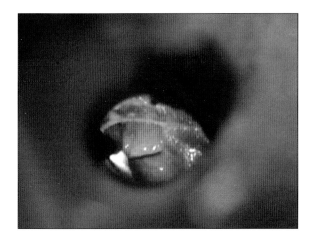

9-2c *With slight downward force and lifting of the tongue the epiglottis edge becomes more visible.*

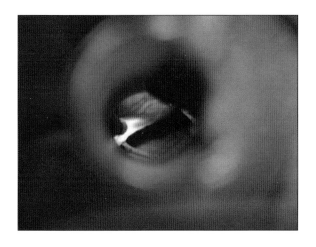

9-2d *Additional lifting and advancement causes the epiglottis edge to lift off the posterior pharyngeal wall.*

Chapter 9   **165**

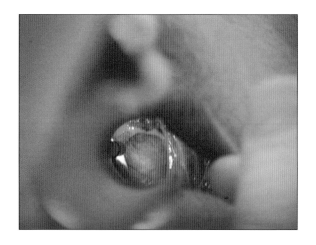

9-2e *Blade has been advanced under the epiglottis edge. The pharyngoepiglottic fold is visible on the right side. Immediately beneath the blade tip is the mucosa of the hypopharynx.*

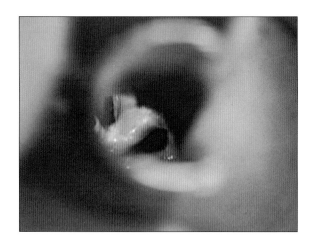

9-2f *With advancement and lifting, the holes of the larynx and esophagus come into view. The esophagus has indistinct posterior borders.*

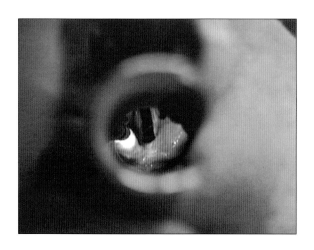

9-2g *In this view of the larynx the true and false vocal cords are distinctly seen, as are the posterior cartilages bilaterally and the interarytenoid notch.*

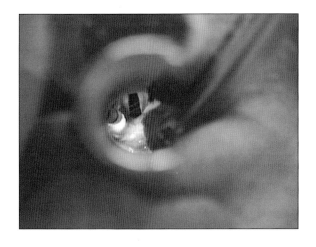

9-2h *The tracheal tube is inserted from the right side without obscuring the view of the larynx.*

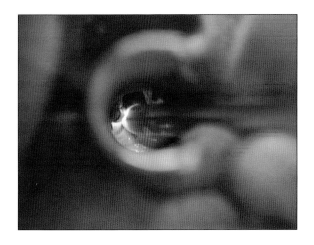

9-2i *Tracheal tube passing through larynx showing posterior cartilages underneath tube.*

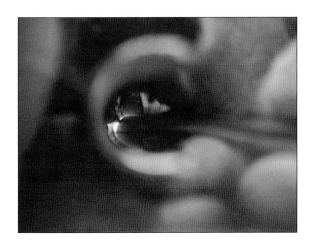

9-2j *Tracheal tube passing through larynx with vocal cords visible above and lateral to tube.*

9-3. Straight blade laryngoscopy with a Miller blade

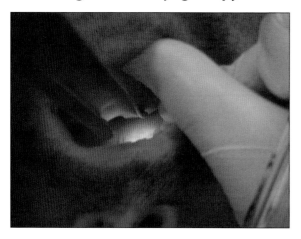

9-3a *Scissor technique with initial insertion of Miller blade.*

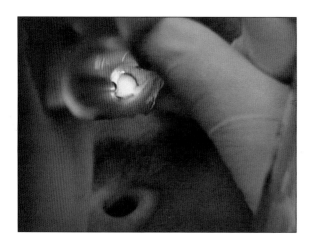

9-3b *Uvula.*

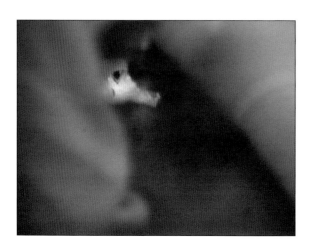

9-3c *The interarytenoid notch and a small portion of the glottic opening. A small portion of tongue is caught on the right side.*

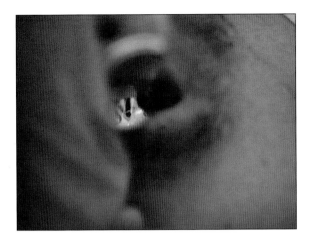

9-3d *True vocal cords and narrow vertical slit of the glottic opening. With blade repositioning the portion of tongue to the right of the blade is now minimal.*

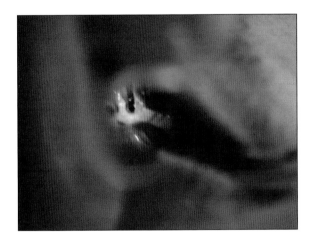

9-3e *Tracheal tube insertion from extreme right corner of mouth permits visualization of the target down the blade lumen as the tube is advanced.*

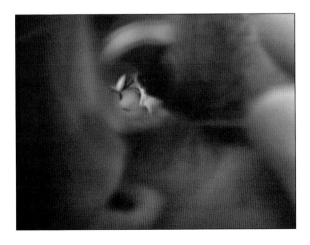

9-3f *Tube passing through the vocal cords.*

9-4. Straight blade laryngoscopy with a Miller blade

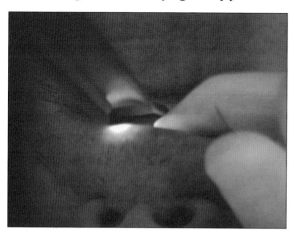

9-4a *Initial blade insertion of Miller blade.*

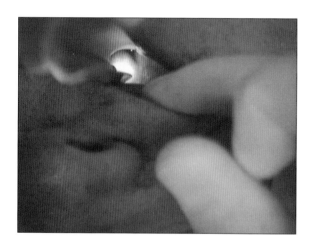

9-4b *Uvula and upper right lip retraction.*

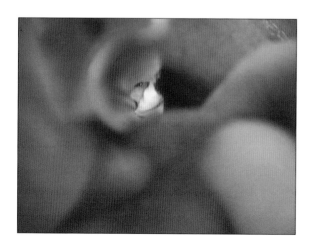

9-4c *The initial view of the glottic opening and interarytenoid notch.*

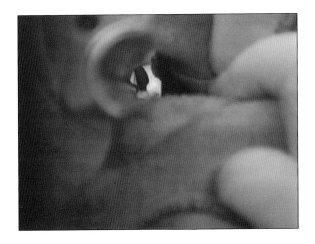

9-4d *Additional lifting exposes more of the glottic opening. The blade is positioned fully to the right of the tongue, in a right paraglossal position. Note the right eye (closed) at the bottom of the image.*

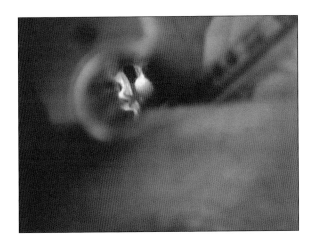

9-4e *Tube is introduced in extreme right corner of mouth and although the working area is very small the tube tip is seen entering the larynx. The tube tip can be seen coming up from below to enter the larynx.*

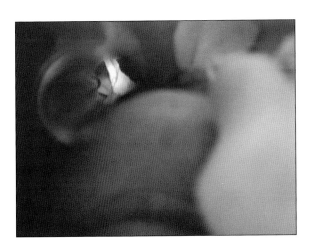

9-4f *Tracheal tube through vocal cords.*

9-5. Straight blade laryngoscopy with a Miller blade

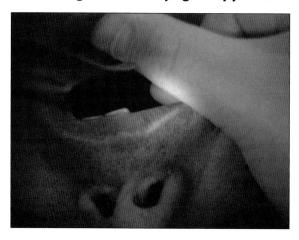

9-5a *Scissor technique with initial blade insertion of Miller blade.*

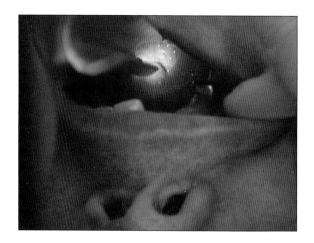

9-5b *The uvula and posterior pharynx. Note the large gap in the upper right dentition. This can be problematic with the large flange of the Macintosh blade that will lock into this position, restricting blade maneuverability, and then limiting visibility of the target as the tube is inserted.*

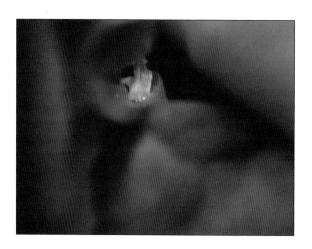

9-5c *Posterior right aspect of larynx and small glottic opening.*

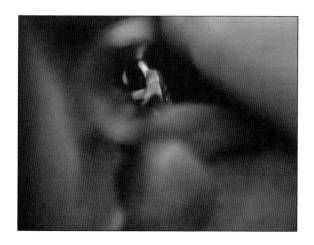

9-5d *Best view of larynx showing the true vocal cords well illuminated. Tracheal rings can be seen through glottic opening.*

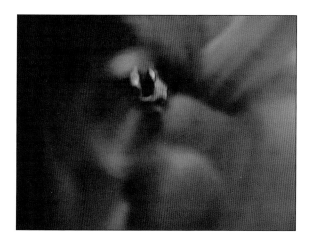

9-5e *Initial tracheal tube insertion through extreme right corner of mouth avoiding narrow lumen of the Miller blade. Tube is directed posteriorly until tip is ready to be advanced toward target.*

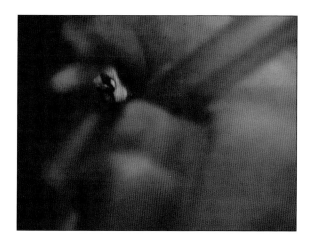

9-5f *Tip of tracheal tube coming up from below is seen as it enters glottic opening.*

9-6. Straight blade laryngoscopy with a Wisconsin blade

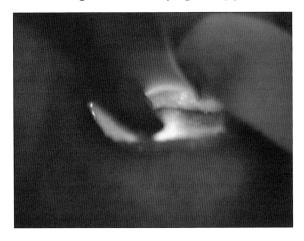

9-6a *Initial blade insertion.*

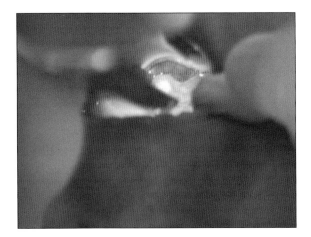

9-6b *Uvula.*

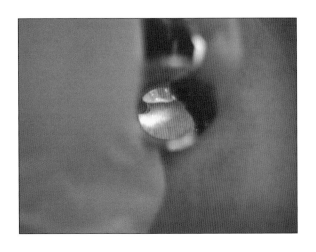

9-6c *Epiglottis edge well delineated. The curved C-shape of the Wisconsin blade is apparent.*

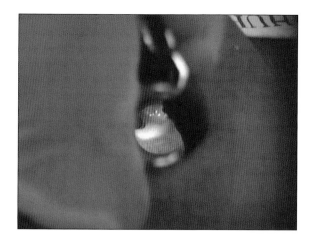

9-6d *After tilting the blade and advancing, the posterior hypopharyngeal wall is visible and there is a poorly defined structure at the top of the lumen of the blade.*

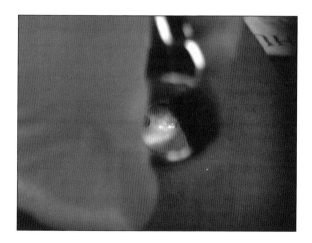

9-6e *The interarytenoid notch and the posterior aspect of the glottic opening come into view.*

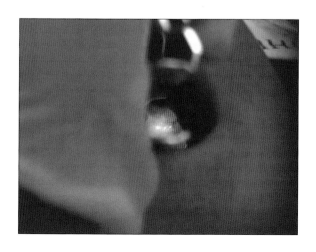

9-6f *With additional elevation more of the glottic opening is exposed, but the vocal cords are not yet seen.*

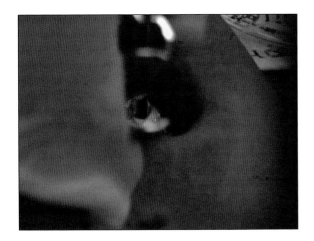

9-6g *A large portion of the glottic opening is seen along with a limited view of the true vocal cords. Note the small section of tongue inadvertently trapped to the right of the blade lumen.*

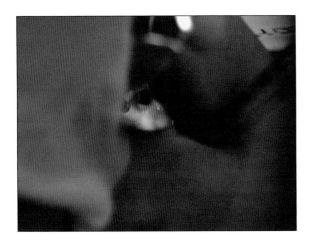

9-6h *Trachea tube introduced using the extreme right corner of the mouth and directed beneath the line of sight and beneath the lumen of the blade.*

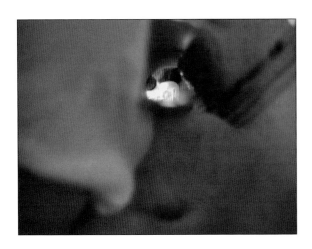

9-6i *Tip of tracheal tube is brought up toward glottic opening.*

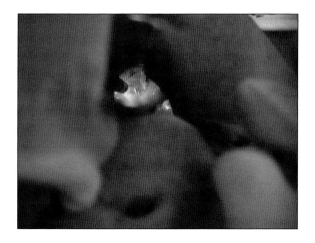

9-6j *Tube is inserted into glottis. Adjacent to the cuff of the tube on the right side are the right posterior cartilages.*

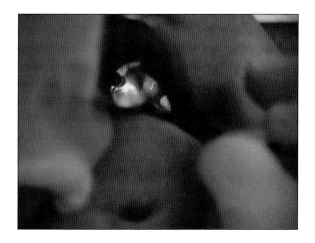

9-6k *The rounded prominence of the right posterior cartilages is well seen adjacent to the tube after the cuff has advanced past the cords.*

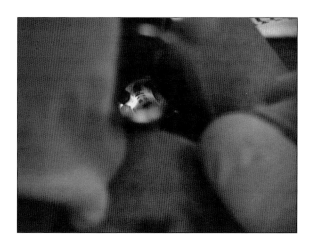

9-6l *Final view of tracheal tube insertion. The left posterior cartilages are underneath the bulb of the blade and adjacent to the tracheal tube.*

9-7. Straight blade laryngoscopy with a Phillips blade

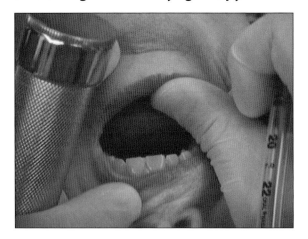

9-7a *Opening the mouth using a scissor technique. Note the laryngoscopist is holding the tracheal tube. This is helpful in field situations and other settings when additional hands may not be available.*

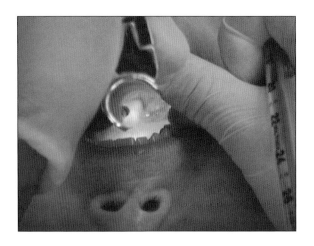

9-7b *Uvula trough lumen of Phillips blade. Phillips blade has a smaller C-shaped flange compared to the Wisconsin blade shown in prior cases 9-2 and 9-6.*

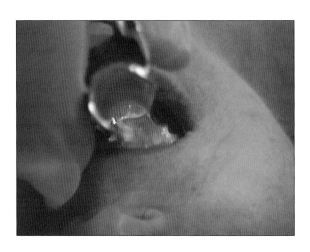

9-7c *Epiglottis edge and posterior pharyngeal wall.*

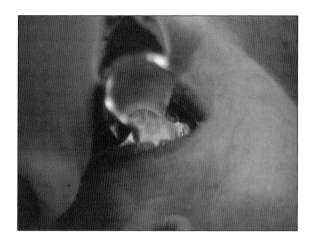

9-7d *After blade tilt and advancement the posterior hypopharynx is visible.*

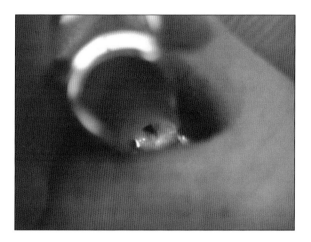

9-7e *With external laryngeal manipulation, the interarytenoid notch, the posterior cartilages, and a very small glottic opening come into view. The laryngoscopist's gloved hand is visible in upper right corner (compare to prior image).*

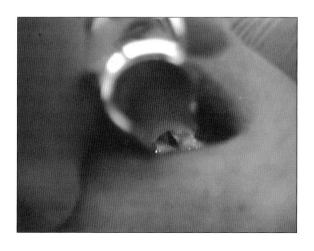

9-7f *The true vocal cords and small glottic opening are visible with continued bimanual laryngoscopy.*

9-8. Straight blade laryngoscopy with a Guedel blade

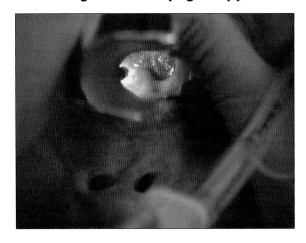

9-8a *The uvula as seen through the large lumen of a Guedel blade.*

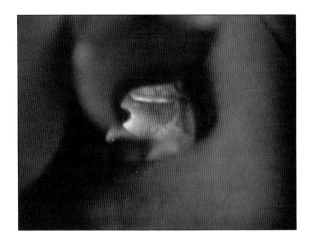

9-8b *Epiglottis edge and posterior pharyngeal wall.*

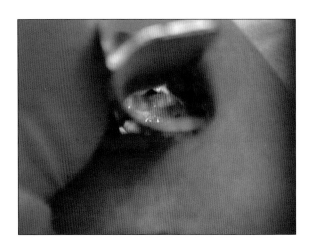

9-8c *Prior to external laryngeal manipulation, only a small portion of the glottic opening is seen. Note the rounded prominences of the posterior cartilages and the interarytenoid notch.*

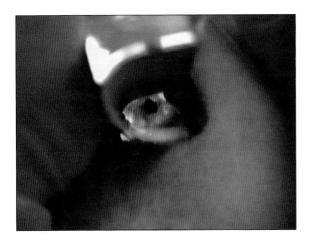

9-8d *With external laryngeal manipulation more of the glottis is seen but the true cords are not yet visible.*

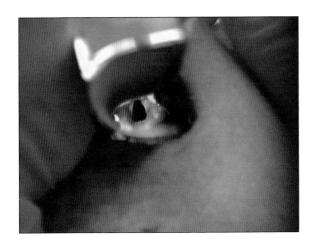

9-8e *Posterior displacement of the larynx (with ELM) brings the true vocal cords into the laryngoscopist's line of sight. The right hand of laryngoscopist can be seen in upper right corner.*

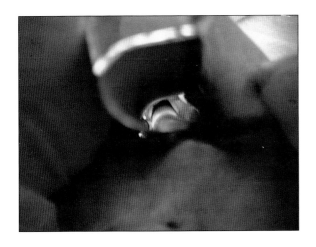

9-8f *Tracheal tube passing through glottis with true vocal cords immediately adjacent. Tube has been advanced until cuff has passed cords. Recommended depth of insertion for orally placed tracheal tubes is 21 cm in women and 23 cm in men measured at the teeth or alveolar ridge.*

9-9. Straight blade laryngoscopy with a Miller blade

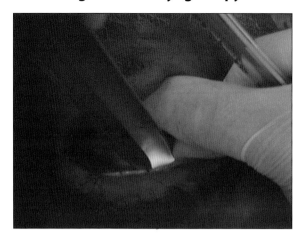

9-9a *Opening the mouth using a scissor technique and introducing the Miller blade.*

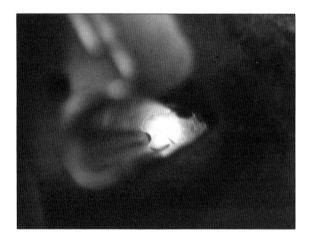

9-9b *Uvula through the narrow lumen of Miller blade.*

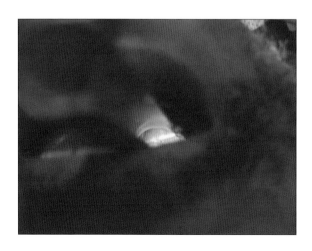

9-9c *The brightly lit epiglottis edge is visible immediately before blade is advanced to go beneath it. Note the orientation of the blade lumen to get under epiglottis in this picture compared to the previous image.*

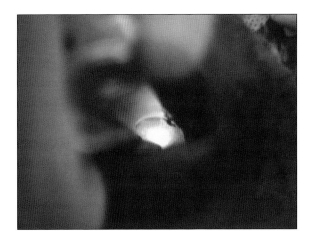

9-9d *After passing epiglottis and advancing blade slightly, the hypopharyngeal wall is exposed.*

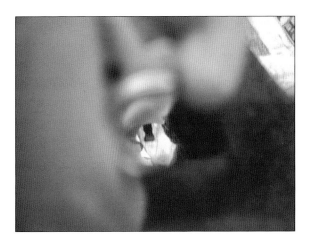

9-9e *As the blade is lifted upward the posterior cartilages, interarytenoid notch and posterior portion of the glottic opening are seen.*

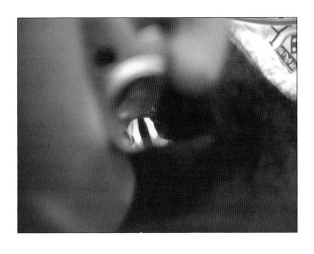

9-9f *The true vocal cords and a large portion of the glottic opening become visible with additional lift.*

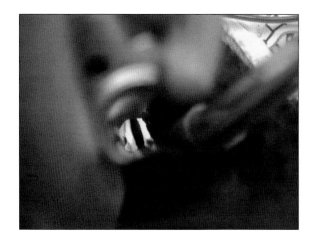

9-9g *Initial tube insertion using the right corner of the mouth.*

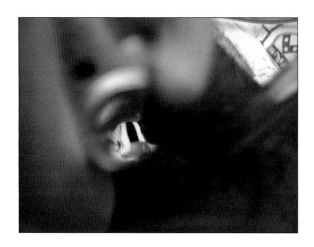

9-9h *Tracheal tube is directed below line of sight and advanced toward glottic opening.*

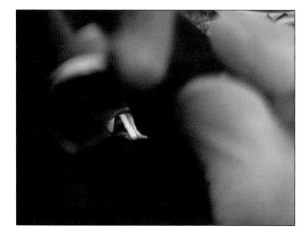

9-9j *Tube insertion through vocal cords.*

Chapter 10

Advanced Concepts in Laryngoscope Blade Design

Traditional Macintosh and Miller designs make up more than 99% of blades used by emergency practitioners. There are some variations within each of these designs, and dozens of other blades have been developed over the years. Alternative devices, most notably fiberoptic scopes, have now replaced the array of different blade designs that were once widely available. Nonetheless, laryngoscopy remains the mainstay of emergency airway management and in the author's opinion, subtle changes in standard designs can have significant impact on blade performance.

Issues in Macintosh Blade Design

American vs. German and English Designs

The primary considerations when comparing Macintosh blades involve the curvatures of the blades, the locations of the bulbs or fiberoptic elements relative to the tip, and the shapes and sizes of the flanges. The author believes that the best performing Macintosh blades have a relatively small flange that runs the full length of the blade, i.e., the "German" fiberoptic designs (Heine, Proper, Sun-Med G-line, Rusch Emerald series), or the English standard bulb designs, as opposed to the tall, straight, proximal flange of the so-called American designs (Figure 10-1). Among some of the American designs, the bulb position in the Macintosh size 4 is much farther back than in the Macintosh size 3 (Figure 10-2). This can cause poor illumination when using the larger size in a smaller patient. With the German design, the fiberoptic light element is positioned in the same place on both the size 4 and the size 3, relative to the tip of the blade (Figure 10-3). This permits bright illumination even if the full length of the longer size is not needed. Also, the flange height is not different between the size 3 and size 4 German (or English) designs (10-3). The American flange design goes straight back from the curvature of the blade, and the large proximal flange on the American size 4 blade can make insertion difficult in a small patient, when mouth opening is

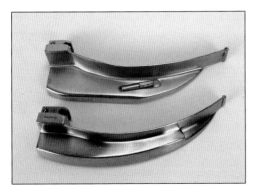

10-1 *Macintosh curved blades. American design (above) and German design (below).*

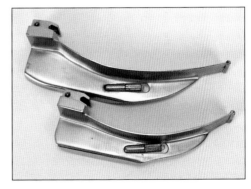

10-2 *American design Macintosh blades (size 3 below, size 4 above) demonstrating different distances from bulb to tip of blade.*

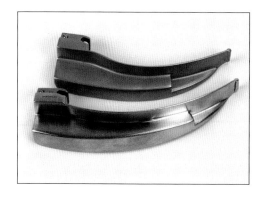

10-3 *German design Macintosh 3 and 4 blades showing similar distances from light to tip.*

restricted, or with prominent dentition. The goal of emergency laryngoscopy is first pass success. Because the amount of blade needed to reach the larynx is not entirely predictable, having a longer blade allows deeper insertion if needed. The size 4 German or English designs can be used on all adult patients (if the laryngoscope is handled correctly, as in Figure 6-17) because they are long enough for reaching the vallecula in large patients or in those with the unexpectedly deep larynx, but their small proximal flanges still allow insertion into smaller adults.

Modifications of the Macintosh Blade

Numerous modifications of the Macintosh blade have involved changing the angle and shape of the distal tip. None of these designs are commonly used today and very few are even available. More recently, the McCoy blade (a.k.a. the CLM blade, the levering laryngoscope, or articulating tip laryngoscope) uses an overall Macintosh design but has a distal tip that can be flipped upward by pressing a lever oriented parallel with the laryngoscope handle. In theory, the distal articulating tip causes elevation of the tissues at the base of the tongue, thereby getting better control of the epiglottis. It has received extensive scrutiny in the anesthesia literature, albeit in relatively small studies, with mixed reviews. The author has imaged this blade using the Direct Laryngoscopy Video System and found that, in fact, it often worsens laryngeal view. This occurs because activation of the blade tip can change the pivot point of the blade, and the mid-section of the blade commonly drops down into the line of sight (Figure 10-4). The author found the articulating blade did not improve laryngeal view nearly as well as external laryngeal manipulation by the laryngoscopist.

A variety of other Macintosh designs have altered the flange height, some eliminating the flange altogether or substantially reducing the proximal flange. The reduced proximal flange minimizes contact with the upper dentition (Figure 10-5), but occasionally this small proximal flange allows the mouth to close during laryngoscopy narrowing the view and working area.

Spatula modifications have included making the spatula tube shaped or expanding the spatula size to help control the tongue better. The "improved vision" Macintosh blade has a tubular shape to the mid-spatula which permits 8 millimeters of additional visualization along the long axis of the blade (Figure 10-6).

The Grandview blade (Hartwell Medical, Carlsbad CA) has a widened spatula that theoretically makes tongue control easier. Although a wider spatula may be helpful in easy

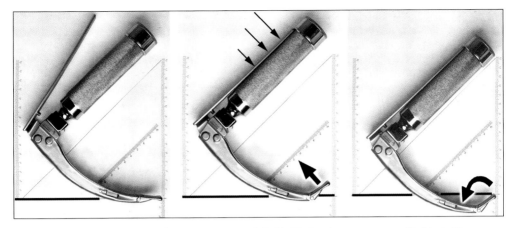

10-4 *McCoy laryngoscope with tip not activated (left). McCoy laryngoscope with blade tip activation (middle), and with blade tip activation causing the blade to pivot about distal tip, moving mid-section of the blade into the line of sight (right).*

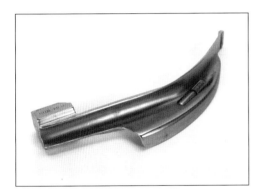

10-5 *Reduced proximal flange Macintosh design. This blade also happens to have a tube shaped, "improved vision" spatula design (see below).*

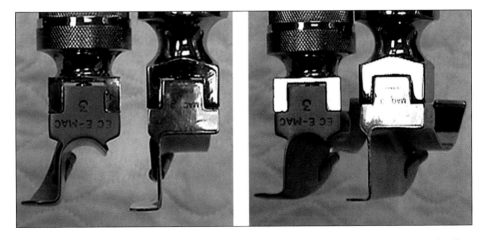

10-6 *View down the tube shaped spatula of "improved vision" blade (left) vs. standard flat spatula Macintosh design (right).*

laryngoscopy patients, anything that increases total displacement volume can make laryngeal exposure more difficult when the patient has a small mouth or large tongue.

In the author's opinion, the single best choice for routine laryngoscopy is the size 4 Macintosh blade made of stainless steel that follows the German or English design. In the disposable line up, the author prefers the Heine XP Blade (Heine USA, Dover NH), because the design matches the German profile (allowing the Mac 4 to be used for all patients), the plastic is not too slippery (as is common with some other plastic blades), and the light transmission is excellent (Figure 10-7). Stainless steel disposable fiberoptic blades that use an acrylic stem for light conduction have just been released by Sun-Med (Largo FL) (Figure 10-8). This product provides a steel blade for EMS and other providers who prefer to work with single patient use equipment.

It is important to note that reusable fiberoptic laryngoscope blades require cold sterilization. They cannot be autoclaved, and improper cleaning will result in loss of light transmission via the fiberoptic channel.

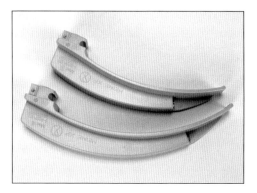

10-7 *Heine XP disposable plastic blade with a fiberoptic light.*

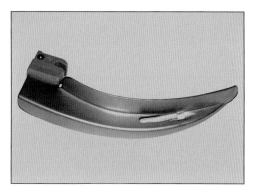

10-8 *Sun Med Greenline D disposable steel blade with acrylic light-conducting bundle.*

Looking Around the Curve

A variety of laryngoscopy adjuncts have been used in the past to look around the curvature of the blade. These include prisms placed down the lumen of laryngoscope blades and mirror devices. The Huffman prism is a small clip-on prism that permits a view around the curvature of the Macintosh blade. The metal clip on these prisms is intended to slide onto the proximal flange and it works best with the flange of an American Macintosh design. The clip is difficult to attach to some fiberoptic blades that have a thick proximal flange. The Siker blade on the other hand, is a curved laryngoscope blade that has a polished mirrored surface underneath the spatula that provides a right-left reversed view of the larynx from the intraoral perspective. Each of these devices potentially has fogging issues and can be rendered useless by secretions, emesis, and blood. Neither is widely used.

Two new variations on this theme are the Rusch ViewMax (Rusch, Duluth GA) and the Sun Med Prism View (Sun Med, Largo FL). The ViewMax is a Macintosh blade with a tubular lens element that is slid down the lumen of the blade and locks into position (Figure 10-9a–b). It provides a view through the lens that is oriented 20 degrees up from the long axis of the blade.

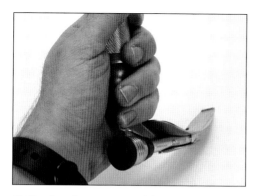

10-9a *Rusch Viewmax. Oblique view.*

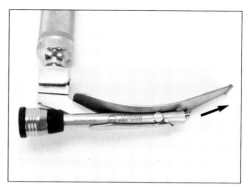

10-9b *Rusch Viewmax. Side view, showing optical path angled 20° above horizontal.*

Theoretically, this will permit a view from below the epiglottis edge upward at the larynx. Optically, it is periscope laryngoscopy, because the relatively long viewing element has a comparatively small viewing area. No clinical trials have been done to date. In the author's experience in the cadaver setting, it clearly improves visualization of tube placement, although the impact on best obtainable laryngeal view is not evident in many cases. The ViewMax does change the optics of the procedure however, because visualization is through the eyepiece on the proximal end of the blade, not directly at the target. The author has noticed in cadaver training courses that some operators with deteriorating visual acuity and focal distance problems find the device very helpful. The insertion technique is like that of a regular curved blade, but after seating the tip in the vallecula the view switches to the eyepiece, which can be viewed from a few inches away.

The recently released Sun Med Prism View also uses a removable optical element on a curved blade. It combines a removable acrylic tube (with a 30 degree optical angle), with a Macintosh blade that has a tubular flange similar to the "improved vision" Macintosh design mentioned above (Figure 10-6).

Issues in Miller Blade Design

The original Miller design had a lumen designed to accept a 37 French Argyle breathing tube. Miller appreciated that placement through the lumen would sometimes be useful. Over the years, the Miller design has had a shrinking flange height, so that current Miller blades will not accept standard adult tracheal tubes through their lumen (Figure 10-10a). As has already been noted, placing the tube through the lumen is generally avoided because it obstructs the line of sight to the target, but having this as a back up means of placement is advantageous. The smaller flange height creates a smaller displacement volume that makes it easier to get to the larynx, but it also compromises the working area. The tip of the Miller blade is upturned to facilitate easier lifting of the epiglottis (Figure 10-10b). This design however, renders the tip invisible to the laryngoscopist after insertion, and sometimes it is difficult to pick up the epiglottis directly, since the tip of the blade cannot be observed to be under the epiglottis. Only after lifting does it become evident whether the epiglottis has in fact been controlled.

Subtle differences in Miller blade design can have significant differences in blade performance. Specifically, the location of the bulb or light relative to the flange is very important. If the bulb is placed on the leading left edge of the flange, it is easily covered by tongue and soft tissues, and provides very poor visualization (Figure 10-11). The original Miller design has a right-sided bulb, and the performance is noticeably better. Alternatively, the bulb can be recessed so that although it is on the left side, it is not at the leading edge of the flange.

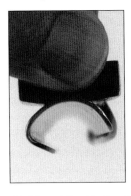
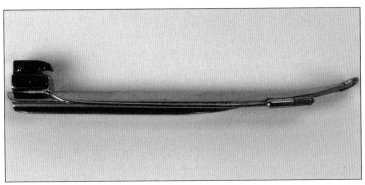

10-10a *Miller blade, view down lumen showing small D-shaped flange (left).*
10-10b *Miller blade, side view showing upturned distal tip (right).*

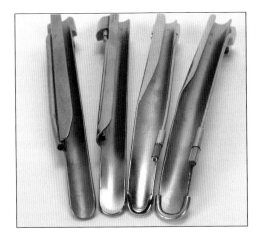

10-11 *Different Miller designs showing variation in tip design and light location. Blade on extreme left has a light that is located at leading edge of flange (light is on left side when looking down the blade). Blade second from left shows better design with light tip recessed underneath flange. Blades at right side of picture have conventional bulb lighting located on right side of blade when looking down the blade with minor differences in flange and tip shapes.*

Other Straight Blade Designs: The Straight Blade Paradox

The optimal size of a straight blade flange is a trade off between the ease of reaching the larynx and the ease of inserting the tube. Increasing the flange size of a straight blade helps with tube insertion but also increases the displacement volume of the blade, making it harder to pass the blade alongside the tongue and to reach the larynx. On the other hand, a smaller flange height and narrower lumen make it easier to get to larynx, but more difficult to pass the tracheal tube.

Prior to the widespread use of fiberoptic scopes, a wide variety of straight laryngoscopes were available. Such designs are primarily of historic interest these days. On one end of the spectrum are blades with flanges even smaller than the Miller (such as the Cranwall that has no side flange), while at the other extreme is the Guedel blade, with a very large flange and full spatula (Figure 10-12). In between these varieties is the Miller with its small D-shaped flange, the Phillips blade with a two-thirds rounded arc, and the Wisconsin with its rounded C-shape (Figure 10-12). In the author's experience, any straight blade gets infrequent use if proper curved blade technique is consistently applied, and although there are some pluses to the larger flange heights, it negates a primary reason for selecting the straight blade in the first place, namely a smaller displacement volume. The Miller is an adequate compromise assuming the light position is on the right side of the blade.

The Henderson Blade

The author believes the best designed straight blade available is the Henderson blade (Karl Storz, Culver City CA), (Figures 10-13a–b, 10-14). It has a relatively small flange height just slightly larger than a Miller, a semi-circular flange shape (approximately half a C-shape when viewed down its long axis from the base), and visible distal tip. The flange height and shape make passage down to the larynx as easy as the Miller, but it does not have the bottom portion of the Miller flange which restricts tube passage. An 8.0 mm non-styletted tracheal tube can be directed down the lumen of the blade if necessary (Figure 10-13a). The distal tip is straight and has a prominent knurled edge that can be seen by the laryngoscopist when looking down the lumen (Figure 10-13b). This visible tip makes epiglottis elevation very easy, without the repetitive lifting and checking required with the Miller blade.

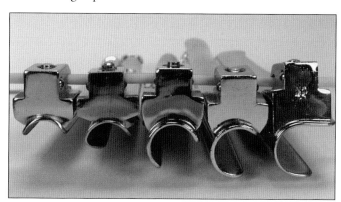

10-12 *Different straight blade designs (from left to right): Cranwall, Miller, Phillips, Wisconsin, and Guedel.*

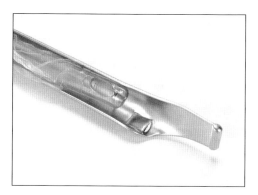

10-13a *Henderson blade showing tracheal tube able to fit within lumen. Note recessed light and knurled distal knob.*

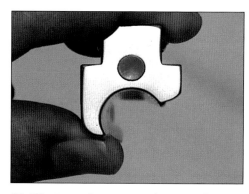

10-13b *Down lumen view shows small proximal flange height and visible distal tip.*

10-14. Sequential imaging of Henderson blade laryngoscopy

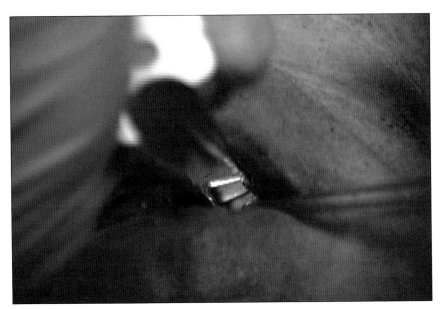

10-14a *Epiglottis edge underneath brightly lit, knurled tip of Henderson blade. Yankauer suction catheter is visible on right side of mouth.*

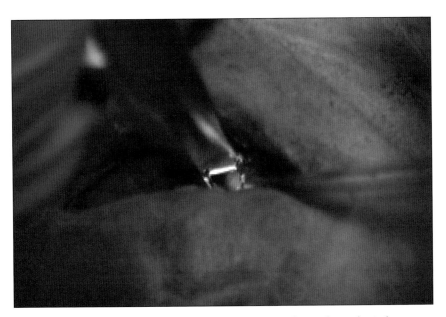

10-14b *Angle of blade has been increased to advance beneath epiglottis (no longer visible). Posterior pharyngeal wall is seen under blade tip. Note tongue to left of blade flange. Technique uses right paraglossal positioning of blade, with no attempt to sweep tongue.*

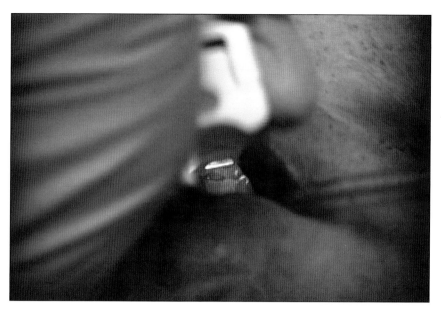

10-14c *After blade tilt and advancement, the laryngoscope is lifted upward revealing the rounded prominences of the posterior cartilages immediately beneath the tip of the blade.*

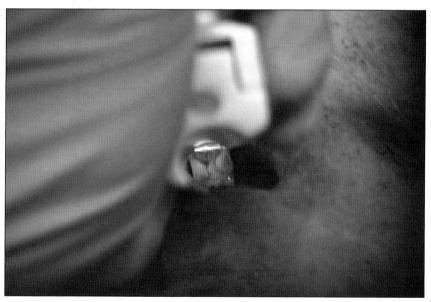

10-14d *With slight incremental lifting more of the posterior cartilages and the interarytenoid notch become visible.*

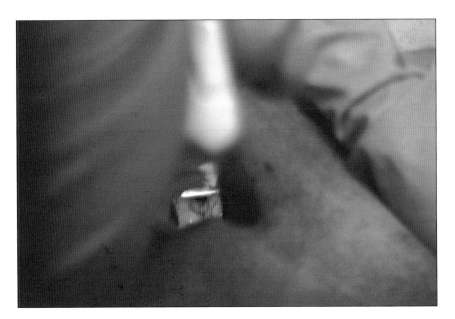

10-14e *Further head elevation and bimanual laryngoscopy (external laryngeal manipulation by laryngoscopist) reveal a small portion of the glottic opening.*

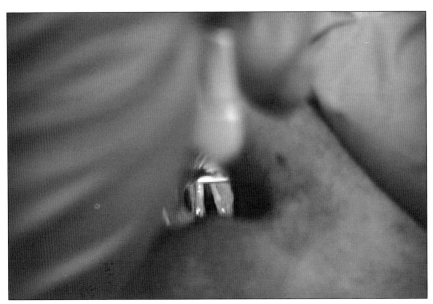

10-14f *Best laryngeal view with full head elevation and external laryngeal manipulation. True and false vocal cords are well seen.*

Chapter 11

Putting it All Together: A Pre-planned Laryngoscopy Strategy for First Pass Success

Having reviewed the elements of laryngoscopy technique, it is important to synthesize these techniques into a pre-planned laryngoscopy strategy to promote first pass success (Figure 11-1). Just as the skydiver has a series of pre-planned and pre-practiced maneuvers that promotes successful primary chute deployment, we as airway managers should have a deliberate and well thought out laryngoscopy strategy.

Pre-planned, step-wise approach to laryngoscopy

1. Macintosh #4, cricoid pressure by assistant

↓

2. Release cricoid – bimanual laryngoscopy

↓

3. Increase head elevation (*not in C-spine precautions*)

↓

4. Straight-to-cuff styletted tube > bougie > optical stylet

> If patient hypoxic > > > VENTILATE!
> Facemask with oral airway
> Lift mandible & submandibular tissues
> Small volume 6-7cc/kg, over 1-2 seconds, low pressure

↓

5. Paraglossal straight blade technique

RESCUE VENTILATION (Facemask, LMA, Combitube)

RESCUE INTUBATION (alternative technique)

11-1 *Pre-planned step-wise approach to laryngoscopy.*

The significance of first pass success in emergency airways cannot be overstated. In a recent study by Mort (Mort TC. Emergency tracheal intubation: Complications associated with repeated laryngoscopic attempts. *Anesth Analg.* 2004; 99:607–13.) analyzing complications associated with 2,833 emergency airways, the incidence of critical hypoxia, aspiration, bradycardia, and cardiac arrest dramatically increased with increasing numbers of laryngoscopy attempts. Hypoxemia associated with one laryngoscopy attempt to four attempts increased as follows: 4.8%, 33.1%, 62%, and 85%. The incidence of aspiration with one laryngoscopy was 0.3% compared to 13% with three or more laryngoscopies. Bradycardia jumped from a 1.3% incidence with one attempt to 18.5% with three or more attempts. Most alarmingly, cardiac arrest occurred in 0.7% of cases with one or two attempts, but was 11% for those with three or more laryngoscopies.

The first decision in a general laryngoscopy strategy is the selection of a starting blade. In the author's opinion, for almost all emergency cases this should be the Macintosh #4 blade. The curved blade's larger flange makes tongue control easier, and the natural stopping point in the vallecula provides for easier depth of placement. In case the epiglottis is difficult to control, the long blade can sometimes be used to directly elevate the epiglottis. A Macintosh #4 blade with a German design has numerous advantages over American design blades and works well in almost all adults.

The initial attempt at laryngoscopy should be with an assistant providing cricoid pressure. Although the efficacy of cricoid pressure is not clear, it is the currently recommended standard of care. Excessive downward pressure, however, will negatively impact on laryngoscopy and tube passage.

If initial laryngoscopy with a Mac #4 and cricoid pressure does not expose the larynx, and assuming the laryngoscopist has not bypassed the epiglottis (a slow methodical march down the tongue with the tip of the blade will prevent this), the next intervention to try is external laryngeal manipulation. This should be done by the laryngoscopist using his or her right hand (bimanual laryngoscopy) and will require the assistant to ease up or let go of cricoid pressure. If the view achieved subsequently permits intubation, the assistant's hand can be directed to the same location to maintain laryngeal exposure while the operator places the tube. Cricoid pressure should only be released under direct vision with suction equipment immediately available.

If the first two steps have failed, the next laryngoscopy intervention is to increase head elevation. This can be done either by an assistant or by the laryngoscopist using his or her right hand placed under the patient's occiput. Increasing head elevation and neck flexion (assuming no cervical spine contraindication), will provide for easier distraction of the mandible and tongue and improved laryngeal exposure. Over aggressive atlanto-occipital extension, by contrast, posteriorly displaces the tongue and worsens laryngoscopy efforts. The importance of proper positioning, particularly in large patients, cannot be overstated, and proper head elevation should be checked beforehand. This means approximating the external auditory canal to roughly the same horizontal line as the sternal notch when viewed from a lateral perspective.

After these steps, if the epiglottis is still obstructing the view, the laryngoscopist must determine if the styletted tube can be successfully placed under the epiglottis edge or more specifically anterior to the interarytenoid notch and posterior cartilages. Recognition of the posterior landmarks of the larynx, even when the cords cannot be seen, will salvage many cases and permit successful intubation. In situations when laryngeal view is poor, proper stylet shaping and careful directional control and observation of the tube tip or introducer is especially important to prevent esophageal placement.

Stylets and introducers can sometimes permit intubation in epiglottis-only views, but there is no guarantee of tracheal placement. If esophageal intubation occurs and the patient's stomach is insufflated, there is a significant risk of regurgitation. With vomitus in the upper airway, laryngoscopy will become even more challenging, and the patient is at grave risk for aspiration and critical hypoxia.

In the previously cited study by Mort, a single esophageal intubation carried a 51% risk of hypoxemia; an 11 times greater risk of hypoxemia compared to patients who did not have an esophageal intubation. With esophageal intubation there was also a 10 times greater risk of regurgitation, an 8 times greater incidence of aspiration, and a 12 times greater risk of bradycardia.

Unlike the standard stylet, the bougie provides some measure of immediate verification of placement. In 60–90% of cases as the tip can be felt bouncing over the tracheal rings as it is advanced. Because of the narrowing of the bronchi there is limitation of advancement between 24 and 40 centimeters. A lighted stylet placed under the epiglottis and into the trachea (as opposed to the esophagus) will generally display bright trans-illumination, depending upon the patient's body habitus and other factors. The safest and potentially most effective means of dealing with the epiglottis-only view on first pass is to use an optical stylet and directly visualize placement through the vocal cords.

Up to this point in our laryngoscopy strategy each of the maneuvers mentioned can be tried upon the first laryngoscopy attempt without switching blades or intervening bagging.

It must be appreciated that effective use of bougies or specialized stylets during first pass laryngoscopy requires pre-planning so that they are immediately available. Lighted stylets and optical stylets require that the tube be placed on the stylet beforehand. Unlike with the bougie or similar introducer, a tracheal tube cannot be passed over the back end of any lighted stylet or optical stylet. If specialized introducers or stylets are not immediately available the next step in tackling the epiglottis-only view is switching to a straight blade. Before switching to a straight blade, or switching operators, adequate oxygenation must be assured.

The paraglossal straight blade technique requires a different approach than the curved blade, as has been previously noted. Because of the smaller spatula of a straight blade, it should not be used when the epiglottis cannot be found, because compared to a curved blade, it is more difficult to find the epiglottis.

If the epiglottis is not identifiable, the curved blade should be reinserted carefully down the midline of the tongue, making sure not to pass the epiglottis. After the epiglottis is located the flange of the blade can be repositioned to control the tongue (with a curved blade) or to achieve a paraglossal right-sided position (with a straight blade).

Apart from slowly moving down the tongue, the other key to locating the epiglottis is to distract the tongue forward enough so that the epiglottis is lifted off the posterior wall and made visible. This recommendation applies to both curved and straight blades when there is difficulty locating the epiglottis. In the author's experience, the curved blade is almost always easier to use for locating the epiglottis because the larger flange and natural stopping point in the vallecula allows for easier tongue control. Sometimes it is helpful to use the tip of the Yankauer suction to help locate the epiglottis, by feel pushing the suction tip down along the tongue. Excess secretions and subtle changes in lighting can contribute to epiglottis camouflage and making the epiglottis edge difficult to identify, especially in larger patients with redundant pharyngeal tissue.

For a select few patients, initial laryngoscopy efforts with a straight blade may be warranted. Straight blades essentially trade the advantages of a large flange and indirect epiglottis control for longer length relative to the flange size and direct control of the epiglottis. Straight blades are generally recommended for children, especially those below eight years of age. They are most useful on patients with a short mandible and relatively small displacement space (i.e., the space between the chin and thyroid cartilage). Straight blades may also be an appropriate first choice in patients with dental gaps, especially if the top three or four central teeth are missing, because the proximal flange of the Macintosh blade sometimes gets locked into this gap and tube passage can be very difficult.

If all of the above interventions (external laryngeal manipulation, head elevation, stylet or introducer placement under the epiglottis, and straight blade rescue), do not result in adequate laryngeal exposure and intubation, the clinician must decide whether the problem can be overcome by repeated attempts. Additional laryngoscopy efforts and switching blades should occur only if oxygenation is adequate, otherwise, rescue ventilation takes priority over persistent intubation efforts. If laryngoscopy is repeated, something should change between attempts, whether that be the operator, positioning, blade choice, etc. Successive laryngoscopy eventually causes deteriorating laryngoscopy conditions and problems with ventilation, due to bleeding and edema from repetitive manipulation. In most instances, laryngoscopy beyond three attempts (with optimal technique) should trigger an alternative intubation approach. Once it is clear that laryngoscopy will not succeed, the oxygenation and ventilation status of the patient will determine whether the patient can tolerate additional efforts at intubation (using an alternative technique), or if rescue ventilation is required.

Conclusions: Laryngoscopy Difficulty and Technique

In the absence of evident anatomic abnormality, laryngoscopy can be conceptualized as having a scale of difficulty that is dependent in large measure upon skills and techniques (Figure 11-2). The simple addition of bimanual laryngoscopy (ELM) drops epiglottis-only views dramatically, from as much as 9% to as low as 1.3%. Combining straight-to-cuff shaping and an intimate knowledge of posterior laryngeal anatomy makes another synergistic improvement, and when coupled to head elevated laryngoscopy positioning (HELP) may reduce the incidence of epiglottis-only views to roughly 1 in 750 (0.2%). In the above laryngoscopy strategy, adding a bougie or the optical stylet can presumably lessen intubation failure even more. Finally, a paraglossal straight blade technique bypasses the mechanical limitations of curved blade laryngoscopy.

In addition to lessening intubation failure, it is hoped that a pre-planned laryngoscopy strategy can minimize the incidence of repeat laryngoscopy. RSI first pass success has been reported to be in the 80–90% range in the ED, and three or more attempts occur in 1.5–5% of ED cases. Historically, failed laryngoscopy has occurred in 0.3–1% of ED cases. There is clearly room for improvement considering that these numbers come from studies that did not use a defined laryngoscopy strategy.

A pre-planned laryngoscopy strategy combines a specific series of techniques (ELM, HELP, paraglossal straight blade) with carefully considered use of appropriate devices (well-designed blades, straight-to-cuff shaping of stylets, bougie, fiberoptic augmentation). It requires a change in practitioner thinking; first pass and overall laryngoscopy success is not a haphazard event but a consequence of techniques, equipment, and understanding.

DIFFICULTY	INCIDENCE	TECHNIQUE
Easy	1st pass success ~ 90% of OR & ED cases by experienced laryngoscopists using RSI	*Recognizing posterior cartilages and interarytenoid notch*
	Epiglottis–only views without bimanual laryngoscopy (ELM) ~ 9%	*Bimanual laryngoscopy (ELM)*
Poor view but 1st pass success	3 or more attempts in ED 1.5–5%

Epiglottis–only with bimanual laryngoscopy (ELM) ~ 1.3% | *Increasing head elevation (HELP)*

Straight-to-cuff stylet shaping |
| **Multiple attempts** | Failed intubation in ED 0.3–1.0% | *Bougie*

Optical stylet |
| **Multiple operators** | Epiglottis–only views with ELM & head elevation (HELP) ~ 0.2% | *Paraglossal straight blade technique* |
| **Impossible** | | |

11-2 *Scale of laryngoscopy difficulty on left, incidence of difficulty in middle, and laryngoscopy technique and equipment used on right.*

Chapter 12

Pediatric Laryngoscopy

Laryngoscopy in infants and small children is a technically easier procedure than in adults. Mouth opening, joint mobility, and dentition are all more favorable for laryngeal exposure and smaller diameter, cuffless tracheal tubes make tube insertion and target visualization easier as well. For emergency care providers who rarely intubate children, however, the procedure can be intimidating. Very few emergency care providers obtain training opportunities on pediatric patients. The limitations of manikin training may also have greater negative impact on skill acquisition with pediatric intubation because of several characteristics of the pediatric airway.

Characteristics of the Pediatric Airway

The pediatric airway differs from adult airways in five main respects. First, the larynx is positioned higher in the neck. At birth the larynx is at the level of the third cervical vertebra. By adulthood it is at the level of the fifth vertebra. This difference, along with other issues, makes it very easy to unintentionally miss the main landmark of laryngoscopy, the epiglottis, with initial blade insertion.

Second, the mandible in infants and small children is under-developed, namely, it is shorter and narrower. This makes the displacement space smaller. A smaller displacement space favors use of a blade with a smaller displacement volume. Along with differences in epiglottis morphology, this is the reason for using a narrow lumen straight blade in small children instead of a large flange, large spatula, curved blade. Many providers familiar with curved blade laryngoscopy in adults do not appreciate the subtleties of straight blade laryngoscopy, especially when the landmarks are much smaller.

The third difference in the pediatric airway is the increased size of the tongue relative to the size of the oral cavity. This redundancy of soft tissue in the upper airway requires very careful, progressive visualization of landmarks. Using a straght blade with a small flange can make effective tongue control challenging. Fortunately, the small diameter of cuffless tracheal tubes relative to the lumen of the laryngoscope blade makes tube passage possible even when the tongue is not optimally controlled.

A fourth difference in the pediatric airway is the relative increased length and stiffness of the epiglottis. The epiglottis is more difficult to control with indirect elevation. This is another reason to use straight blades in small children.

The fifth difference in the pediatric airway involves positioning, the size of the occiput in children, and the resulting head and neck position when small children are supine. The larger occiput size already elevates the head relative to the chest, causing baseline neck flexion in a supine position. This achieves alignment of the external auditory meatus (the ear) and the sternal notch without additional head elevation (Figure 5-2).

In terms of tracheal tube insertion, the pediatric airway has its narrowest point in the subglottic region, not at the vocal cords. This does not affect laryngoscopy, but tube passage may be unsuccessful if the tube selected is too large. Conversely, if the tube selected is too small there will be a significant air leak. Many EMS providers are using cuffed tubes on all but the smallest children because of logistical problems with uncuffed tubes.

The characteristics of the pediatric airway mentioned above diminish with increasing age and for the most part are not significant above the age of eight.

The differences in the sizes of pediatric patients create an entirely different set of challenges compared to adult patients. Length based resuscitation tapes can quickly provide proper sizing for critical airway equipment including tracheal tube sizes and laryngoscopes as well as airway related medications. Proper tracheal tube size is less accurately estimated using the size of the little finger or the nare for proper diameter. The tracheal tube size for a newborn above 2 kilograms is 3.0–3.5 mm ID. Another rule for the proper size of tracheal tubes above the age of two years is 4 plus the age in years divided by 4. A general guide for depth of tube insertion in centimeters at the teeth or alveolar ridge is three times the internal diameter of the tube. Proper laryngoscope size for a newborn to age 6 months is a Miller or Wisconsin 1. A Miller 1.5 or Wisconsin 1.5 can be used to age 2, and a Miller 2 blade covers ages 2–10 years.

The techniques of laryngoscopy already mentioned in this text all apply to pediatric patients, including an emphasis on epiglottoscopy, bimanual laryngoscopy, and recognition of laryngeal landmarks, especially the interarytenoid notch and posterior cartilages (Figures 12-1–12-7). As shown in the laryngoscopy images that follow, tube passage is much less of a challenge due to the size difference between the pencil thin tracheal tubes and the relatively larger lumen of the laryngoscope.

Sequential Images of Pediatric Laryngoscopy

12-1. Straight blade laryngoscopy with a Wisconsin #1 blade on an 11 month old

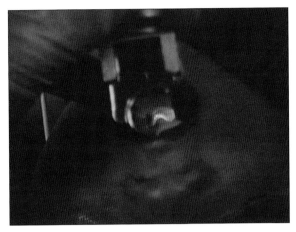

12-1a *The epiglottis.*

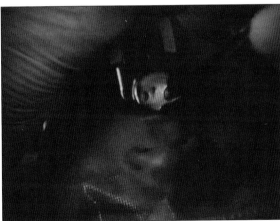

12-1b *The vertical cleft of the interarytenoid notch. The vocal cords are not visible. A small cuffless tracheal tube has been introduced into the right corner of the mouth.*

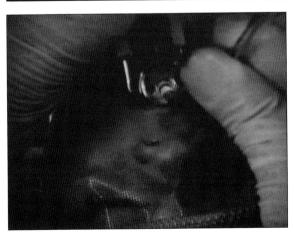

12-1c *The tracheal tube is relatively small compared to the lumen of the blade. The double black lines on the tracheal tube mark the correct depth of insertion.*

12-2. Straight blade laryngoscopy with a Miller #2 blade on a 3 year old

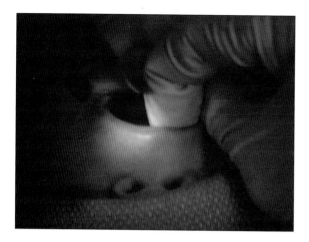

12-2a *Initial blade insertion with scissor technique opening the mouth.*

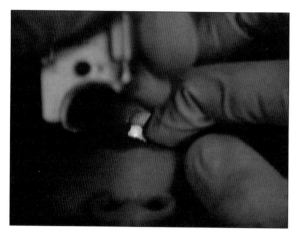

12-2b *The uvula.*

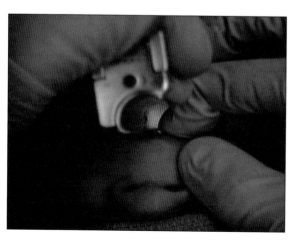

12-2c *The posterior pharynx.*

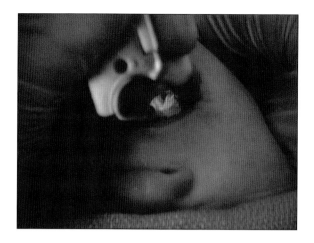

12-2d *The interarytenoid notch and posterior cartilages become visible with bimanual laryngoscopy.*

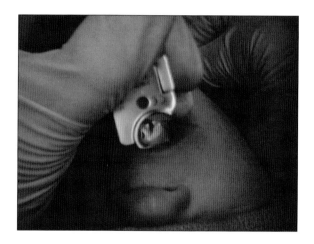

12-2e *A small portion of the true vocal cords can be seen along with the glottic opening.*

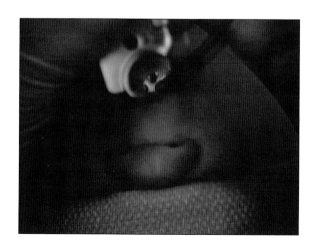

12-2f *Despite the small D-shaped lumen of the Miller blade target visualization with tube insertion is not difficult, due to the even smaller diameter of the cuffless tracheal tube.*

12-3. Straight blade laryngoscopy with a Miller #2 blade on an 8 year old

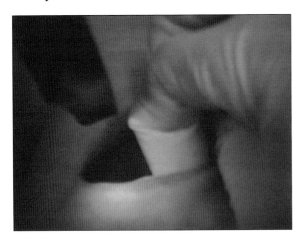

12-3a *Initial insertion and scissor technique opening the mouth.*

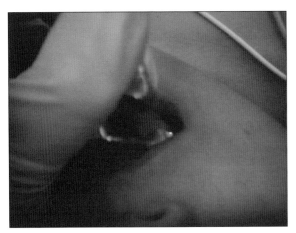

12-3b *The esophagus appears as a round hole without any associated structures.*

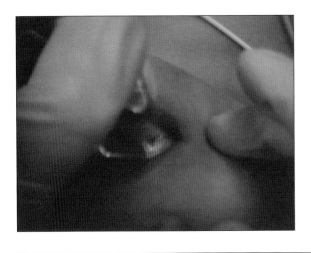

12-3c *The posterior larynx has a V-shape created by the posterior cartilages and the interarytenoid notch. A small section of the glottic opening can be seen.*

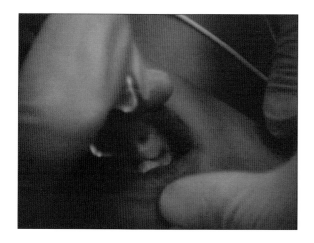

12-3d *The proximity of the larynx and esophagus is apparent in this image. Lip retraction aids visualization.*

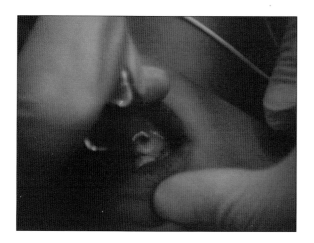

12-3e *In this image the epiglottis has dropped down. Using a Miller blade as a Macintosh (with the tip in the vallecula) is not uncommon in children.*

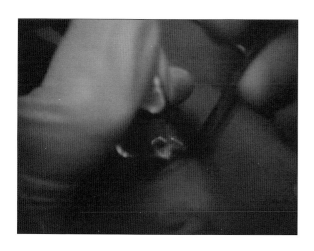

12-3f *Tracheal tube insertion using right corner of the mouth.*

12-4. Straight blade laryngoscopy with a Wisconsin #2 blade on a 5 year old

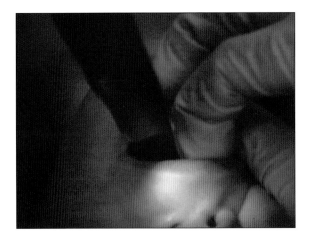

12-4a *Initial blade insertion and opening the mouth.*

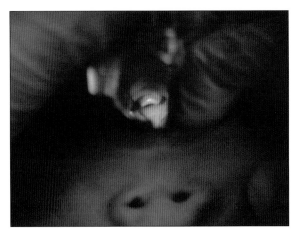

12-4b *The epiglottis.*

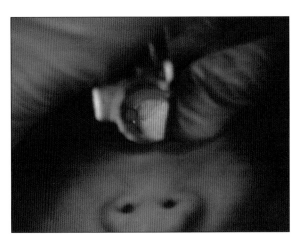

12-4c *The posterior pharynx. The poorly defined round structure in the upper aspect of the lumen of the blade is part of the right posterior cartilages.*

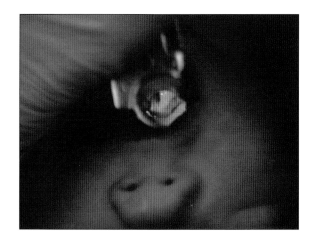

12-4d *The posterior laryngeal structures, the interarytenoid notch, and the glottic opening are well seen in this image. The true vocal cords are not seen.*

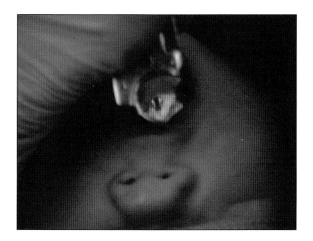

12-4e *The true vocal cords.*

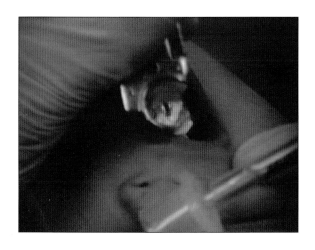

12-4f *Just prior to tube placement retracting the right side of the upper lip creates more room for passing the tube without obscuring the target.*

12-5. Straight blade laryngoscopy with a Miller #2 blade on a 6 year old

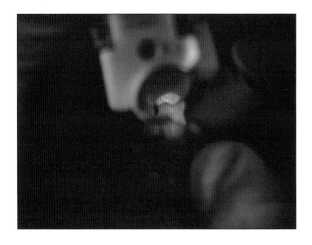

12-5a *The tip of the epiglottis.*

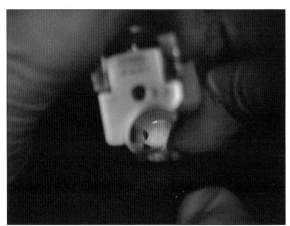

12-5b *The smooth mucosa of the posterior pharynx.*

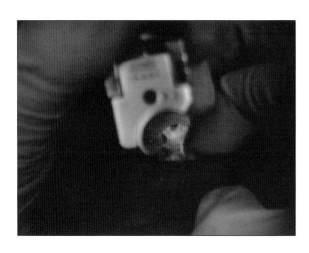

12-5c *The posterior cartilages, the interarytenoid notch, and a small portion of the glottic opening.*

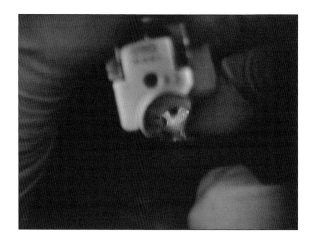

12-5d *More of the glottic opening and posterior laryngeal structures can be seen but the true vocal cords are not yet visible.*

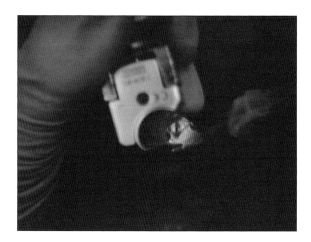

12-5e *The true vocal cords and glottic opening.*

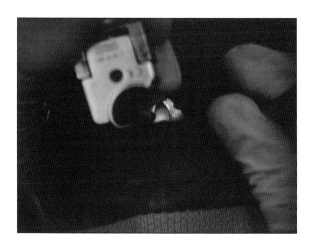

12-5f *The tracheal tube passed through the vocal cords. The right posterior cartilages can be seen lateral to the tracheal tube.*

12-6. Straight blade laryngoscopy with a Miller #1 blade on an 11 month old

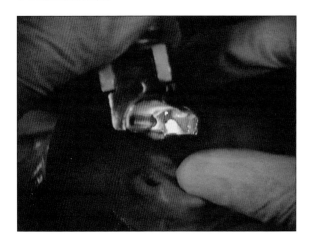

12-6a *The uvula and epiglottis are almost touching in this image. This occurs because of the higher location of the pediatric larynx. The larynx in an infant is at the level of the third cervical vertebra, compared to the fifth vertebra in adults.*

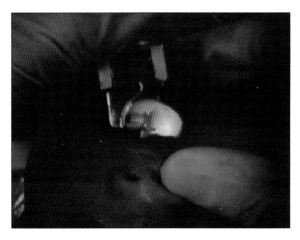

12-6b *The uniform mucosa of the posterior pharynx.*

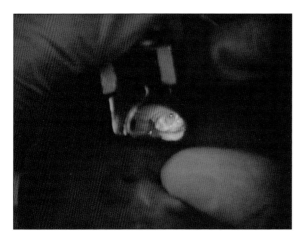

12-6c *The posterior cartilages, interarytenoid notch, and the glottic opening.*

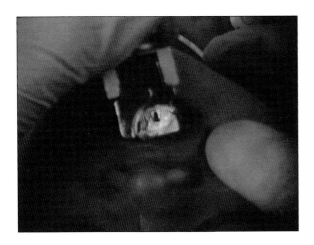

12-6d *An excellent view of the larynx including the true vocal cords.*

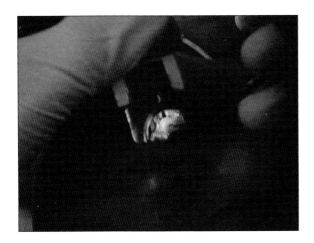

12-6e *Tube insertion with a small cuffless tube. Note the small diameter of the tube relative to the lumen of the Miller #1 blade.*

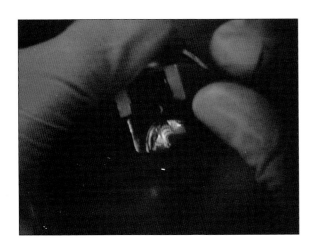

12-6f *Tracheal tube passing through vocal cords.*

12-7. Straight blade laryngoscopy with a Miller #2 blade on a 2 year old

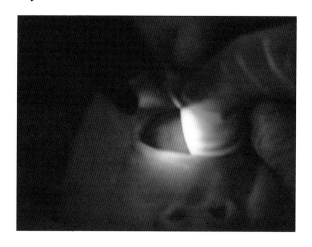

12-7a *Initial blade insertion.*

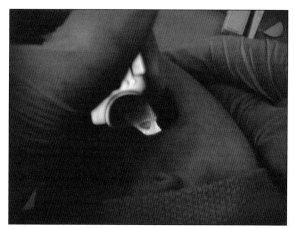

12-7b *A round hole created by inserting the laryngoscope into the upper esophagus. Compared to the larynx there are no associated structures.*

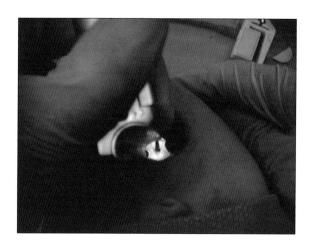

12-7c *The true vocal cords and larynx are brightly illuminated in this image. A small section of tongue is silhouetted on the right side.*

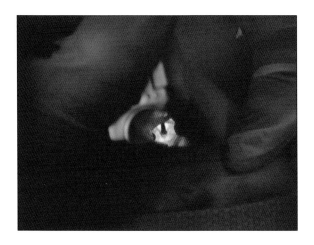

12-7d *Lip retraction helps expand the area for tracheal tube insertion.*

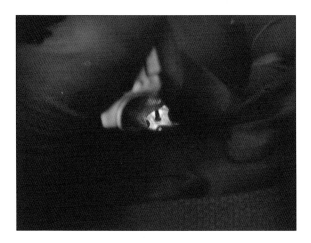

12-7e *Initial tracheal tube insertion using the right corner of the mouth. The tube tip is directed posteriorly, avoiding the lumen of the laryngoscope blade.*

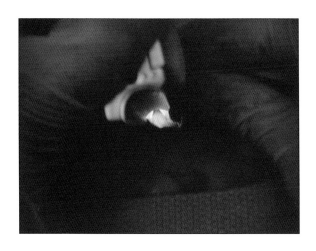

12-7f *Tracheal tube passing through vocal cords.*

Chapter 13

Blind Nasotracheal Intubation

Nasal intubation was once commonplace in emergency departments and pre-hospital care. It was the recommended technique with cervical spine immobilization, and was frequently used in patients with intact muscular tone making laryngoscopy difficult. The technique is now rarely used, as RSI has become standard practice and as laryngoscopy with in-line stabilization is now considered safe in cases of potential cervical spine injury. With or without fiberoptic assistance, nasal intubation remains a valuable technique in some emergency airway situations, despite its overall decline in use. It is best in patients who are not critically hypoxic and who can tolerate the longer time (relative to RSI) that the procedure requires.

Advantages of nasal intubation are that the patient remains awake, direct visualization is not required, and the patient can sit upright if needed. Disadvantages are that, it is difficult to provide supplemental oxygen during nasal intubation attempts, overall success rates are comparatively poor, and complications (especially bleeding and sinusitis) are common. The problems of nasal intubation in the emergency setting, specifically low success rates and bleeding, can be greatly reduced by careful attention to proper technique. Late complications such as sinusitis are usually related to the duration the nasal tube remains in place and dramatically increase after two days.

Numerous patients who cannot be intubated using the oral route require emergency airway management. Examples include severe angioedema, Ludwig's angina, and mechanical obstructions to mouth opening from mandibular fixation or other pathology. The nasal route is often the best choice in this group of patients who have oral pathology. It may also be an appropriate choice when the combination of the 4 Ds of difficult laryngoscopy are so evident that the practitioner is uncomfortable with RSI (Figure 13-1).

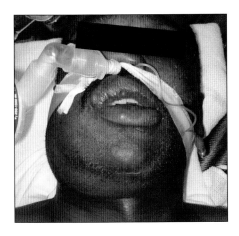 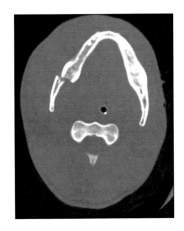

13-1 *Blind nasal intubation in a patient with a right mandible fracture and a large firm hematoma in the floor of mouth causing tongue elevation. RSI was avoided because of concern laryngoscopy down the right side of mouth would be impossible. Patient was intoxicated and could not cooperate for fiberoptic intubation. CT scan showing mandible fracture (right).*

Nasal intubation is relatively contraindicated in patients who are coagulopathic because of the risk of significant hemorrhage. Although possible in cases of apnea, the diminished breath sounds make the procedure much more difficult. Similarly, the decreased air movement in severe asthma or COPD makes nasal intubation more difficult. Midface trauma has traditionally been considered a strong contraindication because of two case reports of intracranial tracheal tube placement. Several large studies of nasotracheal intubation in patients with facial fractures and basilar skull fractures have reported no adverse outcomes, however. If there is evident disruption of the nasopharynx or roof of the mouth, it makes sense that the nasal route be avoided, while conversely, nasal intubation in mandibular fractures is the preferred means of intubation in elective OR repair.

Overview of Nasal Intubation Technique

Proper preparation of the nose and following a specific series of pre-planned steps is essential for success. The author's recommended technique is as follows:

1) Anesthetic spray into nare (2cc of 4% topical lidocaine with oxymetazoline, either via disposable single patient bottle (Afrin bottle) or via disposable spray pump atomizer or syringe (Wolfe-Tory Medical, Figures 2-1, 2-2).

2) Insert nasal trumpet lubricated with 2% lidocaine jelly.

3) Spray anesthetic spray through trumpet and remove trumpet.

4) Insert Endotrol or Parker Flex-Tip tracheal tube to approximately 14–16 cm, keeping the proximal end of the tube directed toward the patient's contralateral nipple (this helps to direct the tip of the tube toward the midline). There should be loud breath sounds audible through the tube.

5) Spray anesthetic once through tube again.

6) Pass tracheal tube through cords when patient coughs and inhales.

7) Confirm placement, sedate, and administer muscle relaxants as needed.

The overall sequence is STSTS: Spray, Trumpet, Spray, Tube, Spray.

Proper Topicalization for Anesthesia and Prevention of Bleeding

Although topical cocaine works effectively as a vasoconstrictor and topical anesthetic, equally effective is a combination of 4% topical lidocaine (liquid solution), and oxymetazoline or phenylephrine. Oxymetazoline (Afrin) or phenylephrine (Neosynephrine) come in small plastic squeeze bottles that are appropriate for single patient use. The lidocaine solution (total volume 2 cc of 4%) can be added to the spray bottle by either taking off the cap or by injecting the solution through the spray-tip hole with a narrow gauge needle. The volume of 4% topical lidocaine solution should not exceed 2 cc total. Excessive use of 4% lidocaine has been associated with lidocaine toxicity and emesis. Wolfe-Tory Medical (Salt Lake City UT) makes a spray pump disposable atomizer as well as bendable spray tubes and syringes useful for anesthetizing the posterior pharynx (Figures 2-1, 2-2).

A second technique to reduce bleeding and ease insertion is to thermo-soften the tube by placing it in a microwaved bottle of water or saline prior to placement in the patient.

Proper topicalization is essential not only for patient comfort, but also to ensure proper placement. Without proper topicalization, the patient will move, gag, and cough, which can prevent the tube from going into the trachea. Therefore, two sprays of the anesthetic/vasoconstrictor solution should first be sprayed into the desired nostril, directed backward (not upward) into the nasopharynx.

External examination cannot be used to determine whether the nare will accept the tracheal tube. Aggressive insertion of a standard tracheal tube can injure the turbinates and may lead to brisk bleeding (Figures 13-2a, 13-2b). For this reason, and also for use as a conduit for additional topical spray, a soft rubber nasal airway or trumpet (28–32 F), should be placed into the chosen nostril.

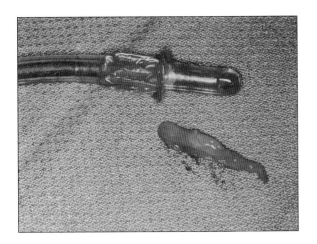

13-2a *Avulsion of the inferior turbinate as a consequence of attempted nasal intubation. (From Norton ML. Atlas of the Difficult Airway, 2nd Ed. Mosby-Yearbook Inc., St. Louis, 1996, with permission of Elsevier.)*

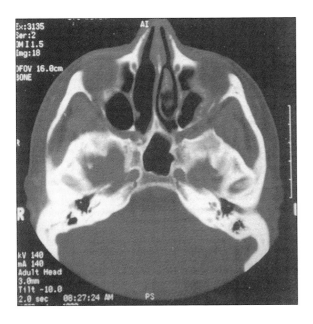

13-2b *CT scan shows absent turbinate in right nasopharynx. (From Norton ML. Atlas of the Difficult Airway, 2nd Ed. Mosby-Yearbook Inc. St. Louis, 1996, with permission of Elsevier.)*

Surgical lubricant can be used to facilitate passage, but 2% topical lidocaine jelly is the preferred lubricant. Lidocaine jelly is not as runny as viscous lidocaine and it adheres better to the trumpet.

The bevel on the trumpet should be oriented facing the turbinates, so that the leading edge moves along the septum and does not bang into the turbinates. The septum is medial and the turbinates lateral. A trumpet inserted on the left side can follow its curvature into the nose (curvature facing downward), while insertion on the right should begin with the trumpet curvature upside down (curvature initially facing upward). The floor of the nasopharynx is straight backwards, i.e., 90 degrees in relation to the face, not upward. The trumpet adds additional anesthesia to the posterior pharynx and hypopharynx, is much softer than the tracheal tube, and demonstrates a patent path toward the larynx. If the trumpet does not pass easily, the other side should be used. A slight pressure, keeping the leading edge of the trumpet downward and toward the septum, is the best way to complete placement. Using trumpets of increasing diameter does not dilate the nostril and only serves to increase bleeding. The trumpet should be fully advanced and kept in place for one minute.

This regimen of nasal spray and rubber trumpet will not anesthetize the larynx, so repeat spraying of the anesthetic solution through the trumpet is recommended. This will cause the patient to buck and cough, which in turn spreads the anesthetic above and below the vocal cords. It is helpful to explain the process to the patient if he or she is awake. Conscious sedation for intubation, using a combination of fentanyl and midazolam, may be appropriate and improve patient comfort, depending on the situation. After the solution has been sprayed through the trumpet it can be removed.

An alternative means of anesthetizing the larynx and trachea is with an acorn nebulizer, mixing 2 cc of 4% lidocaine with 3 cc of normal saline. Another technique is to inject 2 cc of topical lidocaine with a 25 gauge needle through the cricothyroid membrane. Injection through the cricoid membrane should be done only after air has been aspirated, so as to confirm entrance into the trachea. Injection of the solution into the trachea will cause coughing. Regardless of how it is administered, it is important to always keep track of the total lidocaine dose given; no more than 3 cc of the 4% topical solution is necessary; a 5 mg/kg total dose of lidocaine should not be exceeded.

Nasal Tube Insertion and Passage

The tracheal tube (as large as will be tolerated, ideally at least a 7mm ID), lubricated with a small amount of water soluble jelly, should be placed into the nostril like the trumpet, in a manner that prevents the leading edge from banging into the turbinates. Lubrication of the tracheal tube itself should not use lidocaine jelly, as there have been FDA warnings of it drying and causing tracheal tube obstruction. When the tracheal tube is inserted into the nostril, with the curvature of the tube pointing downward, the bevel on a standard tube faces towards the left. Accordingly, tube insertion into the left nostril of the patient follows the curvature of the tube, and the leading edge of the tube will correctly pass alongside the septum. If the right nostril is used, the initial insertion of the tube should be with the curvature upside down (curvature facing upward), until the nasopharynx is passed (approximately 3–4 inches), at which point the tube can be rotated back with its curvature in the standard direction. The path of a nasally placed tracheal tube must make two anterior deflections, first turning down from the nasopharynx, and second coming off of the posterior pharynx into the larynx (Figure 13-3a–b). Because of these deflections, the author prefers to use a trigger tube, or directional-tip tube (Nellcor, Pleasanton CA) (Figure 13-4a–b). The Endotrol tube is made of a softer plastic

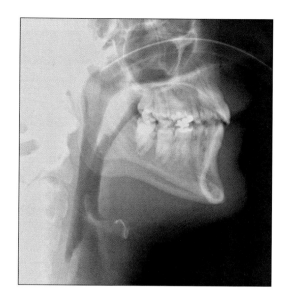

13-3a *Lateral head and neck radiograph showing initial insertion of tracheal tube into nasopharynx. Tube is at 8 cm mark. This is the first point of tube deflection, changing direction from the nasopharynx to pharynx.*

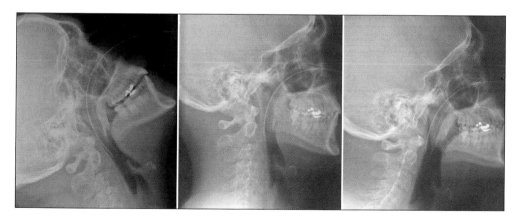

13-3b *Lateral radiographs showing the effect of head movement on the location of the tracheal tube tip relative to the epiglottis and larynx. The second point of tube deflection is directing the tube anteriorly into the larynx. Note that upper airway volume dimension is much greater in the neck flexed position (right) compared to full atlanto-occipital extension (left) or neutral (middle). This is a major reason patients lean forward when in respiratory distress.*

than standard tracheal tubes, which also helps lessen bleeding and trauma. Alternatively, a Parker Medical (Englewood CO) Flex-Tip tracheal tube (Figure 8-6) may be less traumatic for nasal intubation, and is also recommended over standard tracheal tube designs.

Another useful adjunct for nasal intubation is a Beck Airflow Airway Monitor (BAAM) (Great Plains Ballistics, Lubbock TX), attached to the base of the tracheal tube (Figure 13-4a–b). This small plastic whistle accentuates the noise of the air movement through the tube. One must be careful, however, that it does not stick too firmly into the plastic 15 mm connector on the tracheal tube, because after tube passage it will need to be disconnected. Closing the patient's mouth will help accentuate the noise through the tube as well.

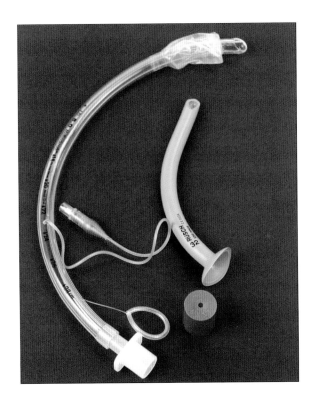

13-4a *Endotrol tube showing proximal trigger, 32 F nasal trumpet, and Beck Airflow Airway Monitor (BAAM whistle).*

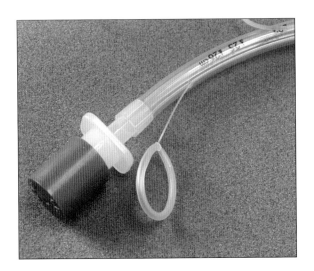

13-4b *Close up of BAAM attached to Endotrol.*

If after trumpet placement and withdrawal the tracheal tube does not easily make the bend from the nasopharynx into the pharynx, gentle steady pressure should be applied, directed slightly medially (staying on the septum), and with the proximal portion of the tube held upright (making sure the tip is heading along the floor of the nasopharynx, perpendicular to the face). As the tube is farther advanced toward the larynx, the back end of the tracheal tube should be oriented toward the patient's contralateral nipple (Figure 13-5). This helps direct the tip toward the midline, otherwise the tube tip will lodge in the ipsilateral piriform recess.

At approximately 14–16 centimeters depth, which is evident by tracheal tube markings, there should be loud air movement through the tube. One spray of the anesthetic solution through the tube at this point adds additional laryngeal anesthesia and elicits coughing. When the patient inhales, passage through the vocal cords and into the larynx is done swiftly. Successful tracheal passage will induce laryngeal reflexes (coughing), loss of phonation, and air movement through the tube. If not already done, it may be necessary to restrain the patient's arms because passage of the tube may elicit arm movement, head turning, and other efforts to remove the tube. The tube should be carefully held in place and then secured with tape, with the tube markings at 26 cm at the nostril for women and 28 cm for men. Care must be taken to avoid pressure necrosis at the nare when securing the tube in place.

If difficulty with tracheal placement occurs, one should determine if the tip is going laterally (into the piriform recess), too anterior (catching on the vallecula), or simply passing posteriorly into the esophagus. Lateral control of the tip is obtained by rotating the base of the tube in the desired direction.

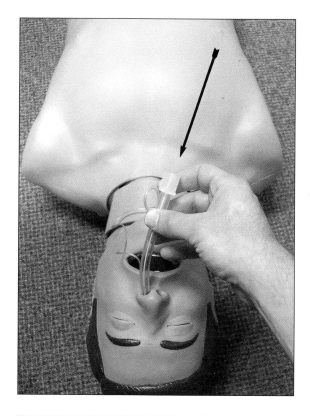

13-5 *Directing the base of the tracheal tube to the contralateral nipple during insertion (after passing nasopharynx) helps direct the leading edge of the tube toward the midline and the larynx, instead of the ipsilateral piriform recess.*

If the tube repeatedly enters the esophagus, adjustment of head positioning, tube twisting, or laryngeal manipulation may assist in directing the tube forward into the trachea.

The best means of directing the tube tip forward into the trachea is to perform the procedure with an Endotrol tube at the outset. Gentle traction on the plastic trigger will direct the tip anteriorly. Use of this tube markedly improves the first pass success rate of nasal intubation. Pulling the trigger should be done gently. Excessive force will impede advancement and cause the tube tip to go into the vallecula or to catch on the tracheal rings.

If a trigger tube is not available, inflation of the tube cuff can help direct the tip anteriorly. The cuff is inflated in the hypopharynx and advanced until resistance is felt at the vocal cords, at which time it is deflated and passed into the trachea. In the conscious patient this may elicit a strong gag or choking response. This blind technique has been shown to be as effective for intubation as use of a fiberscope, but has received limited use outside the OR.

The clinician should be prepared to immediately sedate the patient or administer neuromuscular blockers once the tube is placed. It is the author's practice to have hand restraints in place beforehand if patients cannot follow commands. Even if restraint is not needed initially, extra hands are helpful for restraining the patient as the tube actually enters the trachea. Many patients nasally intubated in emergency settings improve when well oxygenated and ventilated, and then try to forcibly remove the tube.

Successful nasal intubation in the spontaneously breathing patient is not difficult to appreciate. The patient's phonation stops and air is heard moving loudly through the tube and synchronized to respiratory activity. The tube should be advanced to the correct depth, 26–28 centimeters at the nares in adults. End-tidal CO_2 should be confirmed and a CXR should be checked to verify the tube position. Tolerance of the nasal tube is a function of how well the trachea was anesthetized as well as the underlying disease process.

Chapter 14

Alternative Intubation Devices

The role for alternative intubation devices in emergency settings is not clearly established. As previously noted in discussing different non-RSI approaches, there are numerous educational, logistical, and technical challenges to using alternative intubation devices in emergency settings (Figure 2-6). If the oral route is chosen, whether with topical anesthesia and sedation or with RSI, many factors favor using laryngoscopes. A growing array of fiberoptic devices can augment laryngoscopy, and along with increasing use of supraglottic devices for ventilation, fiberoptic augmentation of direct laryngoscopy will become routine. Flexible fiberoptic devices will remain important for a number of reasons. First, they can be used for nasal intubation in spontaneously breathing patients, and second, they are excellent for inspection and diagnostic evaluation of the upper airway. Lastly, through supraglottic devices, they are useful for rescue intubation. Approaches through the neck will also remain necessary, albeit on rare occasion.

In the emergency setting, the potential role of non-laryngoscopy oral devices seems very limited. Lighted stylets may have an advantage over simple stylets as a laryngoscopy adjunct, but it is unclear how much the lighted stylet adds to the malleable stylet and bougie for laryngoscopy. Lighted stylets are neither as versatile nor as effective as optical stylets, which can be used for laryngoscopy, trans-illumination, or fiberoptic intubation independent of laryngoscopy. Many of the same issues are relevant to rigid fiberoptic devices like the Bullard, Wu Scope, and Upsher scope, and other imaging devices like the Glidescope. These devices, which are many times more expensive than optical stylets, cannot be used to supplement laryngoscopy. Each represents a whole new skill set and a commitment to routine use for skill acquisition.

Shikani Optical Stylet

The Shikani stylet (Seeing Optical Stylet, Clarus Medical, Minneapolis MN) is comprised of a long malleable stainless steel stylet coupled to a removal eyepiece. The stylet has a high-resolution 30,000 pixel fiberoptic viewing element with a separate light bundle. At the proximal end of the stylet, coming off at a right angle, is a light guide attachment. This can either be connected to an external light source via a light guide cable, or with a 6 volt battery handle or a standard fiberoptic laryngoscope handle (with an adapter) (Figure 8-12, 8-13). Also at the proximal end of the device is a tube stop that engages the 15 millimeter connection of the tracheal tube, stabilizing the tube on the stylet. A small plastic connector that fits into the tube stop can permit supplemental oxygen attachment, which may help keep the tip of the scope clean and secretion free as it is blown down the inner aspect of the tracheal tube and out the distal end. The stylet can be shaped as desired using an overlying tracheal tube. Breaking the fiberoptic element is possible with extreme force and acute angulation, and that is the rationale for always bending the device with an overlying tracheal tube. Like any fiberoptic viewing device, it cannot be heat sterilized, but since it does not have a working channel, cleaning is a simpler matter and can be done with Steris, glutaraldehyde, or other cold sterilization solutions.

The Shikani stylet can also be used as an independent intubation device without a laryngoscope. The technique involves shaping the device with much more pronounced curvature compared to the shape as a laryngoscopy adjunct (Figure 14-1). The tip should be wiped clean, preferably with an anti-fogging solution. After sliding on the tracheal tube and setting the tip of the scope about 1-2 centimeters behind the tip of the tube, a gradual, relatively large bend (approximately 70–80 degrees total arc) should be made behind the tracheal tube cuff. The light is turned on and the tube and stylet are rocked midline into position. The goal is to identify the epiglottis edge, and then to direct the tip of the tube and stylet into the larynx. Depending on the patient's body habitus, when the tip is properly placed under the epiglottis, trans-illumination of the trachea will occur as is seen with a lighted stylet (Figure 14-2). As with the lighted stylet, it is often helpful to gently rock the device toward the midline to find the correct location. Jaw and tongue distraction (with a gauze pad for added grip) with the non-dominant hand is helpful for lifting the tongue off the posterior pharyngeal wall and enlarging the lumen of the airway. After directing the tip through the vocal cords, the tube is slid off and into the trachea under direct vision.

One of the technically challenging aspects of using the device in this manner is the orientation of the device when it is inserted. Because of the length of the device and the orientation of the eyepiece the operator must drop the head of the bed considerably to have enough height above the patient to view through the eyepiece. This can be challenging for short stature people if the head of the bed cannot be lowered. A camera coupled to the eyepiece overcomes this issue. Like other fiberoptic scopes, it can be difficult to have a view from the scope if the tip cannot be held off of the mucosa. This is often challenging in patients who have no muscular tone (after RSI), but can be overcome with a laryngoscope, a jaw thrust, or pulling on the tongue with a gauze pad.

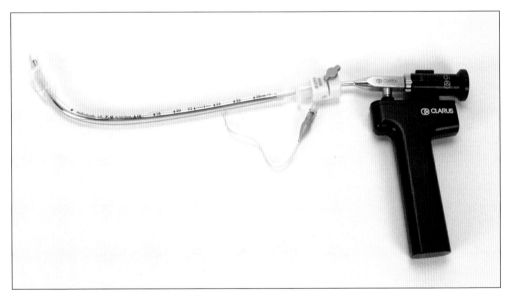

14-1 *Shikani stylet shaped for use as independent intubation device. Note white tube stop at proximal end of stylet, removable black eyepiece, and 6 volt battery handle with Halogen light.*

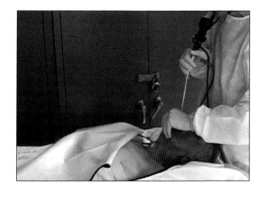

14-2 *Shikani stylet connected to a light conducting cable and external halogen light source creating bright trans-illumination of the neck with the tip of the device in the trachea. An endoscopic camera is connected to the eyepiece.*

Flexible Fiberoptic Rhinolaryngoscopy and Intubation

Short, flexible rhinolaryngoscopes (usually less than 30 cm) are used for diagnostic evaluation of the upper airway while intubating bronchoscopes (approximately 60 cm) are used for tracheal tube placement. Mid-length scopes are also available, and may be the best single device for emergency settings, capable of both diagnostic rhinolaryngoscopy and intubation (using a tube first technique as described below).

The short rhinolaryngoscopes (Olympus ENF-P4: 26 cm length, 3.6 mm outer diameter) have no working channel and are therefore much easier to clean. Scopes with working channels need to be wire brushed prior to sterilization, as well as irrigated during the sterilization process. Tuberculosis and other diseases have been transmitted through improperly cleaned working channels. The mid-range scope (Olympus T3: 36.5 cm working length, 4.8 mm OD, 2.2 mm suction channel) is more resistant to breakage than the long bronchoscope (Olympus LF-2: 60 cm L, 3.8 mm OD, 1.5 mm suction channel), but slightly larger in outer diameter. The larger suction channel is useful for managing blood or secretions and spraying anesthetic, and the shorter length makes it much easier to handle.

Intubation with a bronchoscope can be done either orally or nasally. Examples of clinical situations in which flexible fiberoptic intubation (through the nose) is recommended include severe angioedema and Ludwig's angina. Fiberoptic examination of the larynx is also valuable in patients with upper airway burns and in stridorous patients due to various causes including laryngeal trauma (fractures of the thyroid cartilage), infection (epiglottitis), or cancer. Some authors have advocated the routine use of fiberoptic intubation for proven cervical spine injury, however, direct laryngoscopy with in-line stabilization is generally preferred in the emergency setting because of its proven safety, increased speed and simplicity. Another diagnostic role for the rhinolaryngoscope in the emergency setting is the diagnosis of laryngeal asthma, based on observed paradoxical vocal cord movements.

Fiberoptic endoscopy is easiest when connected to a video camera and displayed on a monitor, as opposed to simply using the eyepiece. The key to acquiring skills with fiberoptic devices is a thorough familiarity with the fiberoptic appearance of landmarks (Figures 14-3a–l). Practice with rhinolaryngoscopes is as effective as long scope practice in terms of fiberoptic intubation skill acquisition. Compared to long scope intubation, which is done very rarely, rhinolaryngoscopy opportunities are routinely available in either the oto-rhino-laryngology clinic or in the emergency department.

14-3. Sequential Landmark Identification During Rhinolaryngoscopy

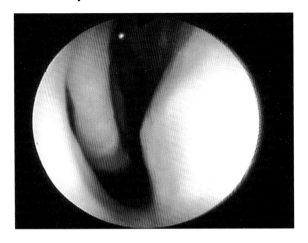

14-3a *Initial insertion of the scope into the right nare displays the inferior nasal turbinate on the left side of image and the septum on the right side. The arrow shaped mark at the top of the screen shows the orientation of the scope and is opposite the articulating lever on the Olympus ENF-P4 rhinolaryngoscope.*

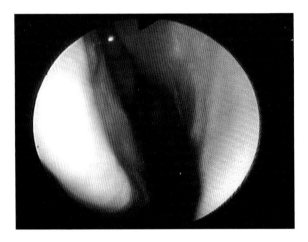

14-3b *The scope is advanced along the septum, following the dark open lumen, and not impacting on the turbinates.*

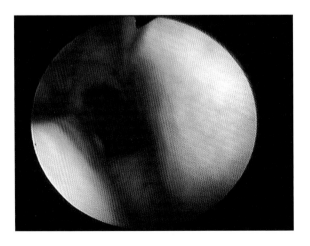

14-3c *The exit of the nasopharynx comes into view.*

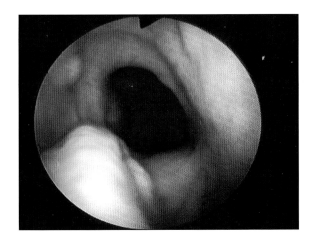

14-3d *Approaching the exit of the nasopharynx.*

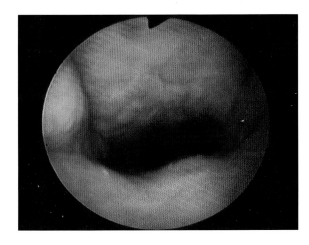

14-3e *The scope has advanced past the inferior turbinate. It is important not to contact the posterior pharyngeal wall upon exiting the nasopharynx. It is helpful if the patient relaxes the palate and protrudes the tongue beginning at this stage of the procedure.*

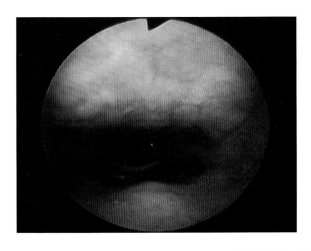

14-3f *Nearing the exit of the nasopharynx the scope tip is deflected downward showing the posterior pharynx and epiglottis edge.*

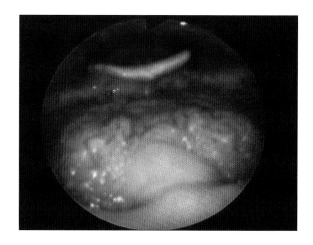

14-3g *Upon exiting the nasopharynx the uvula can be seen at the bottom of the image and the epiglottis edge at the top of the image.*

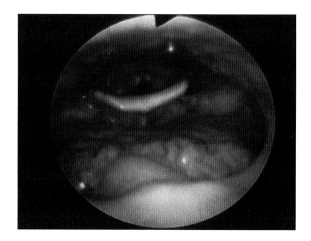

14-3h *Above the epiglottis edge are the posterior cartilages and interarytenoid notch. Below the epiglottis is the vallecula, marking the junction between the tongue and epiglottis.*

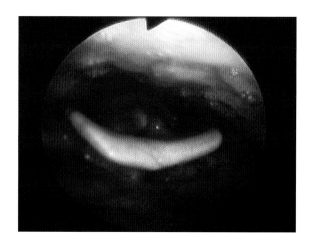

14-3i *Advancing toward the larynx, care must be used not to touch the epiglottis edge anteriorly (below) or the posterior pharyngeal wall (above).*

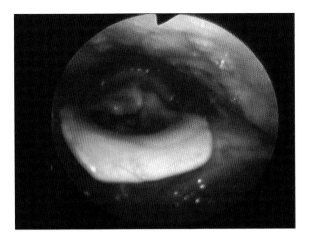

14-3j *An elongated view of the structures of the laryngeal inlet with the epiglottis jutting toward the scope. The posterior cartilages and interarytenoid notch are well seen. The esophagus is located behind the posterior cartilages, but it is collapsed and not visualized.*

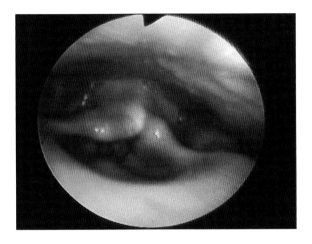

14-3k *With phonation (patient saying "ee") the posterior cartilages come together and the vocal cords shorten.*

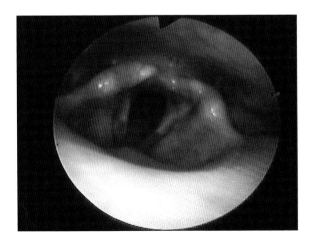

14-3l *Laryngeal view with vocal cord abduction. All of the laryngeal structures can be seen. The patient is inspiring and not phonating.*

Patients undergoing nasal intubation with a bronchoscope should have their noses prepped with sprays of a vasoconstrictant and anesthetic (a combination of oxymetazoline and 4% topical lidocaine), and placement of a nasal trumpet using lidocaine jelly. For those only having rhinolaryngoscopy, anesthetic spray is often not necessary and lidocaine jelly should be avoided, since neither a trumpet nor a tracheal tube will be placed and the jelly may obscure visualization. For rhinolaryngoscopy, the patient should be sitting upright, not leaning backward in a stretcher, nor arching his or her head backward. Establishing a good rapport with the patient is essential if he or she is to tolerate the procedure. The procedure is not truly painful but can be uncomfortable, especially if care is not taken upon initial insertion into the nare. Sitting upright is also advantageous for fiberoptic intubation, because it keeps the tongue and epiglottis off of the posterior pharyngeal wall, a common problem when patients are in a supine position.

While the technical aspects of directing a rhinolaryngoscope or a bronchoscope are the same, controlling the long scope is definitely more difficult. Either scope should always be held out to length, not allowing the mid-portion of the scope to either hang down or loop. If this occurs, the rotation movements applied to the control section will not be transmitted to the tip. Although designed for left hand use only, the author finds it easiest if the dominant hand grips the control section of the scope and the thumb is used to direct the upward and downward movement of the tip. To direct the tip right or left, the dominant hand gripping the handle is rotated (wrist extension/flexion), clockwise or counter-clockwise. The non-dominant hand should be used to advance the tip, and never to twist the scope.

Before inserting the scope into the patient, direct the tip at a target and observe how pressing up or down on the angulation control lever directs the tip. Check the focus and that the lens is clean. Note that the bending of the scope occurs in a small area several centimeters proximal to the tip itself. Bending the distal tip within the tracheal tube, or keeping the tip bent upon withdrawal from the patient, can cause the glass fibers that make up the optical bundle to break. When this occurs, small black dots will permanently appear in the image through the scope.

Often, the most difficult portion of rhinolaryngoscopy is the nasopharynx. It is important not to advance too quickly in the nose. It is critical to go along or below the inferior turbinate, adjacent to the septum. The initial insertion of the scope in the nasopharynx is straight back and medial, followed by a downward direction to exit the nasopharynx. Never advance without seeing the dark open passage you are following. If the image becomes white or pink, the tip of the scope is up against the mucosa. If it gets completely hazy, fog or saliva may be on the lens. This can be addressed by brushing the tip against the mucosa, or if in the pharynx or hypopharynx, by having the patient swallow. If using a bronchoscope, putting lidocaine or saline through the working channel may also help. Connecting the scope to an oxygen source at low flow (1–2 lpm) helps keep the tip clear, but must be used cautiously because of the potential for barotrauma.

After the nasopharynx, it is helpful to have the patient project his or her tongue forward and lean forward so the base of the tongue is off the posterior pharynx. Touching the epiglottis and posterior pharynx should be avoided, as it will stimulate a strong gag response. The piriform fossae should be checked if concerned about a possible foreign body, and the appearance of the cords and epiglottis should be noted. The piriform recess is a blind pouch laterally adjacent to the aryepiglottic fold on either side. Visualization of the piriform recess is facilitated by having the patient puff up his or her cheeks and blow out against closed lips, like playing a trumpet. Examination of the larynx should include phonation testing by having the patient say "ee." An atlas of fiberoptic laryngoscopy is a useful reference for recognizing pathology such as polyps, cancers, and infectious processes.

Nasal Intubation Using a Flexible Fiberscope

As already mentioned, fiberoptic intubation as a rescue technique following failed laryngoscopy may be complicated by bleeding or edema. Also, unconsciousness causes a loss of airway tone, and supine positioning causes the tongue, hypopharynx and epiglottis to fall backward, obstructing the fiberoptic view. Oral intubation with the fiberscope necessitates negotiating a sharp angle from the oropharynx to the larynx. For these reasons, fiberoptic intubation is most easily accomplished in the awake patient as an initial technique, through the nose, sitting upright, or with the head of the bed elevated. Bleeding and secretions make fiberoptic visualization very difficult, and are the most common cause of failed fiberoptic intubation in the emergency setting. Proper topicalization is important to help control bleeding and secretions if the nasal route is chosen.

The author's preferred method of performing fiberoptic intubation in the emergency setting is to place the tracheal tube first, blindly, to a depth of 12–14 centimeters, topicalizing the nares and nasopharynx with oxymetazoline and lidocaine. It is much easier to place the tube first, as opposed to going scope first and then railroading the tube over the scope the entire way from the nares to the cords. This latter approach lengthens the amount of time the scope is at the level of the larynx irritating the patient, and passage of the scope through the nasopharynx does not necessarily mean the tube will follow. When the tube first technique is used however, care should be taken in preparing the nose so that bleeding does not result.

After placing the tracheal tube to a depth of 14 centimeters, the scope is quickly passed down the tube. Upon exiting the tracheal tube, a view of the epiglottis and vocal cords is seen in 85% of cases with minimal or no manipulation of the scope. The larynx may not be exposed due to the epiglottis or other submandibular tissue obstructing the view in patients who are lying supine. This can be overcome by repositioning the head (increasing atlanto-occipital extension), a jaw thrust, or pulling the tongue out using gauze pads or laryngoscope. Once the larynx is identified, the scope is advanced beyond the epiglottis, through the vocal cords, and down the trachea, until the bifurcation at the carina. Topical lidocaine spray can be injected through a syringe connected to the working channel at the vocal cords. This will attenuate the coughing and bucking response upon tube placement. The scope should not be withdrawn until it is clear that the tube has passed the cords and can be advanced to the proper depth for nasal intubation (26 cm in women, 28 cm in men). It is useful to have a nurse standing by with sedative medications so that immediately as the airway is secure the patient can be medicated if necessary.

Tube placement into the larynx, particularly when using a narrow scope, can sometimes be difficult because the diameter of the tube is much larger than the scope. This discrepancy between the two devices can cause the tip of the tube to hang up on the structures comprising the laryngeal inlet. This problem results from the asymmetry of the tip and bevel design of a standard tracheal tube as illustrated with the bougie (Figure 8-9). For this reason, tapered tip tracheal tubes and the Parker Medical tube with its symmetrical tip work better for fiberoptic intubation. With a standard tube tip, rotating the tube 90 degrees counterclockwise as the tube is slid off the scope and through the larynx is recommended as routine practice. This maneuver changes the orientation of the bevel of the tube, allowing the leading edge of the tube tip to be oriented midline and anteriorly, so that the tip does not catch on the laryngeal inlet.

Oral Intubation Using a Flexible Fiberscope

Intubation via the mouth with a fiberoptic bronchoscope is more difficult than nasal intubation because of the sharp angle in the back of the mouth. Particularly in the unconscious person, the tongue and hypopharyngeal structures fall backward, obstructing the view. Jaw thrust, provided by an assistant, along with use of an intubating oral airway, is mandatory when using the oral route. Head extension, if not contraindicated, also helps.

The Berman, Williams, and Ovassapian airways are modified oral airways specifically designed for oral fiberoptic intubation. They each guide the tracheal tube and scope around the tongue and protect the scope should the patient bite down. The Williams airway requires removal of the tracheal tube plastic connector so that after intubation the airway can be slid out over the tracheal tube, while the Berman and the Ovassapian have a specialized groove for this purpose (Figure 14-4). Unless deeply obtunded, topical anesthesia and sedation are necessary for the patient to tolerate an oral airway. A fast and simple technique to anesthetize the tongue and larynx in an awake patient involves a combination of aerosolized lidocaine and lidocaine jelly. The mouth, tongue, and posterior pharynx are first sprayed with topical lidocaine (aerosolized spray, nebulizer, or atomizer). An oral airway is lubricated along its distal lingual surface with lidocaine jelly (2%) and inserted only partially. This is done a second and third time, with repeat application of lidocaine jelly on the distal lingual surface, and with the patient's cooperation, the airway is advanced further. The combination of topical spray and jelly allows the device to be fully inserted without the patient gagging. Once inserted, another spray of topical lidocaine is given down the airway during the patient's inhalation to topicalize the larynx.

After placement of the oral airway, the scope is inserted through the tracheal tube and advanced past the oral airway. The laryngeal structures should be visible, assuming the oral airway has been kept midline. Jaw thrust, atlanto-occipital extension, and tongue traction all help lift the base of the tongue and epiglottis off the posterior pharyngeal wall. The scope is advanced under the epiglottis and into

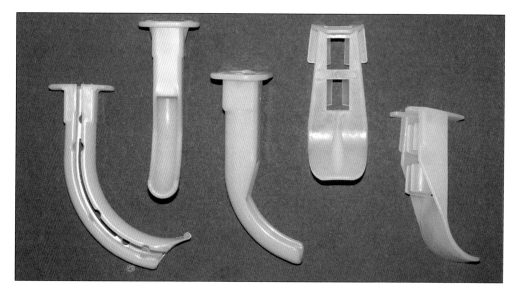

14-4 *Berman intubating airway (left), Williams airways (pink), and Ovassapian airways (right).*

the larynx, down to the carina. With special attention paid to the counterclockwise rotation of the tracheal tube off the scope, placement of the tracheal tube is completed.

The role and use of the flexible fiberscope has been dramatically transformed in the last decade by the increasing use of the LMA, both in elective and emergency settings. In cases of failed RSI, fiberoptic intubation through the LMA is the author's preferred fiberoptic technique compared to those using oral airways because it permits ventilation of the patient while the equipment for fiberoptic intubation is assembled. There are also special facemasks with bronchoscope diaphragm ports for this purpose. These facemasks permit continuous ventilation during intubation, but facemask ventilation compared to LMA ventilation is generally more difficult.

The LMA serves as a tube conduit and positions the end of the scope close to the laryngeal inlet when correctly placed. It may also keep blood and secretions off of the fiberscope. If the LMA Unique (disposable version) is used it is helpful to cut the tube portion of the LMA short, since this will permit a longer section of tracheal tube to advance into the trachea beyond the LMA. The fiberscope should be placed down the LMA to visually confirm location. If none of the laryngeal structures are seen, the LMA should be repositioned. The tracheal tube should advance ahead of the fiberscope when passing through the aperture bars on the LMA or through the epiglottis-elevating bar on the ILMA. The tip of the scope should not be flexed within the tube, nor should the scope be used as a stent to railroad the tracheal tube. Either of these maneuvers can cause damage to the fiberoptic bundles.

After tube placement in the trachea, the LMA should be left in place but deflated. If the mask must be removed, another tracheal tube can serve as a pusher to stabilize the tube in the trachea while removing the mask.

Cleaning and Sterilization, Endoscopic Sheaths

Cases of tuberculosis and other diseases have been transmitted between patients through improperly cleaned bronchoscopes. It is critical that a thin wire brush be passed entirely through the working channel after each use. The working channel must also be flushed during the sterilization process as directed by the manufacturer. Short rhinolaryngoscopes do not have a working channel and therefore do not need wire cleaning or flushing during the cleaning process. Like all fiberoptic instruments, autoclaving and heating will damage the glass fibers and must not be used. A variety of cold sterilization processes can be used, but these are often unavailable in emergency settings. Sending the scope out of the department for cleaning is also a problem.

A new and better means of handling this logistical problem in the ED is to use an endoscopic sheath developed by Vision Sciences, Inc. (Natick, MA) (Figure 14-5). These sterile disposable sheaths are custom built for a variety of scopes and some models even come with a working channel. The tip of the sheath must be fully slid onto the scope so that the special optical element at the end of the sheath is flat against the tip of the scope. After using the sheath, it can be slid off and disposed of without the need to re-sterilize the scope.

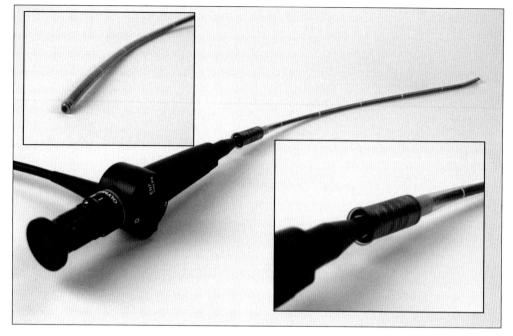

14-5 *Vision Sciences Endo-Sheath on Olympus ENF-P4 rhinolaryngoscope. Close up views of distal tip (above, left) and proximal sheath (below, right).*

Rigid Fiberoptic Devices

The Bullard, Upsher, and Wu-scope each combine rigid metal blades with fiberoptic visualization to achieve oral intubation. Unlike flexible fiberscopes, they cannot be used for nasal intubation, but each requires minimal mouth opening compared to standard laryngoscopes. For oral intubation they are definitely faster and less complicated to use than flexible fiberoptic scopes. Successful intubation with one of these devices is not affected by factors that usually cause difficult direct laryngoscopy. The fiberoptic element in the Bullard and Upsher Scope is completely enclosed by steel. In the Wu-scope there is a removable short, flexible scope that is positioned within the device. Although it has the short length of a rhinolaryngoscope it does not have a distal articulating tip.

Awake insertion of the Bullard, Upsher or Wu-scopes requires full anesthesia of the tongue, pharynx and larynx. From a practical standpoint in emergency situations, this usually limits their use to patients who have received RSI medications.

Each device is rotated along the curvature of the tongue and kept in a midline position. After the larynx is sighted, the tracheal tube slides off a laterally placed stylet on the Bullard scope or through an enclosed central channel on the Upsher and Wu-scope. Like flexible fiberoptic devices, these devices require a thorough familiarity with laryngeal landmarks. The view can be obscured with secretions, blood, or vomitus, although a working channel is provided on each device that can be used for suctioning or oxygen insufflation. Failure with these devices can be due to non-midline placement, problems with visualization at the lens, or inability to trap and elevate the epiglottis. The Bullard and Wu-scopes each have an attachable tip extension to help address this issue.

Glidescope Video Laryngoscope

The Glidescope (Saturn Medical, Vancouver, British Columbia) is a new oral intubation device that does not use a fiberoptic imaging element but instead has a micro-miniature camera built into a specially designed plastic laryngoscope blade (Figure 14-6). The camera location provides an intraoral view of the larynx from just above the laryngeal inlet (Figure 14-7). Compared to a standard Macintosh blade, the blade curvature is more exaggerated (60 degree curvature). The device is very lightweight. At the top of the blade handle is a connection plug to the 7" black and white video monitor. The entire device fits compactly on a small mobile stand and is powered by a single plug and single on/off switch. The device uses a micro-miniature camera (1/4 inch CCD) with a relatively wide-angle lens built directly into the laryngoscope blade. The result is a much larger viewing element, a broader field of view, and a greater depth of focus than is normally seen with fiberoptic devices. The camera lens positioning and orientation seems very resistant to fogging and coverage by secretions, vomitus and blood. The device also has an unusual black and white camera illuminated by one red and one blue LCD light. This system achieves very high contrast and is excellent for defining the laryngeal inlet and glottic structures. Because of the size of the camera and its position within the curvature of the blade, there is essentially no view down the lumen of the plastic blade, even though it appears similar to a laryngoscope.

The recommended insertion technique is to insert the blade less deeply than one would normally insert a standard curved laryngoscope. After visualization of the epiglottis edge, the blade and tip can be manipulated to improve laryngeal exposure as observed on the video monitor (Figure 14-7). Optimal methods of inserting the tracheal tube are still being determined with some users advocating a more midline approach and others using a more lateral technique. The shape of the tracheal tube is a big factor in intubation success. A curvature that matches the device (using a malleable stylet) gets the tube to the target in most cases, but it is often difficult to advance into the larynx because the tube angle catches the anterior tracheal rings. Some users have advocated directional stylets like the Parker Flex-it Stylet (originally the Schroeder stylet). It is probably helpful to keep the end of the stylet at least 2 centimeters from the tube tip so there is more flexibility as the tip is inserted.

Apart from isolated case reports and one study with 15 patients, there is no literature in support of the device, but large trials are reportedly underway in Canada and supposedly have achieved excellent results in both routine and difficult airways. The author has recently tested 16 novice users of the Glidescope (who received minimal training) in three different non-embalmed fresh cadavers. Laryngeal view was excellent in all cases, but overall only 75% of intubation attempts were successful, with a mean intubation time of 76 seconds. Only 7 of 36 successful intubations occurred in less than 30 seconds. The order of cadavers and the ease of direct laryngoscopy had no relationship to successful Glidescope intubation, and skill competence could not be achieved in three attempts despite different stylet shapes and tube insertion techniques.

If the challenges of tube insertion can be solved, the Glidescope has the potential to be widely used because of its similarity of appearance and feel to a standard laryngoscope. Despite outward similarities to a laryngoscope however, the device transforms intubation from a direct visualized procedure into something similar to laparoscopic surgery, i.e., the intubator uses his or her left hand on the Glidescope with the right hand on the tracheal tube, and the procedural field is displayed on a video monitor. For some practitioners this is easy and natural to adopt while others seem to have significant hand-eye coordination issues and feel very uncomfortable with this technique.

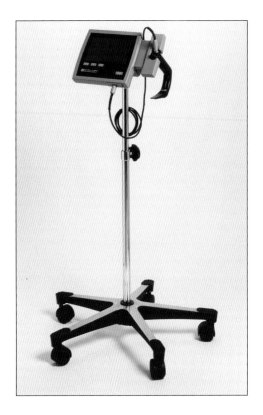

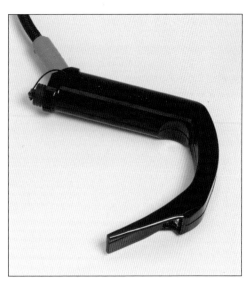

14-6 *Glidescope system (video monitor, laryngoscope, wheeled stand) (left). Closeup of video laryngoscope (above). (Images courtesy of Saturn Biomedical, Burnaby BC.)*

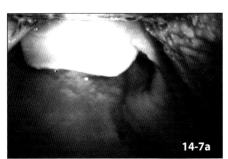

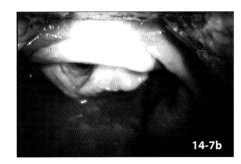

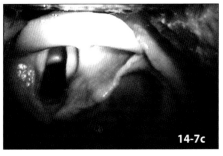

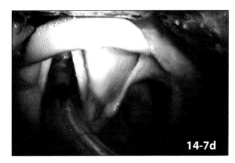

14-7a–d *Sequential intubation images from Glidescope, showing epiglottis (14-7a), posterior cartilages and interarytenoid notch (14-7b), laryngeal view (14-7c), and tube passage (14-7d).*

Lighted Stylets and Trans-Illumination

Lighted stylets can be useful as a laryngoscopy adjunct or as an independent means of intubation. They can also simplify and speed intubation through the LMA or ILMA. Trans-illumination with a lighted stylet is possible because of the trachea's location immediately under the skin of the anterior neck. In this position the lighted stylet produces a bright, localized glow (Figure 14-2). When a lighted stylet is placed in the esophagus, the resultant glow is more diffuse and less intense. In the author's experience, the difference between tracheal and esophageal placement in the same patient is rather evident, however, there is a relatively wide variability in the appearance of tracheal illumination between patients. Obesity and dark skin pigmentation adversely affect trans-illumination, and occasionally the ambient light may need to be reduced or the neck shaded with a towel or hand.

Several different models of lighted stylet are available, varying considerably in cost and complexity (Figure 14-8). The most complicated and costly of these devices is the Trachlight (Laerdal Medical, Wappinger Falls, NY) which has several unique features including a very bright, laterally directed light and a removable wire stiffener. The removable wire stiffener can be partially withdrawn after the lighted tip has been placed in the larynx, allowing the lighted tip to be placed further down the trachea (to the sternal notch). This reportedly makes passage of the tracheal tube easier, however the author has found that using this feature requires practice and significant dexterity. There is no doubt the Trachlight is the best designed of the lighted stylets currently available, but unless practiced regularly, the author recommends use of simpler versions which do not have multiple moving parts.

The following technique, as described by Hung for the Trachlight, can be used with all types of lighted stylets. Ideally the patient's bed should be positioned lower than usual for direct laryngoscopy, or a stool may be helpful to allow the operator to look downward on the anterior neck. If not contraindicated, the patient's head and neck should be fully extended. Note that this is different than direct laryngoscopy, in which the head is extended but the neck is flexed (elevated). The tracheal tube is pre-loaded over the well lubricated lighted stylet until the stylet tip is just at, but not beyond, the tube tip. The stylet, within the tracheal tube, is bent into a 90 degree angle just proximal to the cuff of the tracheal tube. The Trachlight stylet has this area marked, "bend here."

The non-dominant hand is used to distract the mandible and lift upward, while the device and tracheal tube are inserted sideways from the corner of the mouth. After insertion, it is rotated up to midline, into position at the base of the tongue. Rocking the device backward (cephalad) leads the lighted tip into the larynx and should produce a bright glow just beneath the thyroid cartilage. If during advancement at the base of the tongue there is resistance and a glow above the thyroid cartilage, then the tip has hung up at the vallecula. The tip can be directed under the epiglottis by using a jaw thrust and repositioning. If the Trachlight is being used, the wire stiffener is slightly retracted at this point. The tip is advanced further until the bright glow has moved down to the sternal notch and the stylet is then withdrawn. If the lighted stylet does not have this feature, it should be gently advanced as far as possible before the tracheal tube is advanced downward while stabilizing the handle. Sometimes tube advancement can be a problem because the trachea tube tip catches the anterior tracheal rings. While within the trachea, rotating the tube and stylet clockwise may permit the tube to slide off.

Overall, compared to other alternative intubation devices, the lighted stylet is a relatively simple, inexpensive, difficult airway tool that has the potential to be successfully incorporated into emergency airway management. Familiarity with the appearance of trans-illumination of the trachea can initially

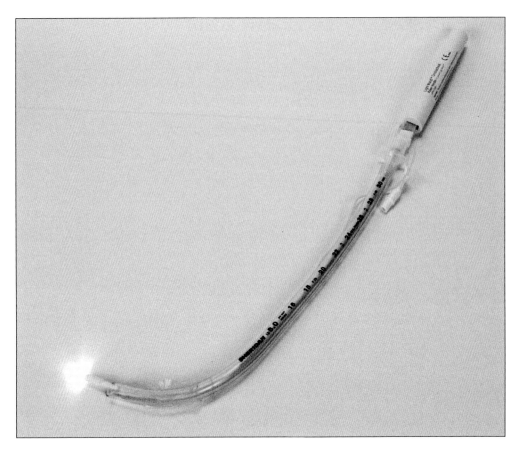

14-8 *Vital Signs (Totawa NJ) Light Wand with reusable handle (3 hour battery life) and disposable stylet within tracheal tube.*

be obtained by using it as a standard stylet. Once confident recognizing tracheal placement, the operator can start using the device as an independent means of intubation.

The major limitation of the lighted stylet is that it frequently works best in the subset of patients who are easiest for laryngoscopy, and conversely, it performs poorly in large patients with short fat necks, a group of patients who often have difficult laryngoscopy. In order for emergency providers to master the device (especially the Trachlight) it must be used routinely instead of the laryngoscope, something that is difficult and uncomfortable for many emergency providers.

Blind Intubation with Neck Palpation

Vacanti has described a method of blind intubation that uses palpation of the cricoid cartilage to assist placement of a styletted tracheal tube. A standard tube stylet is placed within a tracheal tube to within 5mm of the end, and bent at a 60 degree angle (presumably just proximal to the cuff). The patient's head rests on the bed without any additional support, placed in full atlanto-occipital extension. An assistant subluxes the mandible forward by lifting at the angle of the mandible. The intubator stands at the side of the patient and introduces the tracheal tube into the corner of the mouth with his or her dominant hand. The tube and stylet are advanced along the curvature of the tongue while probing with the tube tip; slight pressure is put on the cricoid cartilage with the forefinger and thumb of the other hand. Tracheal placement can be appreciated by palpation and by the clicks felt as the tube is advanced into the trachea. If entry into the trachea is not accomplished, the tube tip can be directed left or right as needed.

Vacanti found that this technique was effective in intubating 49/50 patients in less than a minute. Prior to testing the technique blindly, Vacanti performed fiberoptic evaluation of the technique and concluded that mandible subluxation and cricoid pressure were critical for lifting the epiglottis off of the posterior pharyngeal wall. Tube insertion in the corner of the mouth made for a short distance down to the larynx, and allowed the tube to remain bent appropriately. Although a standard stylet was used, a lighted stylet could also be used in this manner, and would provide the additional benefit of trans-illumination.

Digital Intubation

A tracheal tube can also be placed with direct palpation of the epiglottis or larynx. It is easiest in patients with no teeth and a short distance from the mouth to the larynx. Children and edentulous adults are ideal for this procedure. It should not be attempted unless the patient is in cardiac arrest, is pharmacologically paralyzed, or for some other reason is not capable of biting.

A stiff metal stylet is useful for pre-molding the tube and stylet into a large arc, beginning at the middle of the tube and extending to the tip. The stylet should be well lubricated within the tracheal tube to facilitate removal. The procedure is most easily performed from the patient's left side. Head extension lengthens the distance from the mouth to the trachea and should be avoided. Head and neck flexion may be beneficial, as long as mouth opening is not restricted. Tongue traction may permit further advancement of the fingers.

The index and long fingers of the operator's left hand are slid over the surface of the tongue until the tip of the epiglottis or the posterior cartilages of the larynx is appreciated. The right hand is then used to rotate the pre-molded tracheal tube and stylet downward between the fingers of the left hand. The fingertips help direct the tip anteriorly into the larynx. While the left hand stabilizes the tube, the stylet is withdrawn and the tube advanced into the trachea to the proper depth.

In order to obtain proficiency with digital intubation, the clinician must have a good appreciation of what the epiglottis feels like while wearing a latex glove. Alternatively, being able to palpate the posterior cartilages of the larynx can guide correct placement. Appreciating the feel of the epiglottis or being able to reach the posterior cartilages is quite difficult in many adult patients, especially those with prominent upper dentition. Conversely, this is not the case in small children. In practice, digital intubation is rarely used.

Chapter 15

Surgical Airways

Retrograde Intubation

"Retrograde intubation" describes trans-laryngeal guided intubation in which a wire guide is passed in retrograde fashion from a percutaneous cricoid or tracheal location. The guide is retrieved from either the mouth or nose and a tracheal tube is advanced in anterograde fashion over the guide and into the trachea (Figure 15-1a–k).

Although standard central line wires can be used for this procedure, there is often difficulty in advancing the tracheal tube over the wire. This is caused by the size differential between the wire and the tracheal tube, and by the asymmetric tip of a traditional tracheal tube. A specially designed retrograde intubation kit (Cook Critical Care, Bloomington IN) includes an additional stiffener guide that is threaded down the wire before the tracheal tube is placed. A technique that addresses this issue and also allows for immediate confirmation of tracheal placement, is to use a lighted stylet as a guide within the tracheal tube when the tube is advanced over the wire. The fiberoptic bronchoscope can also be used for this purpose, by passing the scope down the wire using the working channel of the scope. The LMA can also be used as a conduit for tracheal tube placement and ventilation after retrograde wire placement.

Ideal positioning for retrograde intubation involves head extension in a manner that best exposes the cricoid and subcricoid area. The procedure begins with percutaneous entry into the trachea with either a hollow bore needle or catheter. This requires a midline approach aimed in a cephalad direction, and aspiration of air to verify proper depth within the trachea. A small amount of water in the syringe can be helpful for recognizing air aspiration in the syringe.

The best location for percutaneous puncture is a matter of debate. The cricothyroid membrane is usually easily palpable, relatively avascular and superficial. A potential problem with this location however, is that it is only one centimeter below the vocal cords. As the tracheal tube is placed down the wire, the tip of the tube may slip backward out of the trachea. A subcricoid puncture or puncture between the first and second tracheal rings puts more distance between the vocal cords and the puncture location, which allows the tracheal tube to be farther advanced before the wire has to be removed. A small additional amount of length can also be achieved by passing the wire through the Murphy eye of the tracheal tube, instead of through the distal hole.

Once the intra-tracheal location of the needle or catheter is confirmed, the wire is passed through it toward the mouth. Retrieving the wire is sometimes difficult and in the author's experience, it rarely projects spontaneously from the mouth. A sweeping motion of the index finger along the posterior pharynx is helpful in grabbing the wire. Once enough of the wire is advanced out of the mouth (a minimum of 35 cm to accommodate the tube), the lower end of the wire should be clamped where it enters the neck so it is not unintentionally pulled through. The clamp also allows the wire to be held taught.

If a stiff guide catheter with a tapered tip (as supplied in the Cook kit) is available, the guide catheter is directed downward over the wire as far as it will advance. The tracheal tube then follows over this tapered catheter. When it is clear that the tube is advanced as far as possible (resistance is

15-1. Retrograde Intubation Technique

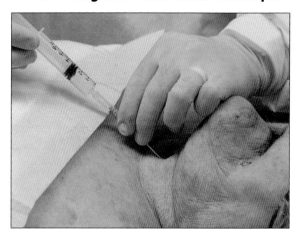

15-1a *Puncturing cricothyroid membrane. Care must be used to avoid puncturing posterior tracheal wall.*

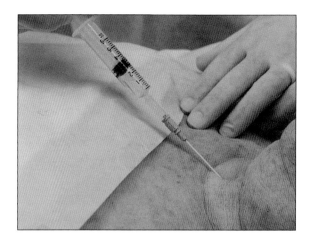

15-1b *Aspirating air through water in syringe to verify intra-tracheal location.*

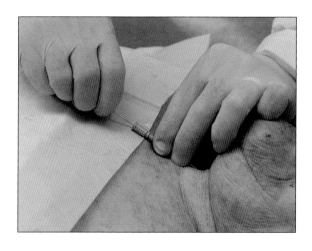

15-1c *Sliding cannula down needle and into trachea.*

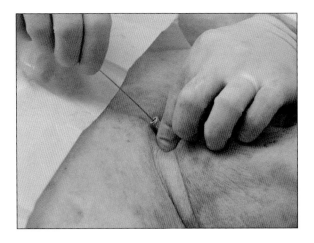

15-1d *Advancing wire through cannula and into trachea.*

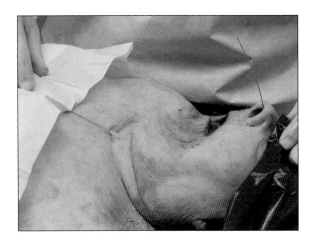

15-1e *Wire may exit nose spontaneously.*

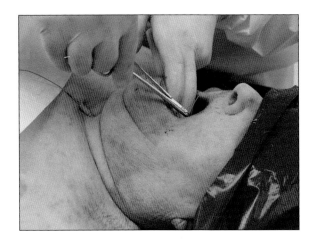

15-1f *Retrieving wire out of mouth can be done by sweeping finger along posterior pharynx or using a small clamp as shown here.*

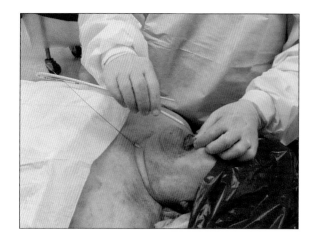

15-1g *Yellow guide catheter is advanced over wire (using wire retrieved out of mouth).*

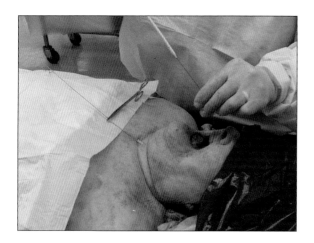

15-1h *Guide catheter is further advanced over wire. Clamp at neck is holding wire and preventing it from accidentally being pulled through neck as guide catheter is advanced.*

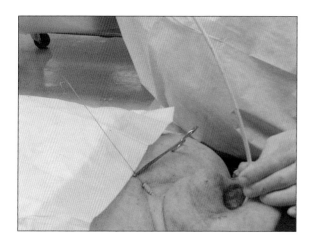

15-1i *Holding proximal end of wire, guide catheter is advanced as far as possible until firm resistance is felt.*

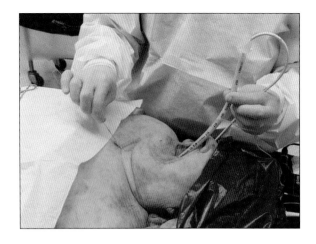

15-1j *Tracheal tube has been advanced over guide catheter until firm resistance is felt. It is helpful to rotate tube counterclockwise as the tube tip passes over laryngeal inlet.*

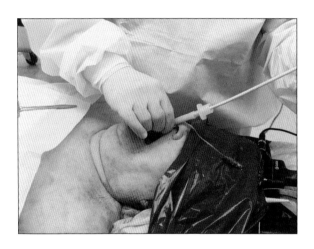

15-1k *Wire has been pulled out from below and cannula used to insert wire has also been removed. Tracheal tube is advanced down catheter and then catheter is pulled from above.*

felt and a bulge is seen as the tube is pushed further down), the bottom end of the wire held by the clamp is either cut at the neck or pulled through from below. The tube is then advanced to the proper depth, depending upon nasal or oral placement.

Retrograde intubation kits are far more likely to yield a successful intubation than use of a wire from a central line kit. Without the stiff catheter supplied in the kit, the tracheal tube (7 or 8 mm internal diameter) is sliding off a very small diameter wire, and frequently gets caught on the laryngeal inlet (specifically at the right aryepiglottic fold). As with the fiberscope, when using a traditional tracheal tube with an asymmetric tip, counterclockwise rotation to 90 degrees is recommended to facilitate tube passage through the laryngeal inlet.

Cricothyrotomy

Cricothyrotomy, as opposed to tracheotomy, is the preferred technique for placing an emergent surgical airway. It has been the traditional end point of the failed emergency airway, although the use of pharmacological adjuncts has caused a sharp decline in its use. The increased use of rescue ventilation devices, particularly the LMA, has dramatically impacted on the use of cricothyrotomy in the OR setting, and will likely further contribute to its declining frequency of use in the emergency setting. The problems with the procedure relate to its high complication rates, the difficulty of skill acquisition and maintenance, and the relatively long time to ventilation. If cricothyrotomy is to be used, it should be initiated early, or only after rescue ventilation has been achieved and the patient is not in immediate danger. If started with the patient already hypoxic and unstable, the outcome is likely to be poor, particularly when performed by inexperienced clinicians. Once the decision to do a cricothyrotomy has been made, the highest priority should be on achieving ventilation quickly to prevent hypoxic brain injury. Apart from brain injury or death due to delayed ventilation, primary short term complications are bleeding and malposition, while long term complications include dysphonia, dysphagia, and subglottic stenosis.

The cricothyroid membrane is superficial and relatively avascular. Its location immediately below the thyroid cartilage generally makes identification straightforward (Figure 15-2). If the thyroid cartilage is not readily identified, the cricoid cartilage can be palpated as the first prominent cartilage coming up from the sternal notch. For cricothyrotomy or tracheotomy, the patient's head should not be elevated, but should be fully extended at the atlanto-occipital joint. In the absence of known or suspected spine pathology, a towel or blanket under the neck and between the shoulders, with the head fully extended backward, will maximize exposure of the critical structures. If time permits, the neck should be prepped and draped. Epinephrine infiltration (lidocaine 1% with epinephrine) may decrease bleeding, however, the procedure is essentially done by palpation, not visualization. Patients with a pulse will likely bleed enough to obscure visualization of any landmarks.

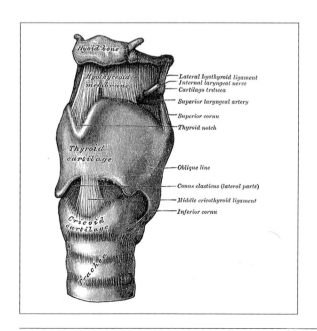

15-2 *The hyoid, thyroid, and cricoid from Gray's Anatomy of the Human Body (1918). The cricothyroid membrane is in the gap between the thyroid and the cricoid cartilages. A common error performing cricothyrotomy is to make the incision too high, mistaking the hyothroid membrane for the proper location. The cricoid ring is the first prominent landmark coming up from the sternal notch. The thyroid cartilage is significantly larger than the other structures, especially laterally. Note the distance between the superior and inferior cornu of the thyroid.*

Traditional vs. 4-step Cricothyrotomy Technique

A number of different methods of open cricothyrotomy have been described including the traditional method and the rapid 4-step technique. They vary in regard to the type of skin incision and the use of a tracheal hook and Trousseau dilator (Figures 15-3, 15-4, 15-6). Both the traditional and 4-step use a trachea hook, and the traditional method also uses the Trousseau dilator. The simplest approach is to use what is immediately available, namely a scalpel, your finger, and a small tracheal tube, instead of a Shiley.

The initial steps involve identifying the cricothyroid membrane and stabilizing the larynx. The larynx should be stabilized with the non-dominant hand while the operator stands at the patient's side facing the neck (Figure 15-5). The tip of the index finger is used to palpate the cricothyroid membrane . The middle finger and the thumb of the non-dominant hand are placed on either side of the larynx, where the thyroid and cricoid cartilages meet posteriorly.

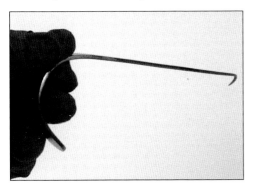

15-3 *Tracheal hook.*

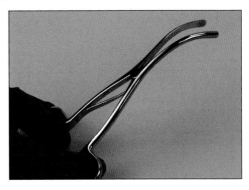

15-4 *Trousseau dilator.*

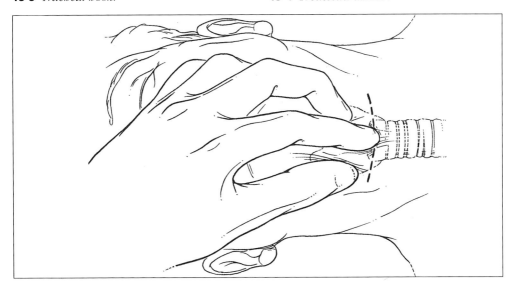

15-5 *Palpating and stabilizing the thyroid cartilage. The thumb and third finger of the non-dominant hand are placed at the lateral borders of the thyroid cartilage and the index finger palpates the cricothyroid membrane. (From Eisele DW and McQuone SJ. Emergencies of the Head and Neck, Mosby Inc., St Louis MO, 2000, with permission of Elsevier.)*

15.6 Traditional Open Cricothyrotomy Technique

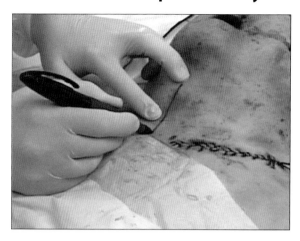

15-6a *Marking midline is helpful in a patient with a large neck.*

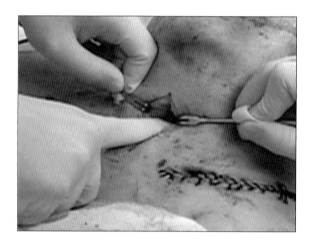

15-6b *Following the vertical skin incision, the cricothyroid membrane is palpated. Skin retractors help keep the incision open.*

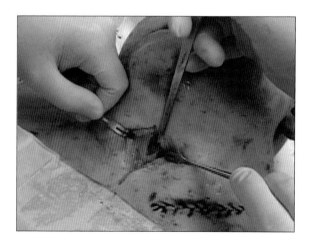

15-6c *The tracheal hook has been inserted into the cricothyroid membrane and upward traction is gently applied to the thyroid cartilage.*

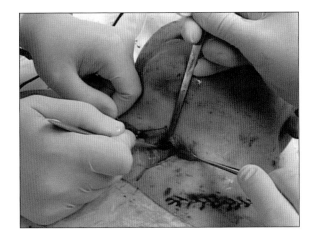

15-6d *Horizontal incision is made through cricothyroid membrane.*

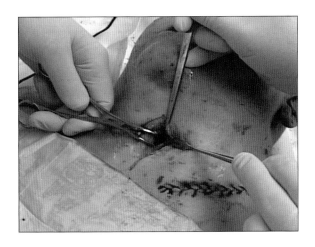

15-6e *The Trousseau dilator expands the opening in the cricothyroid membrane.*

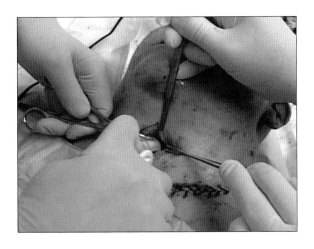

15-6f *A Shiley tracheal tube with inner trocar is inserted. Initial insertion of the Shiley is done with the Shiley turned 90 degrees to the trachea and then rotated into position (this is better seen in Figure 15-7, below).*

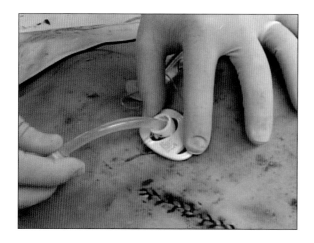

15-6g *The trocar has been removed and the inner cannula is inserted.*

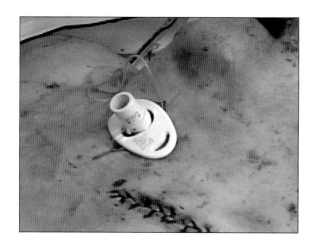

15-6h *With the inner cannula inserted, the Shiley can be connected to the 15 mm fitting of a resuscitation bag.*

With the rapid 4-step technique, the incision through the skin and membrane is done horizontally with a single stab incision (using a larger # 20 blade), and the tracheal hook is used to pull on the cricoid cartilage in a caudal direction (Figures 15-7, 15-8). The traditional technique involves separate skin and membrane incisions, and traction with the tracheal hook is applied to the lower border of the thyroid cartilage in a cranial direction. The incision with the traditional technique is made with a small blade (#11 or 15) and expanded with the Trousseau dilator.

Surgical airways performed on patients making respiratory efforts will cause a strong coughing response when the trachea is entered. The trachea can also drop downward after incision, so it is important that the lumen of the airway be stabilized. If a tracheal hook is not immediately available the non-dominant index finger (from the hand stabilizing the larynx) can be used.

It is easiest in the emergency surgical airway to place a 6.0 mm tracheal tube through the incision and into the trachea. The 6.0 mm tracheal tube has a smaller outer diameter (8.2 mm) than either the #4 Shiley (9.4 mm) or the #6 Shiley (10.8 mm) (Figure 15-9). Shiley tracheotomy tubes

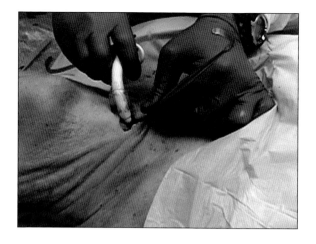

15-7 *The rapid 4-step technique uses traction in a caudal direction on the cricoid ring instead of traction in a cranial direction on the thyroid (as shown in Figure 15-6c). The Shiley with its trocar visible (blunted round tip) is inserted from a sideways direction.*

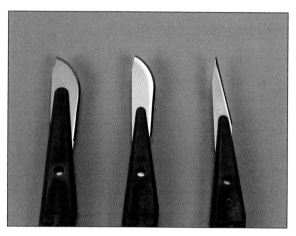

15-8 *Different scalpel designs, from left to right: Large rounded tip of #20, slightly smaller #10, and pointed tip of #11.*

have plastic flanges that obscure tip placement, as well as a rigid shape that requires sideways insertion and subsequent rotation in order to enter the trachea. If a standard tracheal tube is used, it must be carefully secured after placement to prevent dislodgment.

Comparative studies between the traditional technique and the rapid 4-step technique have only been done in cadavers. Among inexperienced operators, the 4-step technique required approximately 43 seconds vs. 134 seconds using the traditional method. In a separate cadaver study involving anesthesiologists (also inexperienced with cricothyrotomy), the average time to ventilation was 102 seconds with the traditional technique. Two separate studies have reported a higher incidence of complications (specifically fracture of the cricoid ring) with the 4-step technique, however.

From the author's experience and observation of many different practitioners with non-embalmed cadavers, the utility of ancillary equipment varies with the specific patient. The dilator is rarely needed since the non-dominant index finger or the base of the scalpel works well for this purpose. A tracheal hook is most helpful in the obese patient with a thick anterior neck. In such cases the trachea is located very deep relative to the skin incision and stabilizing the trachea during the procedure is more difficult. The decision to use a vertical or horizontal incision depends upon the rapid identification of the cricothyroid membrane. If there is no question where the membrane is located a horizontal incision may be appropriate, albeit with the knowledge that it carries a higher incidence of bleeding, especially if it is extended too far laterally. A vertical incision is best when the landmarks are not distinctly palpable through the skin.

For long term use, a tracheotomy tube is obviously preferable and emergency personnel should be familiar with the design and components. Note that tracheotomy tubes have three components: the cuffed tube itself, a removable inner cannula, and a stiff plastic trocar (Figure 15-10). The trocar should always be placed within the tracheotomy tube during insertion. Because of the stiffness of the Shiley and its shape, the tip must be introduced with the device turned 90 degrees to the orientation of the trachea (Figure 15-7). After the tip is introduced, the device is rotated and inserted fully into the trachea. To ventilate the patient, the introducer must be removed and replaced with the inner cannula, which connects to a standard 15 mm connector (Figure 15-6g–h).

The speed to ventilation with cricothyrotomy is dependent upon operator skill, patient's body habitus, and the ability to place the patient in proper position. The procedure is most challenging in cases of cervical immobilization, particularly in obese patients with short necks and non-palpable landmarks. Unfortunately, these are patients who are likely to have difficult laryngoscopy as well, and obesity causes rapid oxygen desaturation. For these patients, rescue ventilation may be crucial, either as a bridge to a surgical airway, or as a means to an alternative intubation technique.

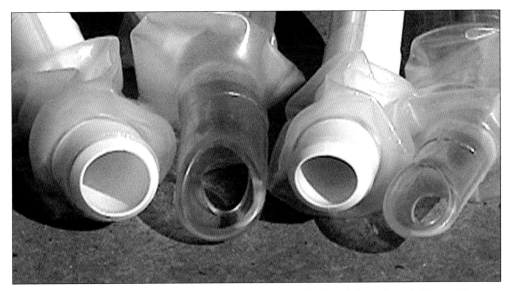

15-9 *Distal ends of Shiley #6 (on left), 8.0 mm ID tracheal tube, Shiley #4, and 6.0 mm ID tracheal tube (far right). Outer diameter of Shiley #6 is 10.8mm, compared to 8.2 mm outer diameter of 6.0 mm ID tracheal tube.*

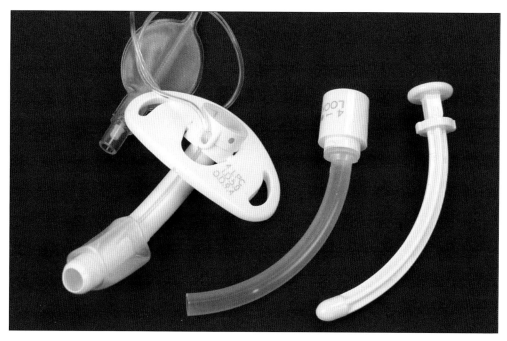

15-10 *Shiley tracheostomy tube and components. Cuffed Shiley with flange (left), removable inner cannula (middle), and trocar used for insertion (right).*

Percutaneous Cricothyrotomy (Melker Kit)

Cricothyrotomy can also be achieved using a guide wire, dilator and tapered airway similar to the Seldinger technique used to place central venous catheters (Melker Cricothyrotomy Kit, Cook Critical Care, Bloomington IN)(Figure 15-11). A small skin incision is made overlying the cricothyroid membrane at the location of wire entry to facilitate subsequent passage of the dilator and airway (Figure 15-12a–e). The wire is inserted in similar fashion to wire insertion for retrograde intubation but in this case, the needle, and subsequently the wire, are directed inferiorly. The dilator, with the tapered airway over it, is advanced over the wire into the trachea. The wire and dilator are then removed, leaving the airway in place.

Because of the familiarity with the Seldinger technique for placing central line catheters, some practitioners have expressed preference for performing cricothyrotomy in this manner. In cadaver studies, this technique has neither higher success rates nor increased speed compared with traditional cricothyrotomy (average time 100 seconds). The biggest challenge is to correctly place the needle into the trachea (not too deep so as to avoid penetrating the posterior tracheal wall), and then to pass the wire. Using a small amount of saline in the aspiration syringe and looking for bubbles upon aspiration may help locate the lumen of the trachea before placing the wire. The Melker Kit now comes in a cuffed version, which is preferable to the original non-cuffed design.

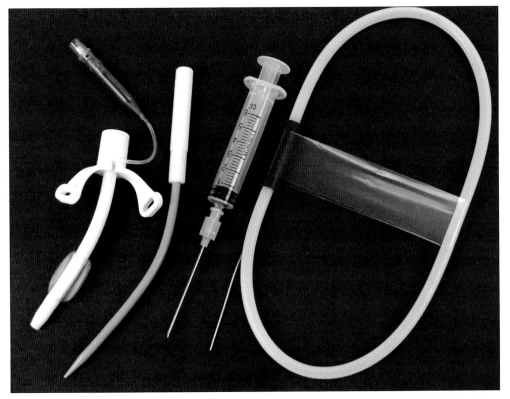

15-11 *Components of Melker percutaneous cricothyrotomy kit. Catheter with cuff and pilot balloon (left), grey dilator, syringe with needle, and wire (right).*

15-12. Melker Percutaneous Cricothyrotomy Technique

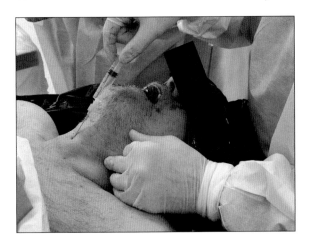

15-12a *Puncturing cricothyroid membrane and directing needle in caudal direction. Care must be taken to avoid puncturing the posterior tracheal wall.*

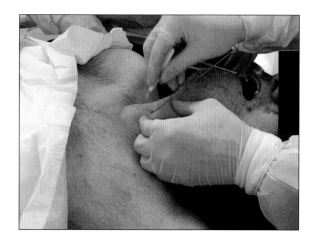

15-12b *Wire has been placed into the trachea. Scalpel is used to create a small skin incision.*

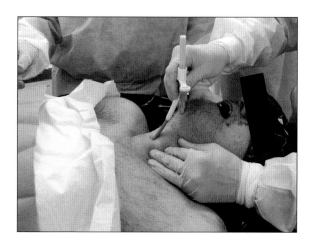

15-12c *Grey tapered dilator and Melker airway catheter are advanced together over the wire.*

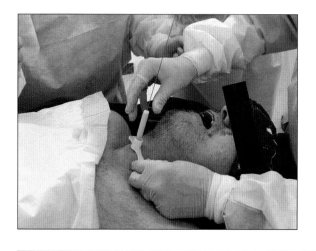

15-12d *With full advancement the base of the Melker catheter is positioned flat against neck.*

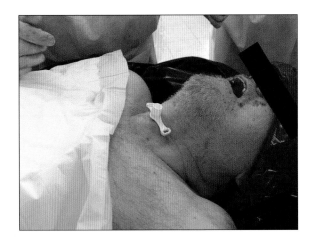

15-12e *Wire and tapered dilator have been removed completing procedure. Small wings on side of catheter can be used to secure device around neck.*

Tracheotomy

Tracheotomy is rarely performed in the emergency setting. Cricothyrotomy is technically easier to perform, markedly faster, and has significantly fewer complications. The only indications for tracheotomy on an emergent basis are when a cricothyrotomy cannot be done or when a cricothyrotomy is not below the level of the pathology. In rare instances, infection or neoplasm may make the airway lumen at the level of the cricoid too small for cannulation. Severe laryngeal trauma or tracheal transection can require tracheotomy as a primary means of airway management.

The traditional technique involves dissection, exposure, and division of the thyroid gland (clamping the area for incision with two clamps and then using a scalpel to divide it), followed by creation of a window in the third and fourth tracheal rings through which the tube is placed. Percutaneous tracheotomy, using a guide wire with progressively larger dilators, is now commonly done in the intensive care setting, though there are no reports of its use in emergency settings. In the emergency setting, patients who require tracheotomy may not have time for dissection and ligation, and instead, a slash approach is sometimes used to gain rapid entry into the trachea. Brisk bleeding should be anticipated and locating the trachea will be done by feel, not sight. Once ventilation has been achieved, the wound can be packed or repaired as needed to achieve hemostasis. Pneumothorax is a common complication of emergent tracheotomy, and should be suspected if ventilation problems or hemodynamic instability occur immediately after the procedure.

Chapter 16

Special Clinical Challenges

Angioedema

Angioedema involves swelling of the lips, soft palate, tongue and larynx, and can result in rapidly life-threatening airway obstruction (Figure 16-1). The etiology is most frequently drug related, specifically angiotensin converting enzyme inhibitors, although hereditary forms also exist. Therapeutic measures that may prevent progression and intubation include intravenous steroids and antihistamines. The efficacy of racemic epinephrine is unproven. Subcutaneous epinephrine must be used cautiously in older patients with coronary artery disease (many of the same patients who have isolated tongue swelling from ACE inhibitors), but it is first line therapy for the young patient with anaphylaxis and angioedema. Thankfully, few patients progress to warrant intubation in the face of treatment. The need for airway intervention is determined by the clinical status of the patient, oropharyngeal examination, and fiberoptic laryngeal examination. Progression of swelling despite treatment is a serious sign. Patients with increased work of breathing and lingual and laryngeal edema (dysphonia, stridor) should be intubated via the nose or the neck as soon as possible.

If the patient is cooperative and time permits, a fiberoptic nasal intubation is ideal. Fiberoptics work poorly if the patient is agitated and hypoxic. A blind nasal technique, as previously described, is warranted if the patient is uncooperative or if fiberoptic equipment or expertise is not available. If nasal intubation fails, a surgical approach should be rapidly undertaken to prevent hypoxic injury. Rapid sequence intubation is contraindicated with significant angioedema of the tongue and involvement of the larynx, since mask ventilation, in addition to laryngoscopy, may be impossible once muscular tone is lost. Awake laryngoscopy, with sedatives or topical agents, is a high-risk procedure (bleeding, emesis) with a very slim chance of success and should be avoided. Assuming the problem is confined to the anterior tongue and does not involve the larynx, the LMA or Combitube may be useful as a temporary means of ventilating the patient if necessary. Trans-tracheal ventilation may be possible, but if exhalation is compromised due to high grade obstruction, high pressure and high volume ventilation will be catastrophic.

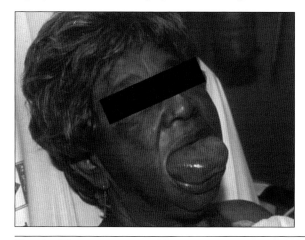

16-1 *Marked angioedema of the tongue secondary to an angiotensin converting enzyme inhibitor. Patient was in no respiratory distress and intubation was not required. Swelling resolved with steroids and antihistamines. Photograph courtesy of Edward Dickinson, MD.*

Ludwig's Angina: Deep Space Infection of the Floor of the Mouth

Ludwig's angina is a potentially life-threatening infection of the floor of the mouth that can progress quickly and obstruct the airway. It is almost always odontogenic in origin, and is usually seen in the ED several days after tooth extraction or other dental procedure. As the infection spreads it elevates and posteriorly displaces the tongue causing marked trismus and may lead to airway obstruction (Figure 16-2). Diagnosis on physical exam requires palpation of the submandibular space and intraoral palpation of the floor of the mouth.

In the author's experience, few patients with Ludwig's require ED airway management. Emergency department interventions include starting antibiotics and steroids and obtaining a CT scan to delineate the infection. An oral or ENT surgeon consultation is mandatory, as almost all patients require operative drainage. As with angioedema, signs of impending obstruction that mandate securing the airway include stridor, difficulty managing secretions, anxiety, and increased work of breathing. Either awake tracheotomy or awake nasal intubation (with a flexible fiberscope and the patient sitting upright) is recommended. In the operating room, with tracheotomy ready to be performed, intubation with a laryngoscope has been reported to be feasible once trismus has been relieved with inhalational anesthesia. If laryngoscopy is attempted, a straight blade with a small flange using a paraglossal approach is suggested. A bougie or introducer may be useful if visualization is poor. The need for a surgical airway must be expected. Rapid sequence intubation in the emergency setting is contraindicated because of the mechanical obstacles to laryngoscopy and ventilation and the real potential for catastrophic loss of the airway. The laryngeal mask airway (assuming it can be inserted), or trans-tracheal ventilation, have been reported to be useful as a temporary means of ventilation if necessary.

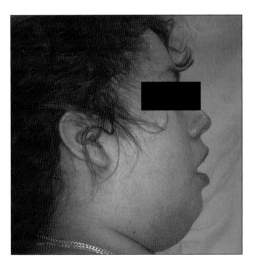 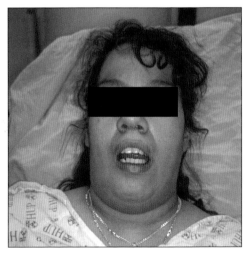

16-2a   16-2b

16-2a–b *Ludwig's angina following a lower tooth extraction four days earlier. Patient has elevation of the tongue, fullness of the floor of the mouth, and trismus. The patient did not require intubation in the ED, but was taken to the operating room and received a tracheotomy prior to neck drainage. Photograph courtesy of Steve Larson, MD.*

Penetrating Neck and Lower Facial Trauma, Blast Injuries

Penetrating wounds of the neck and lower face can produce airway compromise by direct injury or by compression from hematoma. Management is dictated by the clinical status of the patient, and also by the specific areas of the neck involved. As opposed to Ludwig's angina or angioedema, which usually do not progress to need ED intervention, aggressive early ED airway management is warranted because of the likelihood of increased swelling and urgent surgical management (Figures 16-3a–b, 16-4a–b, 16-5a–c, 16-6, 16-7).

In the obtunded patient with no gag response or those in cardiac arrest, immediate laryngoscopy is recommended (Figure 16-3a–b). Patients with evident laryngeal or tracheal injury, i.e., subcutaneous emphysema, dysphonia, stridor, inability to tolerate a supine position, etc., may warrant immediate tracheotomy. When there is evident tracheal violation RSI is contraindicated because the tube may not be passable from the mouth and ventilation from above will be impossible (the redundancy of safety does not exist). In these cases, a surgical airway should be done initially. Alternatively, a tube can sometimes be placed directly through the violated trachea (Figure 16-5a–c). In all other patients, laryngoscopy with rapid sequence intubation and preparation for a surgical airway if laryngoscopy fails is the preferred technique.

Penetrating or blast injuries to the upper airway well above the larynx are usually manageable by direct laryngoscopy, but they often have extensive bleeding and tissue disruption of the tongue and floor of the mouth. Feasibility of laryngoscopy should be determined by whether the tongue can be followed to the epiglottis. If this bridge is disrupted, laryngoscopy should not be attempted. Forward distraction of the mandible during laryngoscopy may be very easy if the mandible is broken bilaterally. If the supporting structures of the midface, mandible and hyoid are disrupted, however, it may be impossible to mask ventilate even with oral and nasal airways. A supraglottic device (LMA or Combitube) may work if the pathology is confined well above the larynx and hypopharynx, but these devices are relatively contraindicated with distorted anatomy. In the author's experience, RSI is appropriate in the vast majority of facial trauma cases, except those in which the floor of the mouth and the base of the tongue are severely affected. If RSI is used in major lower face and neck trauma, an immediate surgical airway may be required if laryngoscopy fails.

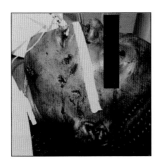 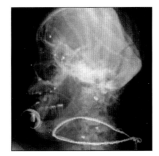

16-3a   **16-3b**

16-3a *Multiple gunshot wounds to face in patient with agonal respirations and hypotension. Patient was intubated without any medications. The tongue was involved and there was a large amount of bleeding, but intubation was successful on first pass.*
16-3b *Radiograph of head and neck shows large number of metallic fragments from bullets.*

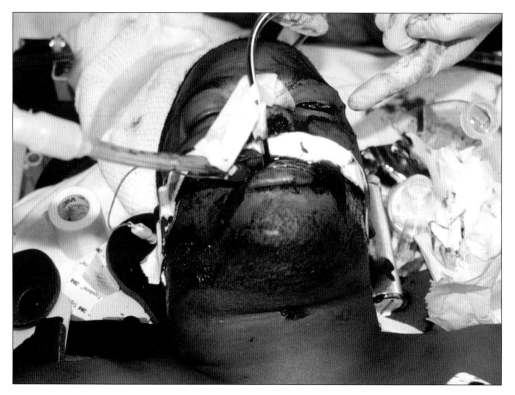

16-4a *Gunshot wound and resulting right neck hematoma. Bullet entered behind left eye (finger pointing to entrance). After traversing across sinus and palate it lodged beneath the angle of the mandible and injured the jugular vein on the right side. Patient was intubated on presentation. Large neck hematoma developed approximately 30 minutes after arrival.*

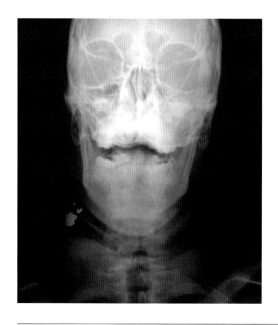

16-4b *Radiograph showing location of bullet beneath right mandible. Photograph and radiograph courtesy of Edward Dickinson, MD.*

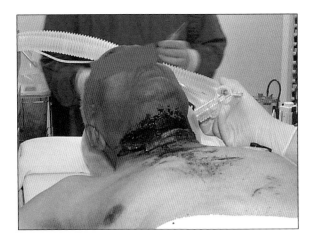

16-5a *Gaping neck wound in man who fell through a plate glass window and presented to the ED several hours after injury. Bleeding had stopped and patient was in no respiratory distress breathing through wound.*

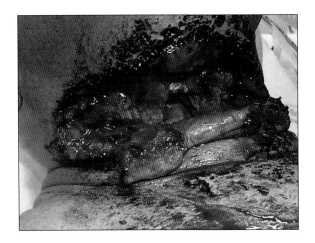

16-5b *Close up of neck wound. Dried blood is evident at wound margins. Wound is at the level of the cricothyroid membrane.*

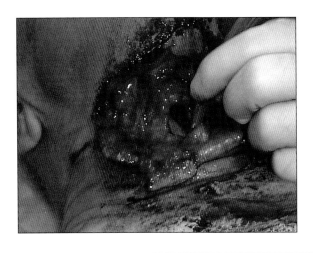

16-5c *Direct tracheal intubation through wound. Photographs courtesy of Bryan Cotton, MD.*

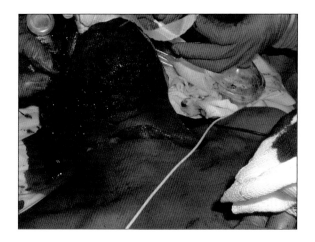

16-6 *Large slash wound to neck. Prior to intubation the wound was inspected and trachea palpated. No violation was evident and the patient did not have phonation problems or intraoral bleeding. RSI laryngoscopy was successful on first pass.*

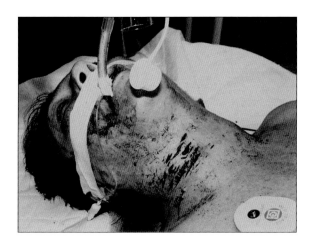

16-7 *Multiple self-inflicted stab wounds. Patient was non-cooperative with exam and agitated. RSI was used to secure the airway with an understanding that the potential of tracheal violation existed and that a surgical airway might be rapidly required. Laryngoscopy was easy and intubation succeeded on first pass. Subsequent CT and neck exploration showed no tracheal violation.*

Fiberoptic evaluation and airway management in trauma cases should be reserved for patients who are clinically stable, cooperative, and without significant bleeding. For purposes of laryngoscopy, cervical spine precautions are not needed in isolated gunshot wounds to the head or neck in which the spine is not directly involved (as evidenced by location of the wound, trajectory, or neurological findings).

Burns

Burns can cause direct airway injury and compromise the airway through resultant edema. The overriding principle of airway management in burns is to intubate the patient early in any case where edema might ensue (Figure 16-8). Clues that a significant thermal injury to the airway has occurred include loss of nasal hairs, compromised voice, or respiratory distress. The author has seen

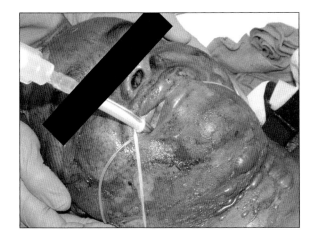

16-8 *Facial burns to entrapped driver following a front-end collision. Patient initially had no respiratory difficulty. Evidence of potential thermal injury to airway includes singed nasal hairs and proximity of blistering to nose and mouth. Patient became stridorous shortly after arrival and had evident airway edema upon laryngoscopy.*

many cases of smoke exposure with carbonaceous material in the mouth and nares without thermal burns. Intubation for smoke exposure alone is not needed unless the patient has associated respiratory distress or altered mental status (from hypoxia or toxin exposure, such as carbon monoxide or cyanide).

When thermal burns are present, debris and edema may cause marked distortion of normal anatomy. An epiglottis first approach with careful landmark identification is required. Succinylcholine is not contraindicated for RSI in acute burns.

Blunt Laryngo-Tracheal Injury

Blunt injuries to the thyroid cartilage, larynx and trachea are problematic because of the possibility that intubation from above may be technically impossible, exacerbate the injury, or result in a false passage. They are very rare, occurring in approximately one in 15,000 trauma cases. Clinical signs include subcutaneous emphysema, dysphonia, stridor, and inability to tolerate a supine position (Figure 16-9). Some tracheal injuries, however, may have minimal to no presenting symptoms because the disruption may be reduced by the patient's position and then become evident only when the neck is extended. If stable, fiberoptic examination and CT will define the extent of injury (Figure 16-10). Management options for the unstable patient are preferentially, in order: immediate tracheotomy, intubation over the fiberscope if time permits, and direct laryngoscopy with an understanding of its attendant risks and limitations. Use of an LMA, Combitube, or trans-tracheal jet ventilation, is discouraged in the presence of a disrupted airway and subcutaneous emphysema. Ventilation from above or under pressure may exacerbate the injury, produce massive subcutaneous emphysema, and lead to cardiac arrest from barotrauma. An early surgical airway–below the larynx, i.e., a tracheotomy as opposed to a cricothyrotomy–is an appropriate choice in any patient with a significant laryngeal fracture.

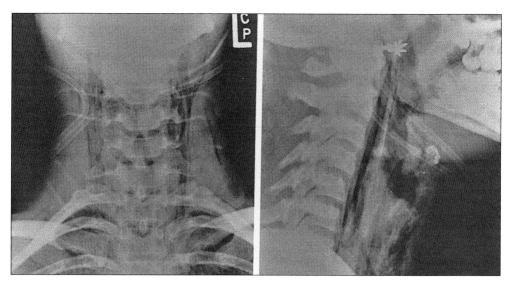

16-9 *AP and lateral neck radiographs on young woman who was riding a scooter in the dark and received a blunt clothesline injury to the neck. Free air can be seen tracking through neck and there is significant soft-tissue swelling evident on the lateral film. Patient had no respiratory distress and a normal voice at the time the films were taken. She was subsequently intubated using a fiberoptic bronchoscope. (Reprinted from Eisele DW, McQuone SJ. Emergencies of the head and neck. Mosby Inc. St. Louis, 2000, used with permission of Elsevier.)*

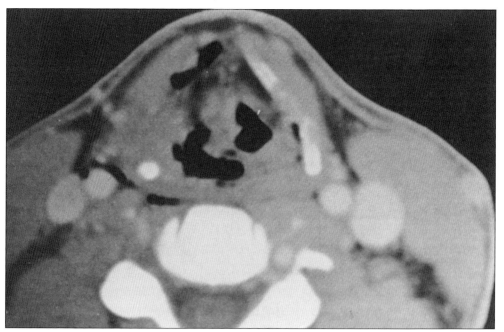

16-10 *CT image of laryngeal fracture in young man kicked in the neck. He was acutely short of breath and had hemoptysis immediately following injury but his symptoms rapidly cleared. He had a normal voice and no airway complaints at the time of his awake tracheostomy. (Reprinted from Eisele DW, McQuone SJ. Emergencies of the head and neck. Mosby Inc. St. Louis, 2000, with permission of Elsevier.)*

Obstructing Intrinsic Lesions

Neoplasm and infection can cause problems at the level of the epiglottis and larynx (Figures 16-11, 16-12a–b). Dysphonia, dysphagia, and inability to lay flat are warning signs that should not be ignored. If stable, both fiberoptic examination and radiographic studies should be done to define the pathology. CT is best for the evaluation of neoplasm, while lateral neck radiographs can be helpful for quickly identifying epiglottitis (Figure 16-13). The feasibility of fiberoptic intubation hinges on the degree of obstruction, the skill of the operator, and the cooperation of the patient (Figure 16-11). Racemic epinephrine, steroids, and sitting the patient upright may improve symptoms. In patients who present with increased work of breathing and other obstructive symptoms, the airway will need intervention. If surgical consultation is available and time permits, these cases are best handled in the OR with either an awake tracheotomy or fiberoptic intubation. On rare occasion, tracheotomy will need to be done in the ED if fiberoptic intubation fails or is unavailable. In cardiac arrest or near arrest, laryngoscopy may be warranted while the surgical airway is initiated, but under no circumstances should these patients receive RSI. Small tracheal tubes (5.0 mm and 6.0 mm ID) should be available in case the glottic opening is restricted and also for placement through the neck as needed. Trans-tracheal ventilation may serve as a bridging device, but this must be done cautiously in high grade obstruction due to the risk of barotrauma. Supraglottic devices (LMA and Combitube) are contraindicated with hypopharyngeal and laryngeal pathology.

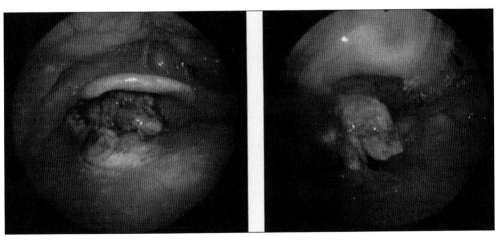

16-11 *Obstructing laryngeal carcinoma. Patient was successfully intubated (right) with fiberscope. (Reprinted from Ovassapian A. Fiberoptic endoscopy and the difficult airway. 2nd ed., Lippincott-Raven, Philadelphia, 1996, with permission of Elsevier.)*

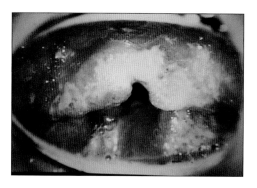
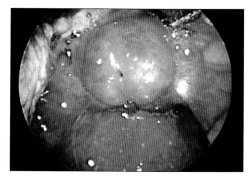

16-12a   **16-12b**

16-12a *Exudative epiglottitis.* **16-12b** *Marked epiglottic edema from epiglottitis in a small child. Pin-hole sized glottic opening is at the center of image. Patient was able to be mask ventilated and intubated with direct laryngoscopy in the OR. Photographs courtesy of Steven Handler, MD.*

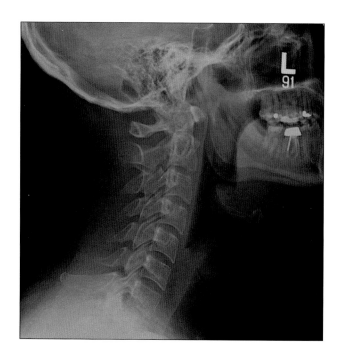

16-13 *Rounded appearance of swollen epiglottis on lateral neck radiograph in a young man with fever and throat pain. Patient had trouble with swallowing and phonation but no respiratory distress. Lumen of airway was not compromised on rhinolaryngoscopy. Adult epiglottitis is rarely associated with airway problems compared to epiglottitis in children. Laryngoscopy in epiglottitis is feasible as long as the landmarks are appropriately recognized, but whenever there is distorted laryngeal anatomy it is safest to avoid RSI.*

Cervical Halo and Fixed Kyphosis of the Cervical Spine

Either of these two conditions prevents proper positioning for laryngoscopy by restricting atlanto-occipital extension. Oral intubation is often possible, but is a function of other variables, i.e., mouth opening, tongue size, upper dentition, ability to prognath the lower jaw forward, etc.

In extreme situations (cardiac arrest and near arrest) immediate laryngoscopy is appropriate as is use of a rescue ventilation device if mask ventilation is not effective. Under less urgent conditions, intubation is best performed with avoidance of laryngoscopy, using an awake nasal approach. Alternatively, options through the mouth include awake laryngoscopy, a rigid optical device, or a lightwand, but these may be difficult without muscular relaxation and will also require topical anesthesia. Surgical airways may be especially difficult in extreme cervical kyphosis because of restricted access to the anterior neck. Laryngoscopy has been successful in ankylosing spondylitis with extreme reverse Trendelenberg positioning, elevating the foot of the bed dramatically, and supporting the head with pillows (having the neck flexed on the chest). If laryngoscopy is attempted, a straight blade may be better suited to deal with the small displacement space created by the marked degree of neck flexion.

Hanging

Hanging can cause fractures to the cervical spine, hyoid bone, and thyroid cartilage but most hanging victims are injured by asphyxiation (Figure 16-14). Spine fractures and cartilaginous neck injuries are extremely rare in patients who have strangled themselves without a significant drop from height. Apart from patients who are found in cardiac arrest, neurologic outcome is not related to initial presentation, and some patients initially with a GCS 3 will recover. The airway does not need intervention in patients who are awake, alert, not hypoxic, and not exhibiting signs of airway obstruction. Fiberoptic evaluation and CT may be useful for identifying laryngeal injury, and plain films or CT may be useful for evaluation of hyoid injury. In patients requiring airway management, this should be done by direct laryngoscopy, with or without RSI as needed.

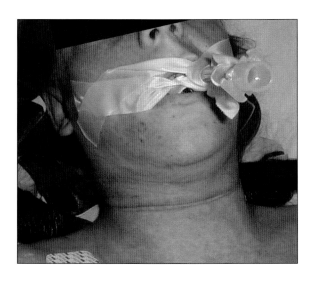

16-14 *Ligature marks in young woman who presented in cardiac arrest after hanging herself with a small diameter cord. (Photograph courtesy of Bryan Cotton, MD).*

Special Clinical Challenges and RSI Pharmacology

The above cases illustrate specific airway and intubation challenges in emergency care. The instances in which RSI should be avoided have been extensively reviewed in this text, although the vast majority of emergency airways are handled in routine fashion with oral intubation using RSI. In a recent study of ED intubations over three years at the author's institution, RSI was used in 98% of non-cardiac arrest cases. With rare exception, almost all RSI cases used 0.3 mg/kg of etomidate and 1.0–1.5 mg/kg of succinylcholine. With hypotension and volume depletion (systolic BP below 90), and depending on the mental status of the patient, the etomidate dose is occasionally reduced. Succinylcholine is the primary neuromuscular agent for RSI unless there is an evident contraindication, in which case vecuronium is given (0.2 mg/kg for faster onset). Succinylcholine has many features that make it ideal in emergency cases including fast onset time (approximately 60 seconds), reliable intubating conditions, and rapid plasma metabolism. Following a standard 1.0 mg/kg intravenous dose, the patient will not have full respiratory recovery for 9 minutes, so the use of succinylcholine does not eliminate the need for rescue ventilation should intubation fail.

Succinylcholine, Hyperkalemia, and Exaggerated Hyperkalemic Response

Succinylcholine causes muscle depolarization and a mild elevation of potassium (approximately 0.5–1.0 mEq/L). This rise could be dangerous if the potassium level is already elevated, especially when the elevation is acute. Exaggerated hyperkalemic response leading to cardiac arrest has been reported in burns, crush injury, serious intra-abdominal infections, and extensive denervation of skeletal muscle from myopathies and upper and lower motor neuron injury. The onset of this response is as short as two days after injury and usually peaks at 7–10 days, but the duration of risk has been reported as long as several years following injury. Succinylcholine is considered safe for use within the first twenty-four hours of burns and other acute injuries. Succinylcholine has been associated with hyperkalemia and cardiac arrest in children with undiagnosed, mild, or asymptomatic muscular dystrophies. Because of these case reports manufacturers and the FDA have added warnings about this risk and many pediatric institutions have stopped using succinylcholine altogether.

The author's preferred approach to managing RSI in situations of potential hyperkalemia and contraindications to succinylcholine noted above is to use double dose vecuronium (0.2 mg/kg). Alternatively, rocuronium (at a dose of 0.6–1.2 mg/kg) may also be used. Although non-depolarizing agents have slower onset times than succinylcholine, the time to intubation can be shortened by using the "timing principle." In this technique, the non-depolarizer is given first as a single bolus, and the induction agent (etomidate, for example) is given after the onset of clinical weakness. This approach will provide muscle relaxation approximately 60 seconds after the onset of clinical weakness. In patients who are awake and alert, they should be warned that they may feel weak immediately before going to sleep. A small dose of midazolam helps facilitate amnesia in these patients. Vecuronium has a duration of action of approximately 30 minutes, but this is lengthened with double dosing.

Safety of Succinylcholine in Myasthenia Gravis vs. other Neuromuscular Diseases

Myasthenia gravis is unlike other neuromuscular diseases, such as Guillain-Barré Syndrome, in which denervation of muscle leads to upregulation of acetylcholine receptors. In GBS and other diseases up-regulation of acetylcholine receptors creates the risk of an exaggerated hyperkalemic response and cardiac arrest with succinylcholine administration. Non-depolarizing agents are recommended in these conditions and succinylcholine is contraindicated. Myasthenia is unique among the neuromuscular diseases because the disease itself involves destruction of acetylcholine receptors. Because there are fewer receptors, in myasthenia there is resistance to succinylcholine and increased sensitivity to non-depolarizing agents. Compared to normal patients, the same level of muscular relaxation for a patient with myasthenia requires 2.6 times the dose of succinylcholine and only 0.4–0.55 times the dose of vecuronium. RSI can be safely performed in myasthenic crisis with succinylcholine (1.5–2.0 mg/kg), or low doses of vecuronium (approximately 0.05 mg/kg). An excellent review of myasthenia and the anesthetic considerations is by Able and Eisenkraft (Abel M, Eisenkraft JB. Anesthetic implications of myasthenia gravis. *Mt Sinai J Med.* 2002; 69:31–7.).

Safety of Succinylcholine in Head Injury and Open Eye Injury

Two other clinical situations in which RSI pharmacology has been controversial include head injury and eye injuries with an open globe. Initial studies with succinylcholine showed an ICP rise that could be prevented by a defasciculating dose of a non-depolarizer, but the clinical significance of the ICP effect was never defined. More recent studies have suggested the rise does not occur or is not consequential. The benefit of intravenous lidocaine 3–4 minutes prior to laryngoscopy, another pre-treatment intended to minimize the ICP rise during the procedure, is also unproven. Current practice at the author's institution and other leading trauma centers is to use succinylcholine in head injury without defasciculation or pre-treatment with lidocaine.

Succinylcholine is considered contraindicated in open globe injuries according to many sources, though this dictum is not supported by literature review or common practice at numerous major eye centers that have extensively reported its safe use. An excellent review of the literature is by Vachon (Vachon CA, Warner DO, Bacon DR. Succinylcholine and the open globe. Tracing the teaching. *Anesthesiology.* 2003; 99: 220–3.). Coughing, bucking, and mask ventilation have all been shown to raise intraocular pressures significantly (much more so than succinylcholine), and it is appropriate that when the eye is salvageable every effort should be made to achieve first pass intubation success using RSI (with succinylcholine).

Special Clinical Challenges Post-Intubation

Tracheal intubation in most patients with respiratory distress improves oxygenation and clinical status. Mechanical ventilation and RSI can cause post-intubation hypotension, however, through reduced venous return (secondary to positive intrathoracic pressure), and the pharmacologic effects of muscle relaxants and induction agents (from direct vasodilation and reduced sympathetic tone). Patients with problems getting air out are at increased risk for hemodynamic compromise and cardiac arrest from mechanical intubation. This group primarily comprises patients with COPD and asthma. In an ED series of life threatening hypotension following emergency intubation, COPD patients had a ten times greater risk of complications than all other ED intubated patients.

In COPD and asthma, ventilation is the problem, specifically exhalation. These patients get intubated when they become too weak to effectively ventilate themselves. They all experience significant hypercarbia, and may or may not have hypoxia. Hypoxia is generally the rule in COPD, however, this is not the case with asthma unless there is extensive mucous plugging. Prior to intubation COPD patients and asthmatics have small tidal volumes at rapid rates. Even though they are tachypnic, the minute ventilation, calculated by multiplying the tidal volume by the rate, is still very low. A COPD patient breathing at 30 times per minute, but with a tidal volume of only 200 cc, has a minute ventilation of only 6 liters. With intubation it is possible to deliver a significantly greater minute volume. A standard adult resuscitation bag has a volume of 1000 cc. If following intubation the laryngoscopist squeezes the bag 15 times per minute, and assuming 800 cc is delivered with every squeeze, the minute ventilation post-intubation is double what it was beforehand; 800 cc times 15 breaths per minute, or 12 liters. The problem becomes getting this increased volume of air out. The tracheal tube in COPD and asthma facilitates air entry but does nothing for exhalation. Through a variety of causes, the exhalation time (or expiratory flow) in COPD and asthma is prolonged. With intubation and bag ventilation, the inspiratory phase begins before the expiratory phase finishes. This breath "stacking" or "dynamic hyperinflation" causes a significant rise in lung volumes and pressures. With additional bagging on top of incomplete emptying with each breath, the lungs get more and more distended, and pressures rise. This is noticeable by marked resistance with squeezing the bag. As the pressure and size of the lungs increase within the closed space of the thorax, the heart gets compressed and ultimately cannot fill. Decreased venous return leads first to hypotension and quickly to pulseless electrical activity.

With dynamic hyperinflation, treatment for hypotension and cardiac arrest immediately post-intubation involves transiently discontinuing ventilation for 10–30 seconds to see if this improves blood pressure and causes a return of circulation. Squeezing the chest may also help get air out while ventilation is suspended. Prevention of dynamic hyperinflation involves: 1) reducing tidal volumes (initiate at 6 cc/kg) and respiratory rates (start at 10 breaths per minute); 2) relieving expiratory flow resistance (beta agonists, suctioning), and 3) decreasing inspiratory time. The decrease in tidal volume and rate will not correct the hypercapnia that is present in COPD and asthma, but CO_2 levels to 100 and acidosis to 7.15 are well tolerated. Bicarbonate can be given for pH values below this level, but should not be used to fully correct the acidosis. Allowing the CO_2 to be elevated, which is also known as "permissive hypercapnia" or "controlled hypoventilation," has dramatically lessened the mortality rates of mechanically ventilated asthmatics. It is also recommended practice for COPD patients, though there are fewer studies of its impact on mortality.

Chapter 17

Confirmation of Tracheal Tube Placement

Following intubation, tracheal placement should be immediately confirmed through clinical signs and carbon dioxide monitoring. Clinical signs include bilateral axillary breath sounds, absence of gurgling over the stomach, and chest rise. Unfortunately, clinical signs alone do not reliably exclude esophageal intubation, regardless of operator training or expertise.

Etiology of Esophageal Intubation

Esophageal intubation can occur through improper recognition of critical structures, restricted visualization, mis-shaping of the stylet obscuring the target, or from lack of concentrated focus on where the tip of the tracheal tube is being placed (Figure 17-1, 17–2a–d).

Novice intubators can easily misinterpret a round hole as the target, especially if unfamiliar with laryngeal landmarks and if the epiglottis is not sighted. This often happens when the blade is inserted too deeply (Figure 17-1).

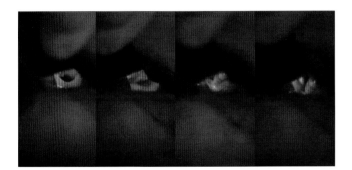

17-1 *The round hole of the esophagus (far left) after blade was inserted too deeply and upward force applied. Withdrawal of the blade in subsequent images exposes posterior structures and then glottic opening (far right).*

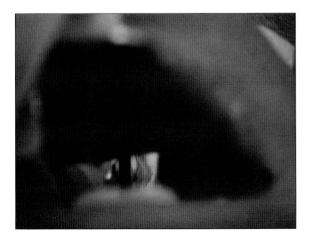

17-2a *An excellent view of the larynx including true vocal cords and glottic opening, but the tongue is poorly controlled. A large section of tongue is visible on the right side. This will limit the working area for tube insertion and target visualization.*

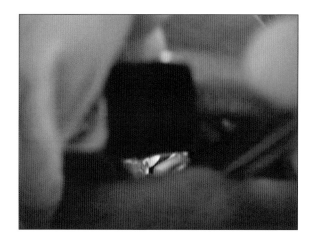

17-2b *As tube is introduced, the lifting force on laryngoscope is relaxed slightly. The tip of the epiglottis is seen just under the left side of the spatula. The tracheal tube has been poorly shaped and the cuff and distal third of the tracheal tube block the line of sight to the target. The vocal cords are no longer seen.*

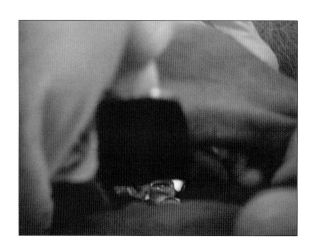

17-2c *The cuff of the tracheal tube has now passed the epiglottis. Underneath the right side of the laryngoscope spatula there is a small section of the epiglottis tip that is brightly lit. Note the section of tongue hanging down on the right side of the spatula.*

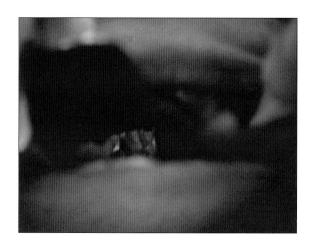

17-2d *After tube has been advanced further there is a partial view of the empty larynx. Immediately under the right edge of the laryngoscope spatula is a small section of the glottic opening. The posterior cartilages and the interarytenoid notch are well seen. On the right edge of the picture can be seen the proximal section of the tracheal tube.*

If the operator is not confident of laryngeal landmarks, the tube should never be blindly advanced under the epiglottis. Although the vocal cords or glottic opening may sometimes not be visible, the tip should be watched carefully as it passes anterior to the posterior cartilages and interarytenoid notch. The location of the esophagus immediately behind the larynx, and the posterior inferior tilt of the laryngeal inlet, make passage of the tracheal tube backward into the esophagus likely if the tube tip is not carefully observed. It is worth noting that prior to the mandatory use of pulse oximetry and monitoring of end-tidal CO2 in the operating room, unrecognized esophageal intubation was a leading cause of anesthesia related death and injury. It remains a common occurrence in EMS and non-operating room settings, with incidences from 1–15%.

The consequences of esophageal intubation may be significant even when immediately recognized. First, it delays the time to ventilation and puts the patient at greater risk of critical hypoxia. Secondly, when ventilation is done through the misplaced tracheal tube, this will distend the stomach and promote regurgitation. In a recent study by Mort, esophageal intubation was associated with a 10 times greater risk of regurgitation compared to patients in whom esophageal intubation did not occur (Mort TC. Emergency tracheal intubation: Complications associated with repeated laryngoscopic attempts. *Anesth Analg.* 2004; 99:607–13.). It also carried a 60% incidence of hypoxemia. If during laryngoscopy the tip cannot be confidently directed into the trachea, it is probably best not to pass the tube. Regardless of the quality of laryngeal view, or the confidence of the intubator, verification of tracheal placement must be performed on every patient.

End-tidal CO2 Detection Devices

The American Society of Anesthesiologists has stated that monitoring of end-tidal CO2 is the standard of care throughout the hospital, regardless of location. The National Association of Emergency Medical Services Physicians has recommended the routine use of CO2 detection devices and esophageal intubation devices in the EMS setting. Carbon dioxide detection can be performed either with qualitative colormetric devices (Figure 17-3a–b), or handheld quantitative

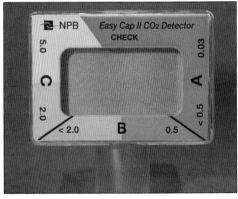
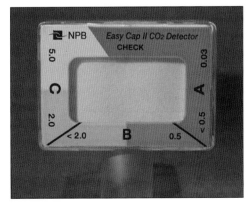

17-3a   **17-3b**

17-3a *Colormetric end-tidal CO2 detector (Easy Cap, Nellcor Puritan Bennett, Pleasanton CA). Purple color of Easy Cap upon opening device and with low CO2 level.*
17-3b *Yellow color of Easy Cap after several exhalations. Tan color (at lower right corner of device) can occur in cardiac arrest and low perfusion states even when tracheal tube is correctly located in trachea.*

devices with or without capnographic waveforms. CO_2 production precedes return of spontaneous circulation following cardiac arrest. In cases of poor perfusion, as long as there is a pulse, some CO_2 will be detectable, though there may be incomplete color change with colormetric devices. It is important to appreciate the initial purple color of the colormetric device. If the packaging of the device was opened or accidentally exposed to air for a prolonged time the the color indicator will turn beige. If this is not appreciated when the device is used an esophageal intubation may be erroneously interpreted as being in the trachea.

Esophageal Intubation Detectors

In cardiac arrest end-tidal CO_2 may be undetectable, even if the tube is correctly located, because no CO_2 is being produced. This may occur in as many as 30% of emergency department cardiac arrests, in which case esophageal intubation detectors (EIDs) can be used. Such devices create negative pressure, either through a large syringe or a self-inflating bulb (Figure 17-4a–d).

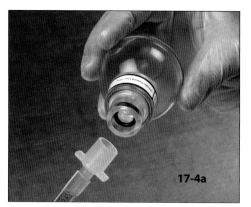
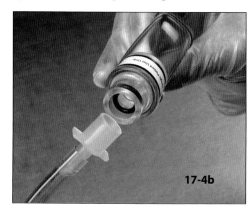
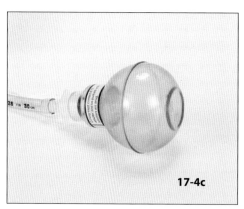
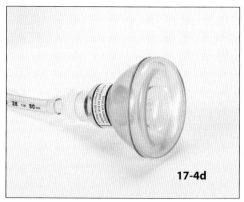

17-4a *Esophageal Intubation Detector (EID) (Wolfe-Tory, Salt Lake City UT). EID showing inner rubber ring that contacts tracheal tube connector to ensure proper seal. If device is incompletely connected a false positive result can occur.*
17-4b *EID is deflated prior to attachment to tracheal tube connector. This creates negative pressure at the end of the tracheal tube once the bulb is attached.*
17-4c *If tube is in the trachea, the bulb will self-inflate (pop-up). Slow inflation has been reported in obesity, pulmonary edema, and severe asthma.*
17-4d *If tube is in esophagus, the bulb will not inflate.*

The differences in the morphology of the trachea and the esophagus create different effects when negative pressure or suction is applied to a tracheal tube placed in these two structures. The trachea is an open structure, supported by the tracheal rings, while the esophagus is flat and collapsed. A tube in the trachea will have no resistance to aspiration with the syringe, or there will be immediate (<4 seconds) self-inflation of the bulb. In the esophagus, negative pressure or suction at the end of a tube causes the esophageal mucosa to seal around the holes of the tracheal tube. There will be strong resistance to aspiration with the syringe, or if the bulb type device is used, it will not self-inflate.

The EID has nearly 100% specificity and sensitivity for detecting esophageal intubation in adults, but false negatives and false positives can occur. Numerous factors have been identified which can cause delayed filling of EIDs, i.e., the tube is in the trachea but the bulb does not inflate (a false negative test). Delayed filling occurs in morbid obesity, pulmonary edema, and severe asthma. Some authors have recommended that 10 seconds, instead of 4 seconds, be used as the time limit for inflation of the self-inflating bulb to decrease the incidence of false negative results. The incidence of false negatives, particularly in morbid obesity, can also be reduced if the bulb is attached to the tube and then squeezed, as opposed to being squeezed first and then attached. The latter method creates mores suction at the end of the tube and presumably more false negatives. False positive results, i.e. self-inflation even though the tube is in the esophagus, can occur if the seal between the tube and the EID is not tight. This may explain reported errors with the device, particularly with the syringe model, which is very cumbersome to use while stabilizing the tracheal tube. Neither the presence of a nasogastric tube nor deliberate inflation of the stomach has been shown to affect the reliability of EIDs.

End-tidal CO2 detection should be used in all patients and should be demonstrable on all patients in whom a pulse is palpable. If there is no palpable pulse, verification of tube placement should be done first by end-tidal CO2, then if this test is negative, with an EID or with repeat laryngoscopy. Posterior displacement of the tracheal tube or external laryngeal manipulation may permit visualization of the tube passing anterior to the posterior cartilages, or adjacent to the vocal cords. Repeat laryngoscopy by itself is not reliable for verifying tube placement. In a study done by the author involving 768 previously placed tracheal tubes in fresh cadavers, the overall correct identification rate for physicians (allowed 10 seconds for checking tube placement) was only 86%. (Levin WJ, Levitan RM, Kinkle WC. Confirming the location of previously placed tracheal tubes by direct laryngoscopy. [Abstract] *Acad Emerg Med*, 2004;11:491–2).

End-tidal CO2 devices and EIDs may erroneously confirm tracheal placement in one other situation in addition to the limitations mentioned already. If the tube is located above the vocal cords, the end-tidal CO2 will be positive and the EID will have immediate inflation. A quantitative CO2 device may detect a lower than expected exhaled CO2 level, and a capnographic device will have an abnormal curve. It is always necessary when confirming tube location to also check tube depth. For oral tubes this should be 21 cm in women and 23 cm in men, while for nasal tubes it should be 26 and 28 centimeters, respectively.

Chapter 18

Airway Equipment Kits for Emergency Settings

The goal of creating an emergency airway kit is to assemble in one location all the devices necessary to ensure safe airway management. Individual providers of advanced airway management, especially those that use RSI, should take personal responsibility for appropriately stocking and checking the equipment upon which their patients' lives depend. Emergency physicians have often inappropriately abdicated this responsibility to department administrators, nurses, or purchasing managers, who do not have a thorough knowledge of the equipment. Nor do they bear the ultimate responsibility for airway outcomes.

Apart from assuming responsibility for the equipment, providers of emergency airway management need to be honest about their skills and capacity for using different equipment. The number of different devices should be limited for educational, logistical, and financial reasons. No provider can master all currently available airway devices. Transporting the entire array of available airway devices requires an enormous equipment cart that is difficult to stock and to have accessible at the head of the bed.

An emergency airway kit must address the need for solutions through the mouth, the nose and the neck. This begins with mask ventilation equipment, including oral and nasal airways, and a well selected curved laryngoscope. The author's preference is for a Macintosh #4 blade that has a German profile and a fiberoptic light. Several manufacturers offer models in steel and plastic. If conventional blades are to be used instead, the English version Macintosh design has a flange, profile, and light position similar to the German designs.

Next come malleable stylets and the bougie (introducer). Straight-to-cuff stylet shaping minimizes the need for a bougie, but the bougie is inexpensive (especially the disposable variety) and has many characteristics that make it ideal for emergency airway use. It is simple to use, inexpensive, easy to store, and has a well proven record of assisting in difficult laryngoscopy, especially in the epiglottis-only situation. A straight blade is a requirement, although it will get minimal use once external laryngeal manipulation is incorporated into routine curved blade technique. The ideal straight blade is the Henderson, but this blade is currently proprietary to Storz and very expensive. A Miller 3 or Phillips 2 is a less expensive substitute. To assist with nasal intubation, the Endotrol tracheal tube (sizes 7.0, 8.0) is invaluable. Its directional tip and soft plastic make it function significantly better than standard tubes for this purpose. A Beck Airflow Airway Monitor (BAAM whistle) makes an inexpensive and nice addition for nasal intubation. Finally, for going through the neck, a scalpel is needed for surgical airways, or alternatively, the Melker percutaneous cricothyrotomy kit. Rescue ventilation devices are mandatory, including the LMA (adult sizes 4, 5) and the Small Adult Combitube. This collection of devices is inexpensive and compact, and from a patient safety perspective it incorporates the essential equipment for safe practice.

For departments with the resources to acquire and maintain other devices, as well as the commitment to practice them regularly, many other devices are available. Intubating laryngeal mask airways are a good investment as both rescue ventilation devices and rescue intubation devices. It is anticipated that plastic disposable versions of these will be available shortly. From a difficult laryngoscopy perspective, the next step up involves an optical stylet that can be used to augment laryngoscopy and for rescue intubation. In order for this investment to be warranted, it requires a commitment of routine use so that the practitioner can master the challenges of recognizing laryngeal anatomy and manipulating the scope in a timely and direct manner when it is truly needed.

A greater commitment still is a flexible fiberoptic scope. Practically speaking, this type of instrument is only for hospital use, as opposed to the optical stylet and the intubating LMA, which can easily be adapted for the field. In the ED, the fiberoptic scope can be used diagnostically on a routine basis, even if rescue intubation with the scope is rarely needed. For departments willing to make the financial commitment to acquire one flexible scope, a single scope for overall use is the 36.5 cm working length ENT scope (i.e., Olympus Endoscopy ENF-T3 scope). Although it does require more sophisticated cleaning because of its working channel, the device can be used for rhinolaryngoscopy examination as well as for intubation (with a tube first approach). Mid-length ENT scopes are significantly more durable and easier to use in emergency settings than long intubating bronchoscopes. Routine use of a scope for fiberoptic examination is necessary to achieve competency using the device for intubation. An especially useful adjunct for a flexible scope in the emergency department are single use fiberoptic sheaths that eliminate the need for cold sterilizing or sending the scope out for cleaning.

The above devices meet the clinical challenges of emergency airway management. Educational programs face different challenges in terms of supervising providers in training, especially under emergency situations. Additional equipment that can be useful in these settings include endoscopic cameras and monitors for use with optical stylets and the flexible fiberscope. This set-up can provide residents the opportunity to intimately learn laryngeal anatomy. Newer imaging devices that will permit routine fiberoptic imaging from the standard curved laryngoscope are also being developed. The advantage of these devices, compared to the optical stylets for example, is that they permit observation of laryngeal landmarks and intubation without in any manner changing the way the operator (trainee) performs the procedure. Conversely, these devices are less versatile for rescuing difficult laryngoscopy, since the fiberoptic image is coming from the laryngoscope and not from a separate instrument that can be manipulated under the epiglottis.

Figure 18-1 outlines the components of different airway kits designed for emergency settings. The Practical Emergency Airway Kit is inexpensive, compact, and appropriate for individual acquisition (Figure 18-2). The Advanced Practical Emergency Airway Kit represents a substantial expenditure (approximately $3,000), but is still compact, easily transportable, and may be appropriate for individual practitioners. This is what the author brings to work for every shift in the ED. In the Comprehensive Practical Emergency Airway Kit the flexible scope adds much greater expense (approximately $5,000–$10,000 depending upon specific model), and adds significant logistical complexity (education and skill acquisition, storage, cleaning, etc.). It clearly requires a departmental commitment, as does the additional monitoring equipment for teaching settings.

The above equipment recommendations must be coupled with a commitment to the fundamentals of emergency airway management. Mask ventilation skills and the immediate availability of rescue ventilation devices are the cornerstones of patient safety. An appreciation of the risks of RSI and an awareness of when it should be avoided will prevent "cannot intubate," "cannot ventilate" catastrophes. As mastery of laryngoscopy increases, the need for alternative intubation devices decreases. Adding alternative intubation devices will not improve outcomes if first pass laryngoscopy success rates are poor and hypoxic injury is not prevented.

The Practical Emergency Airway Kit

1. Mask ventilation devices, oral & nasal airways
2. Laryngeal Mask Airways (size 4, 5)
3. Combitube, Small Adult (37F)
4. Macintosh #4 German or English design
5. Two laryngoscope handles
6. Styletted straight-to-cu/ tracheal tubes (6–8.0 mm ID)
7. Straight blade (Henderson, Miller 3, or Phillips 2)
8. Bougie (tube introducer)
9. Endotrol tracheal tubes, BAAM whistle
10. Scalpel or percutaneous Melker Kit
11. End-tidal CO2 device & Esophageal Intubation Detector

The Advanced Practical Emergency Airway Kit (plus above)

1. Intubating Laryngeal Mask Airways
2. Optical stylet

(Additional items to consider: lighted stylet, retrograde intubation kit.)

The Comprehensive Practical Emergency Airway Kit (plus above)

1. Flexible fiberoptic scope with endoscopic sheaths
2. Light source for scope (either built in or external)
3. Intubating airways for oral fiberoptic intubation

Equipment for Teaching Settings

1. Endoscopic cameras & monitors
2. Optical elements built into laryngoscope

18-1 *Airway equipment kits for emergency settings.*

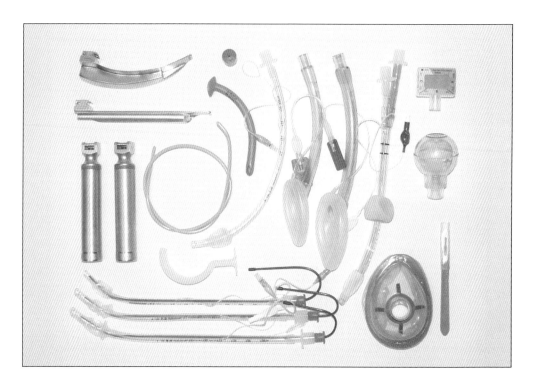

18-2 *The Practical Emergency Airway Kit. Includes devices for intubation via the mouth, nose or neck, as well as rescue ventilation via facemask, LMA and Combitube. See text for details.*

References

Patient Safety and Airway Algorithms

1. Abernethy LJ, Allan PL, Drummond GB. Ultrasound assessment of the position of the tongue during induction of general anesthesia. *Br J Anesth.* 1990; 65:744.

2. American Society of Anesthesiologists Policy Statement, October 16, 2002. Available at: http://www.asahq.org/publicationsAndServices/DifficultAirway.pdf. Accessed June 6, 2004.

3. Bair AE, Filbin MR, Kulkarni RG, et al. The failed intubation attempt in the emergency department: Analysis of prevalence, rescue techniques, and personnel. *J Emerg Med.* 2002; 23: 131–140.

4. Benumof JL, Dagg R, Benumof R, Critical hemoglobin desaturation will occur before return to an unparalyzed state following 1 mg/kg intravenous succinylcholine. *Anesthesiology.* 1997; 87:979–82.

5. Benumof JL. Preoxygenation: Best method for both efficacy and efficiency? *Anesthesiology.* 1999; 91: 603–5.

6. Benumof JL: Management of the difficult airway: With special emphasis on awake tracheal intubation. *Anesthesiology.* 1991; 75:1087–110.

7. Berthoud MC, Peacock JE, Reilly CS. Effectiveness of preoxygenation in morbidly obese patients. *Br J Anaesth.* 1991; 67:464–6.

8. Caplan RA, Benumof JL, Berry FA, Blitt CD, Bode RH, Cheney FW, Connis RT, Guidry OR, Ovassapian A. Practice guidelines for management of the difficult airway: A report by the ASA Task Force on Management of the Difficult Airway. *Anesthesiology.* 1993; 78:597–602.

9. Caplan RA, Posner KL, Ward RJ, Cheney FW. Adverse respiratory events in anesthesia: A closed claims analysis. *Anesthesiology.* 1990; 72:828–33.

10. Crosby ET, Cooper RM, Douglas MJ, et al. The unanticipated difficult airway with recommendations for management. *Can J Anaesth.* 1998; 45:757–76.

11. Hawthorne L, Wilson R, Lyons G, Dresner M. Failed intubation revisited: 17-yr experience in a teaching maternity unit. *Br J Anaesth.* 1996; 76:680–4.

12. Heidegger T, Gerig HJ, Ulrich B, Kreienbuhl G. Validation of a simple algorithm for tracheal intubation: Daily practice is the key to success in emergencies—an analysis of 13,248 intubations. *Anesth Analg.* 2001; 92: 517–22.

13. Jense HG, Dubin SA, Silverstein PI, O'Leary-Escolas U. Effect of obesity on safe duration of apnea in anesthetized humans. *Anesth Analg.* 1991; 72:89–93.

14. Levitan RM. Patient safety in emergency airway management and rapid sequence intubation: metaphorical lessons from skydiving. *Ann Emerg Med.* 2003;42: 81–7.

15. Levitan RM. Myths and realities: the "difficult airway" and alternative airway devices in the emergency setting. [Editorial] *Acad Emerg Med.* 2001; 8:829–32.

16. Rose DK, Cohen MM: The incidence of airway problems depends on the definition used. *Can J Anaesth.* 1996; 43:30–4.

17. Williamson JA, Webb RK, Szekely S, Gillies ERN, Dreosti AV. Difficult intubation: An analysis of 2000 incident reports. *Anaesth Intens Care.* 1993; 21:602–7.

Emergency Airway Management Studies

1. Adnet FA, Jouriles NJ, Le Toumilien P, et al. Survey of out-of-hospital emergency intubations in the French prehospital medical system: A multicenter study. *Ann Emerg Med.* 1998; 32: 454–60.

2. Afilalo M, Guttman A, Stern E, Lloyd J, Colacone A, Tselios C, Dankoff J. Fiberoptic intubation in the emergency department: A case series. *J Emerg Med.* 11: 387–91, 1991.

3. Bair AE, Filbin MR, Kulkarni RG, et al. The failed intubation attempt in the emergency department: Analysis of prevalence, rescue techniques, and personnel. *J Emerg Med.*2002; 23: 131–140.

4. Brunette DD. Twelve years of emergency medicine at Hennepin County Medical Center. Changing critical care experience. *Minnesota Medicine.* 1999; 82:42–8.

5. Bushra JS, McNeil B, Wald D, et al. A comparison of trauma intubations managed by anesthesiologists and emergency physicians [abstract]. *Acad Emerg Med.* 2002; 9: 404–5.

6. Calderon Y, Gennis P, Martinez C, Gallagher EJ. Intubations in an emergency medicine residency: The selection and performance of intubators [abstract]. *Acad Emerg Med.* 1995; 2: 411–412.

7. Chang RS, Hamilton RJ, Carter WA. Declining rate of cricothyrotomy in trauma patients with an emergency medicine residency: Implication for skills training. *Acad Emerg Med.* 1998; 5: 247–51.

8. Davis DP, Ochs M, Hoyt DB, et al. Paramedic-administered neuromuscular blockade improves prehospital intubation success in severely head-injured patients. *J Trauma.* 2003; 55: 713–9.

9. Delaney KA, Hessler R. Emergency flexible fiberoptic nasotracheal intubation: A report of 60 cases. *Ann Emerg Med.* 1988; 17: 919–26.

10. Jaberi M, Mitchell K, MacKenzie C. Cricothyrotomy: Good, bad, or ugly? [Abstract]. *Trauma Care* (Journal of the International Trauma and Critical Care Society). 2001; 11: 13.

11. Jones JH, Weaver CS, Rusyniak DE, Brizendine EJ, McGrath RB. Impact of emergency medicine faculty and an airway protocol on airway management. *Acad Emerg Med.* 2002; 9: 1452–6.

12. Levitan RM, Everett WW, Ochroch AE. Limitations of difficult airway prediction in emergency department intubated patients. *Ann Emerg Med.* 2004; 44: 307-13.

13. Levitan RM, Rosenblatt B, Meiner EM, Reilly PM, Hollander JE. Alternating day EM and anesthesia resident responsibility for management of the trauma airway: A study of laryngoscopy performance and intubation success. *Annals Emerg Med.* 2004; 43: 48–53.

14. Li J, Murphy-Lavoie H, Bugas C, Martinez J, Preston C. Complications of emergency intubation with and without paralysis. *Am J Emerg Med.* 1999; 17: 141–3.

15. Mort TC. Emergency tracheal intubation: Complications associated with repeated laryngoscopic attempts. *Anesth Analg.* 2004; 99:607–13.

16. Ochs M, Davis D, Hoyt D, Bailey D, Marshall L, Rosen P. Paramedic-performed rapid sequence intubation of patients with severe head injuries. *Ann Emerg Med.* 2002; 40: 159–67.

17. Omert L, Yeaney W, Mizikowski S, Protech BS. Role of the emergency physician in airway management of the trauma patient. *J Trauma.* 2001; 51: 1065–8.

18. Retondo MF, McGonigal MD, Schwab CW, et al. Urgent paralysis and intubation of trauma patients: Is it safe? *J Trauma,* 1993; 34: 242–6.

19. Sakles JC, Laurin EG, Rantapaa AA, Panacek EA. Airway management in the emergency department: A one year study of 610 tracheal intubations. *Ann Emerg Med.* 1998; 31:325–332.

20. Tayal VS, Riggs RW, Marx JA, et al. Rapid-sequence intubation at an emergency medicine residency: Success rate and adverse events during a two-year period. *Acad Emerg Med.* 1999; 6: 31–7.

21. Vissers RJ, Barton ED, Sagarin MJ, et al. Success and complication rates of rapid-sequence vs. non-rapid-sequence intubation in 1,200 emergency intubations [abstract]. *Acad Emerg Med.* 1998; 5: 481.

22. Walls RM, Gurr DE, Kulkarni RG, Sakles J, Pollack C. 6,294 Emergency department intubations: Second report of the ongoing national emergency airway registry (NEAR) II Study. *Ann Emerg Med.* 2000; 36(4) part 2, A196.

23. Wang HE, Kupas DF, Paris PM, Bates RR, et al. Multivariate predictors of failed prehospital endotracheal intubation. *Acad Emerg Med.* 2003; 10: 717–24.

Mask Ventilation, Cricoid Pressure, and Aspiration Prevention

1. Abernethy LJ, Allan PL, Drummond GB. Ultrasound assessment of the position of the tongue during induction of general anesthesia. *Br J Anesth.* 1990; 65:744.

2. Admani M, Yeh TF, Jain R, Mora A., Pildes RS. Prevention of gastric inflation during mask ventilation in newborn infants. *Critical Care Medicine.* 1985; 13: 592–3.

3. Boidin MP. Airway patency in the unconscious patient. *Br J Anesth.* 57:306; 1985.

4. Bowman FP, Menegazzi JJ, Check BD, et al. The lower esophageal sphincter pressure during prolonged cardiac arrest and resuscitation. *Ann Emerg Med.* 1995; 26: 216–9.

5. Brimacombe JR, Berry AM. Cricoid pressure. *Can J Anaesth*. 1997;44: 414–25.

6. Cook WP., Schultetus RR. Lower esophageal sphincter integrity is maintained during succinylcholine-induced fasciculations in dogs with "full" stomachs. *Anesth Analg*. 1990; 70: 420–3.

7. Dorges V, Wenzel V, Knacke P, Gerlach K. Comparison of different airway management strategies to ventilate apneic, non-preoxygenated patients. *Crit Care Med*. 2003; 31:800–4.

8. Hartsilver EL, Vanner RG. Airway obstruction with cricoid pressure. *Anaesthesia*. 2000; 55: 208–11.

9. Howells TH, Chamney AR, Wraight WJ, Simons RS. The application of cricoid pressure: An assessment and survey of its practice. *Anaesthesia*. 1983; 38:457–60.

10. Kron, SS. Questionable effectiveness of cricoid pressure in preventing aspiration [letter]. *Anaesthesia*. 1995; 50:912–3.

11. Mac G, Palmer JH, Ball DR. The effect of cricoid pressure on the cricoid cartilage and vocal cords: An endoscopic study in anaesthetised patients. *Anaesthesia*. 2000; 55: 263–8.

12. Nandi PR. Effect of general anesthesia on the pharynx. *Br J Anesth*. 1991; 66:157.

13. Petito SP, Russell WJ. The prevention of gastric inflation—a neglected benefit of cricoid pressure. *Anaesth Intensive Care*. 1988; 16: 139–43.

14. Ralph SJ, Wareham CA. Rupture of the oesophagus during cricoid pressure. *Anaesthesia* 1991; 46:40–1.

15. Schwartz DE, Cohen NH. Questionable effectiveness of cricoid pressure in preventing aspiration [letter]. *Anesthesiology*. 1995; 83: 432.

16. Schwartz DE, Mathhay MA, Cohen NH. Death and other complications of emergency airway management in critically ill adults. *Anesthesiology*. 1995; 82: 367–76.

17. Sellick BA. Cricoid pressure to control regurgitation of stomach contents during induction of anesthesia. *Lancet*. 1961; ii: 404–6.

18. Shorten GD, Opie NJ, Graziotti P, et al. Assessment of upper airway anatomy in awake, sedated, and anaesthetised patients using magnetic resonance imaging. *Anaesth Intensive Care*. 1994; 22: 165.

19. Smith KJ, Ladak S, Choi PT, Dobranowski J. The cricoid cartilage and the esophagus are not aligned in close to half of adult patients. *Can J Anaesth*. 2002; 49:503–7.

20. Thibodeau LG, Verdile VP, Bartfield JM. Incidence of aspiration after urgent intubation. *Am J Emerg Med*. 1997; 15: 562–5.

21. Tournadre JP, Chassard D, Berrada K, Bouletreau P. Lower oesophageal sphincter pressure during application of cricoid pressure in conscious volunteers. *Br J Anaesth*. 1996; 76: A50.

22. Tournadre JP, Barclay M, Bouletreau P, Chassard D. Lower oesophageal sphincter tone increases after induction of anaesthesia in pigs with full stomach. *Can J Anaesth*. 1998; 45: 479–82.

23. Vanner RG, O'Dwyer JP, Pryle BJ, Reynolds F. Upper oesophageal sphincter pressure and the effect of cricoid pressure. *Anaesthesia.* 1992; 47: 95–100.

24. Wenzel V, Idris AH, Dorges V, et al. The respiratory system during resuscitation: A review of the history, risk of infection during assisted ventilation, respiratory mechanics, and ventilation strategies for patients with an unprotected airway. *Resuscitation.* 2001; 49: 123–134.

25. Wenzel V, Idris AH, Banner MJ, Kubilis PS, Williams JL Jr. Influence of tidal volume on the distribution of gas between the lungs and stomach in the non-intubated patient receiving positive-pressure ventilation. *Critical Care Medicine.* 1998; 26: 364–8.

26. Whittington RM, Robinson JS, Thompson JM. Fatal aspiration (Mendelson's) syndrome despite antacids and cricoid pressure. *Lancet.* 1979; ii: 28–30.

Laryngeal Mask Airway

1. Alexander R, Hodgson P, Lomax D, Bullen C. A comparison of the laryngeal mask airway and Guedel airway, bag and facemask for manual ventilation following formal training. *Anaesthesia.* 1993; 48:231–4.

2. Asai T, Barclay K, Poer I, et al. Cricoid pressure impedes placement of the laryngeal mask airway and subsequent tracheal intubation through the mask. *Br J Anaethesia,* 1994; 47: 72.

3. Aye T, Milne B. Use of the laryngeal mask prior to definitive intubation in a difficult airway: A case report. *J Emerg Med.* 1995; 13: 711–4.

4. Barker P, Langton JA, Murphy PJ, Rowbotham DJ. Regurgitation of gastric contents during general anaesthesia using the laryngeal mask airway. *Br J Anaesth.* 1992; 69:314–5.

5. Barnes TA, MacDonald D, Nolan J, et al. Airway devices. *Ann Emerg Med.* 2001; 37: S145–151.

6. Benumof JL. Use of the laryngeal mask airway to facilitate fiberscope-aided tracheal intubation. *Anesth Analg* 1992; 74:313–5.

7. Brain AJ. The laryngeal mask: A new concept in airway management. *Br J Anaesth* 1983; 55:801.

8. Breen PH. Simple technique to remove laryngeal mask airway "guide" after endotracheal intubation. *Anesth Analg.* 1996; 82: 1302.

9. Brimacombe J, Berry A, van Duren P. Use of a size 2 laryngeal mask airway to relieve life threatening hypoxemia in an adult with quinsy. *Anaesth Intens Care* 1993; 21: 475–6.

10. Brimacombe J, Berry A. Insertion of the laryngeal mask airway: A prospective study of four techniques. *Anaesth Intensive Care* 1993; 21:89.

11. Brimacombe J, Keller C. Water flow between the upper esophagus and pharynx for the LMA and COPA in fresh cadavers. Laryngeal mask airway, and cuffed oropharyngeal airway. *Can J Anaesth.* 1999; 46:1064–6.

12. Brimacombe J. The advantages of the LMA over the tracheal tube or facemask: A meta-analysis. *Can J Anaesth.* 1995; 42:1017–23.

13. Brimacombe J, White A., Berry A. Effect of cricoid pressure on ease of insertion of the laryngeal mask airway. *Br J Anaesth.* 1993; 71: 800–2.

14. Brimacombe JR, Berry A. The incidence of aspiration associated with the laryngeal mask airway: A meta-analysis of published literature. *J Clin Anesth.* 1995; 7:297–305.

15. Brimacombe JR, Brimacombe JC, Berry AM, Morris R, Mecklem D, Clarke G, Barry J, Kirk T. A comparison of the laryngeal mask airway and cuffed oropharyngeal airway in anesthetized adult patients. *Anesth Analg.* 1998; 87: 147–52.

16. Carey MF, Smith J, Cooney CM, Laryngeal mask to aid tracheal intubation. *Anaesthesia* 1991; 46:1083.

17. Davies PRF, Tighe SQM, Greenslade GL, Evans GH. Laryngeal mask airway and tracheal tube insertion by unskilled personnel. *Lancet.* 1990; 336:977–9.

18. E Mikatti N, Luthra A, Healy T, et al. Gastric regurgitation during general anaesthesia in the supine position with the laryngeal and face mask airways. *Br J Anaesth.* 1992; 68:529–30.

19. Ezri T, Ady N, Szmuk P, Glanz L, Shklar B, Katz J, Geva D. Use of cuffed oropharyngeal vs. laryngeal mask airway in elderly patients. *Can J Anaesth.* 1999; 46: 363–7.

20. Frerk CM. Intubation through the laryngeal mask. *Anaesthesia* 1991; 46:985–6.

21. Gabbott DA, Sasada MP. Laryngeal mask airway insertion using cricoid pressure and manual in-line neck stabilisation. *Anaesthesia.* 1995; 50: 674–6.

22. Greenberg RS, Brimacombe J, Berry A, et al. A randomized controlled trial comparing the cuffed oropharyngeal airway and the laryngeal mask airway in spontaneously breathing anesthetized adults. *Anesthesiology.* 1998; 88: 970–7.

23. Hasham F, Kumar CM, Lawler PG. The use of the laryngeal mask airway to assist fibreoptic orotracheal intubation. *Anaesthesia.* 1991; 46:891.

24. Heath ML, Allagain J. Intubation through the laryngeal mask. A technique for unexpected difficult intubation. *Anaesthesia.* 1991; 46:545–8.

25. Heringlake M, Doerges V, Ocker H, Schmucker P. A comparison of the cuffed oropharyngeal airway (COPA) with the laryngeal mask airway (LMA) during manually controlled positive pressure ventilation. *J Clin Anesth.* 1999; 11: 590–5.

26. Higgins D, Astley BA, Berg S. Guided intubation via the laryngeal mask. *Anaesthesia.* 1992; 47:816.

27. Ivens D, Verborgh C, Phan Thi HP, Camu F. The quality of breathing and capnography during laryngeal mask and facemask ventilation. *Anaesthesia.* 1995; 50:858–62.

28. John RE, Hill S, Hughes TJ. Airway protection by the laryngeal mask: A barrier to dye placed in the pharynx. *Anaesthesia.* 1991; 46:366–7.

29. Keller C, Brimacombe J, Radler C, Puhringer F. Do laryngeal mask airway devices attenuate liquid flow between the esophagus and pharynx? A randomized, controlled cadaver study. *Anesth Analg.* 1999; 88:904–7.

30. King CJ, Davey AJ, Chandradeva K. Emergency use of the laryngeal mask airway in severe upper airway obstruction caused by supraglottic oedema. *Br J Anesth.* 1995; 75:785–6.

31. Lim SL, Tay DH, Thomas E. A comparison of three types of tracheal tube for use in laryngeal mask assisted blind orotracheal intubation. *Anaesthesia.* 1994; 49:255–7.

32. Lowinger D, Benjamin B, Gadd L. Recurrent laryngeal nerve injury caused by a laryngeal mask airway. *Anaesthesia & Intensive Care.* 1999; 27:202–5.

33. Martin PD, Cyna AM, Hunter WAH, Henry J, Ramayya GP. Training nursing staff in airway management for resuscitation: A clinical comparison of the facemask and laryngeal mask. *Anaesthesia.* 1993; 48:33–7.

34. Martin SE, Ochsner MG, Jarman RH, et al. Use of the laryngeal mask airway in air transport when intubation fails. *Journal of Trauma-Injury Infection & Critical Care.* 1999; 47:352–7.

35. Oczenski W, Krenn H, Dahaba AA, Binder M, El-Schahawi-Kienzl I, Kohout S, Schwarz S, Fitzgerald RD. Complications following the use of the Combitube, tracheal tube and laryngeal mask airway. *Anaesthesia.* 1999; 54:1161–5.

36. Osborn IP, Soper R. It's a disposable LMA, just cut it shorter—for fiberoptic intubation. *Anesth Analg.* 2003; 97:299–300.

37. Owens TM, Robertson P, Twomey C, Doyle M, McDonald N, McShane AJ. The incidence of gastroesophageal reflux with the laryngeal mask: A comparison with the face mask using esophageal lumen pH electrodes. *Anesth Analg.* 1995; 80:980–4.

38. Parmet JL, Colonna-Romano P, Horrow JC, Miller F, Gonzales J, Rosenberg H. The laryngeal mask airway reliably provides rescue ventilation in cases of unanticipated difficult tracheal intubation along with difficult mask ventilation. *Anesth Analg.* 1998; 87:661–5.

39. Pennant JH, Walker MB. Comparison of the endotracheal tube and laryngeal mask in airway management by paramedical personnel. *Anesth Analg.* 1992; 74:531–4.

40. Reinhart DJ, Simmons G. Comparison of placement of the laryngeal mask airway with endotracheal tube by paramedics and respiratory therapists. *Ann Emerg Med.* 1994; 24:260–3.

41. Rumball CJ, MacDonald D. The PTL, Combitube, laryngeal mask, and oral airway: A randomized prehospital comparative study of ventilatory device effectiveness and cost-effectiveness in 470 cases of cardiorespiratory arrest . *Prehospital Emergency Care.* 1997; 1:1–10.

42. Smith JE, Sherwood NA. Combined use of laryngeal mask airway and fibreoptic laryngoscope in difficult intubation. *Anaesthesia & Intensive Care.* 1991; 19:471–2.

43. Stone BJ, Leach AB, Alexander CA, et al. The use of the laryngeal mask airway by nurses during cardiopulmonary resuscitation—Results of a multicentre trial. *Anaesthesia.* 1994; 49:3.

References

44. Tanigawa K, Shigematsu A. Choice of airway devices for 12,020 cases of nontraumatic cardiac arrest in Japan. *Prehospital Emergency Care*. 1998; 2:96–100.

45. Verghese C., Brimacombe JR. Survey of laryngeal mask airway usage in 11,910 patients: Safety and efficacy for conventional and nonconventional usage . *Anesth Analg*. 1996; 82:129–33.

Intubating Laryngeal Mask Airway

1. Agro F, Brimacombe J, Carassiti M, Marchionni L, Morelli A, Cataldo R. The intubating laryngeal mask. Clinical appraisal of ventilation and blind tracheal intubation in 110 patients. *Anaesthesia*. 1998; 53(11):1084–90.

2. Avida MS, Harvey A, Chitkara N, Ponte J. The intubating laryngeal mask airway compared with direct laryngoscopy. *British Journal of Anesthesia*. 1999; 83: 615–7.

3. Brain AI, Verghese C, Addy EV, Kapila A, Brimacombe J. The intubating laryngeal mask. II: A preliminary clinical report of a new means of intubating the trachea. *Br J Anaesth*. 1997; 79(6):704–9.

4. Choyce A, Avidan MS, Patel C, Harvey A, Timberlake C, McNeilis N, Glucksman E. Comparison of laryngeal mask and intubating laryngeal mask insertion by the naive intubator. *Br J Anaesth*. 2000: 84(1):103–5.

5. Frappier J, Guenoun T, Journois D, Philippe H, Aka E, Cadi P, Silleran-Chassany J, Safran D. Airway management using the intubating laryngeal mask airway for the morbidly obese patient. *Anesth Analg*. 2003; 96(5):1510–5.

6. Fukutome T, Amaha K, Nakazawa K, Kawamura T, Noguchi H. Tracheal intubation through the intubating laryngeal mask airway (LMA-Fastrach) in patients with difficult airways. *Anaesthesia & Intensive Care*. 1998; 26(:387–91.

7. Inoue Y, Koga K, Shigematsu A. A comparison of two tracheal intubation techniques with Trachlight and Fastrach in patients with cervical spine disorders. *Anesth Analg*. 2002; 94(3):667–71.

8. Joo H, Rose K, Fastrach—a new intubating laryngeal mask airway: Successful use in patients with difficult airways. *Can J Anaesth*. 1998; 45(3):253–6.

9. Joo HS, Kapoor S, Rose DK, Naik VN. The intubating laryngeal mask airway after induction of general anesthesia versus awake fiberoptic intubation in patients with difficult airways. *Anesth Analg*. 2001; 92(5):1342–6.

10. Joo HS, Rose DK. The intubating laryngeal mask airway with and without fiberoptic guidance. *Anesth Analg*. 1999; 88:662–6.

11. Kapila A, Addy EV, Verghese C, Brain AI. The intubating laryngeal mask airway: An initial assessment of performance. *Br J Anaesth*. 1997: 79:710–3.

12. Keller C, Brimacombe J, Keller K. Pressures exerted against the cervical vertebrae by the standard and intubating laryngeal mask airways: A randomized, controlled, cross-over study in fresh cadavers. *Anesth Analg*. 1999; 89:1296–300.

13. Langeron O, Semjen F, Bourgain JL, Marsac A, Cros AM. Comparison of the intubating laryngeal mask airway with the fiberoptic intubation in anticipated difficult airway management. *Anesthesiology*. 2001; 94:968–72.

14. Levitan RM. Myths and realities: The "difficult airway" and alternative airway devices in the emergency setting. [editorial] *Acad Emerg Med*. 2001; 8:829–32.

15. Levitan RM, Ochroch EA, Stuart S, Hollander JE. Use of the intubating laryngeal mask airway by medical and non-medical personnel. *American J Emerg Med*. 2000; 18: 12–6.

16. Martel M, Reardon RF, Cochrane J. Initial experience of emergency physicians using the intubating laryngeal mask airway: A case series. *Acad Emerg Med*. 2001; 8:815–22.

17. Messant I, Lenfant F, Chomel A, et al. Evaluation of the learning curve of a new intubation technique: Intubating laryngeal mask. *Ann Fr Anesth Reanim*. 2002; 21:622–6.

18. Murashima K, Fukutome T, Brimacombe J. A comparison of two silicone-reinforced tracheal tubes with different bevels for use with the intubating laryngeal mask. *Anaesthesia*. 1999: 54:1198–2000.

19. Reardon RF, Martel M. The intubating laryngeal mask airway: Suggestions for use in the emergency department. *Acad Emerg Med*. 2001; 8:833–8.

20. Reeves MD, Skinner MW, Ginifer CJ. Evaluation of the Intubating Laryngeal Mask Airway used by occasional intubators in simulated trauma. *Anaesth Intensive Care*. 2004; 32: 73–6.

21. Rosenblatt WH, Murphy M. The intubating laryngeal mask: Use of a new ventilating-intubating device in the emergency department. *Ann of Emergency Medicine*. 1999; 33:234–8.

22. Schuschnig C, Waltl B, Erlacher W, Reddy B, Stoik W, Kapral S. Intubating laryngeal mask and rapid sequence induction in patients with cervical spine injury. *Anaesthesia*. 1999; 54:793–7.

23. Wong JK, Tongier WK, Armbruster SC, White PF. Use of the intubating laryngeal mask airway to facilitate awake orotracheal intubation in patients with cervical spine disorders. *J Clin Anesth*. 1999; 11:346–8.

Combitube

1. Agro F, Frass M, Benumof JL, Krafft P. Current status of the Combitube: A review of the literature. *J Clin Anesth*. 2002; 14:307–14.

2. Davis DP, Valentine C, Ochs M, Vilke GM, Hoyt DB. The Combitube as a salvage airway device for paramedic rapid sequence intubation. *Ann Emerg Med*. 2003; 42: 697–704.

3. Della Puppa A, Pittoni G, Frass M. Tracheal esophageal combitube: A useful airway for morbidly obese patients who cannot intubate or ventilate. *Acta Anaesthesiol Scand*. 2002; 46:911–3.

4. Atherton GL, Johnson JC. Ability of paramedics to use the Combitube in prehospital cardiac arrest. *Ann Emerg Med.* 1993; 22:1263–7.

5. Butler BD, Little T, Drtil S. Combined use of the esophageal-tracheal Combitube with a colorimetric carbon dioxide detector for emergency intubation/ventilation. *Journal of Clinical Monitoring.* 1995; 11:311–6.

6. Frass M, Frenzer R, Mayer G, Popovic R, Leithner C. Mechanical ventilation with the esophageal tracheal combitube (ETC) in the intensive care unit. *Archives of Emergency Medicine.* 1987; 4:219–25.

7. Frass M, Frenzer R, Rauscha F, Schuster E, Glogar D. Ventilation with the esophageal tracheal combitube in cardiopulmonary resuscitation. Promptness and effectiveness. *Chest.* 1988; 93:781–4.

8. Frass M, Frenzer R, Rauscha F, Weber H, Pacher R, Leithner C. Evaluation of esophageal tracheal combitube in cardiopulmonary resuscitation. *Critical Care Medicine.* 1987; 15:609–11.

9. Frass M, Frenzer R, Zdrahal F, Hoflehner G, Porges P, Lackner F. The esophageal tracheal combitube: Preliminary results with a new airway for CPR. *Ann Emerg Med.* 1987; 16:768–72.

10. Frass M. The Combitube: Esophageal/tracheal double-lumen airway. In: Benumof JL, ed. Airway management principles and practice. Philadelphia: *WB Saunders*, 1996:444–55.

11. Gaitini LA, Vaida SJ, Mostafa S, et al. The Combitube in elective surgery: A report of 200 cases. *Anesthesiology.* 2001; 94:79–82.

12. Hagberg CA, Vartazarian TN, Chelly JE, Ovassapian A. The incidence of gastroesophageal reflux and tracheal aspiration detected with pH electrodes is similar with the Laryngeal Mask Airway and Esophageal Tracheal Combitube—a pilot study. *Can J Anaesth.* 2004; 51:243–9.

13. Hartmann T, et al. The oesaphageal Combitube Small Adult. *Anaesthesia.* 2000; 55: 670–5.

14. Krafft P, Nikolic A, Frass M. Esophageal rupture associated with the use of the Combitube [letter]. *Anesth Analg.* 1998; 87:1457.

15. Lefrancois DP, Dufour DG. Use of the esophageal tracheal combitube by basic emergency medical technicians. *Resuscitation.* 2002; 52:77–83.

16. Ochs M, Vilke GM, Chan TC, Moats T, Buchanan J. Successful prehospital airway management by EMT-Ds using the combitube. *Prehosp Emerg Care.* 2000; 4:333–7.

17. Oczenski W, Krenn H, Dahaba AA, Binder M, El-Schahawi-Kienzl I, Kohout S, Schwarz S, Fitzgerald RD. Complications following the use of the Combitube, tracheal tube and laryngeal mask airway. *Anaesthesia.* 1999; 54:1161–5.

18. Paventi S, Liturri S, Colio B, Santevecchi A, Ranieri R. Airway management with the Combitube during anaesthesia and in an emergency. *Resuscitation.* 2001; 51:129–33.

19. Rumball CJ, MacDonald D. The PTL, Combitube, laryngeal mask, and oral airway: A randomized prehospital comparative study of ventilatory device effectiveness and cost-effectiveness in 470 cases of cardiorespiratory arrest . *Prehospital Emergency Care.* 1997; 1:1–10.

20. Rabitsch W, Schellongowski P, Staudinger T, et al. Comparison of a conventional tracheal airway with the Combitube in an urban emergency medical services system run by physicians. *Resuscitation.* 2003; 57:27–32.

21. Rumball C, Macdonald D, Barber P, Wong H, Smecher C. Endotracheal intubation and esophageal tracheal Combitube insertion by regular ambulance attendants: A comparative trial. *Prehosp Emerg Care.* 2004;8:15–22.

22. Urtubia RM, Aguila CM, Cumsille MA, Combitube: A study for proper use. *Anesth Analg.* 2000; 90:958–62.

23. Vezina D, Lessard MR, Bussieres J, Topping C, Trepanier CA. Complications associated with the use of the Esophageal-Tracheal Combitube. *Can J Anaesth.* 1998; 45:76–80.

24. Vezina D, Trepanier CA, Lessard MR, Bussieres J, Esophageal and tracheal distortion by the Esophageal-Tracheal Combitube: A cadaver study . *Can J Anaesth.* 1999; 46:393–7.

25. Wafai Y, Salem MR, Baraka A, Joseph NJ, Czinn EA, Paulissian R. Effectiveness of the self-inflating bulb for verification of proper placement of the Esophageal Tracheal Combitube. *Anesth Analg.* 1995; 80:122–6.

26. Walz R, Davis S, Panning B. Is the Combitube a useful emergency airway device for anesthesiologists?*Anesth Analgesia.* 1999; 88:233.

27. Wong JK, Tongier WK, Armbruster SC, White PF. Use of the intubating laryngeal mask airway to facilitate awake orotracheal intubation in patients with cervical spine disorders. *J Clin Anesth.* 1999; 11:346–8.

28. Yardy N, Hancox D, Strang T. A comparison of two airway aids for emergency use by unskilled personnel. The Combitube and laryngeal mask. *Anaesthesia.* 1999; 54:181–3.

Definition, Incidence, and Prediction of the Difficult Airway

1. Arne J, Decoins P, Fusciardi J, et al. Preoperative assessment for difficult intubation in general and ENT surgery: predictive values of a clinical multivariate risk index. *Br J Anaesth.* 1998; 80: 140–6.

2. Benumof JL. Definition and incidence of the difficult airway. In: Benumof JL, ed. Airway management: Principles and practice. *Mosby-Yearbook.* St. Louis, 1996: 121–25.

3. Bellhouse CP, Dore C. Criteria for estimating the likelihood of difficulty of endotracheal intubation with the Macintosh laryngoscope. *Anaesthesia and Intensive Care.* 1988; 16: 329-37.

4. Butler PJ, Dhara SS. Prediction of difficult laryngoscopy: an assessment of thyromental distance and Mallampati predictive tests. *Anaesthesia and Intensive Care.* 1992; 20: 139–42.

5. Calder I. Predicting difficult intubation. *Anaesthesia.* 1992; 47: 528–9.

6. Cohle SD, Jones DH, Puri S. Lingual tonsillar hypertrophy causing failed intubation and cerebral anoxia. *American Journal of Forensic Medicine & Pathology*. 1993 ; 14:158–61.

7. Davies S, Ananthanarayan C, Castro C. Asymptomatic lingual tonsillar hypertrophy and difficult airway management: A report of three cases. *Can J Anaesth*. 2001; 48: 1020–4.

8. el-Ganzouri AR, McCarthy RJ, Tuman KJ, Tanck EN, Ivankovich AD. Preoperative airway assessment: Predictive value of a multivariate risk index. *Anesthesia and Analgesia*. 1996; 82: 1197–204.

9. Ezri T, Medalion B, Weisenberg M, et al. Increased body mass index per se is not a predictor of difficult laryngoscopy. *Can J Anaesth*. 2003; 50: 179–83.

10. Frerk CM. Predicting difficult intubation. *Anaesthesia*. 1991; 46: 1005–8.

11. Hawthorne L, Wilson R, Lyons G, Dresner M. Failed intubation revisited: 17-yr experience in a teaching maternity unit. *Br J Anaesth*. 1996; 76: 680–4.

12. Jones DH. Cohle SD. Unanticipated difficult airway secondary to lingual tonsillar hyperplasia. *Anesth Analg*. 1993; 77:1285–8.

13. Juvin P, Lavaut E, Dupont H, Lefevre P, Demetriou M, Dumoulin JL, Desmonts JM. Difficult tracheal intubation is more common in obese than in lean patients. *Anesth Analg*. 2003; 97: 595–600.

14. Karkouti K, Rose DK, Ferris LE, Wigglesworth DF, Meisami-Fard T, Lee H. Inter-observer reliability of ten tests used for predicting difficult tracheal intubation. *Can J Anaesth*. 1996; 43: 5549.

15. Karkouti K, Rose DK, Wigglesworth D, Cohen MM. Predicting difficult intubation: A multivariable analysis. *Canadian Journal of Anesthesia*. 2000; 47: 730–9.

17. Mallampati SR, Gatt SP, Gugino LD, et al. A clinical sign to predict difficult intubation; A prospective study. *Canadian Anaesthetists' Society Journal* 1985; 32: 429–34.

18. Mallampati. SR. Recognition of the difficult airway. In: BenumofJL, ed. Airway management: Principles and practice. *Mosby-Yearbook*. St. Louis, 1996:126–42.

19. Nath G, Sekar M. Predicting difficult intubation - a comprehensive scoring system. *Anaesthesia and Intensive Care*. 1997; 25: 482–6.

20. Oates JD, Macleod AD, Oates PD, Pearsall FJ, Howie JC, Murray GD. Comparison of two methods for predicting difficult intubation. *Br J Anaesth*. 1991; 66: 305–9.

21. Ovassapian A, Glassenberg R, Randel GI, et al. The unexpected difficult airway and lingual tonsil hyperplasia: A case series and a review of the literature. *Anesthesiology*. 2002; 97: 124–32.

22. Rose KD, Cohen MM. The incidence of airway problems depends on the definition used. *Can J Anaesth*. 1996; 43: 30–4.

23. Samsoon GLT, Young JRB. Difficult tracheal intubation: A retrospective study. *Anaesthesia*. 1987; 42: 487–90.

24. Savva D. Prediction of difficult tracheal intubation. *Br J Anaesth*. 1994; 73: 149–53.

25. Schmitt HJ, Kirmse M, Radespiel-Troger M. Ratio of patient's height to thyromental distance improves prediction of difficult laryngoscopy. *Anaesth Intensive Care.* 2002; 30: 763–5.

26. Tse JC, Rimm EB, Hussain A. Predicting difficult endotracheal intubation in surgical patients scheduled for general anesthesia: A prospective blind study. *Anesthesia and Analgesia.* 1995; 81: 254–8.

27. Tham EJ, Gildersleve CD, Sanders LD, et al. Effects of posture, phonation and observer on Mallampati classification. *BJ Anaesth.* 1992; 68:32–8.

28. Ulrich B, Listyo R, Gerig HJ, Gabi K, et al. The difficult intubation. The value of BURP and 3 predictive tests of difficult intubation. *Anaesthesist.* 1998; 47: 45–50.

29. Voyagis GS, Kyriakis KP, Dimitriou V, Vrettou I: Value of oropharyngeal Mallampati classification in predicting difficult laryngoscopy among obese patients. *Eur J Anaesthesiol* 1998; 15:330–4.

30. Wilson ME, Spiegelhalter D, Robertson JA, Lesser P. Predicting difficult intubation. *Br J Anaesth.* 1988; 61: 211–16.

31. Yamamoto K, Tsubokawa T, Shibata K, Ohmura S, Nitta S, Kobayashi T. Predicting difficult intubation with indirect laryngoscopy. *Anesthesiology.* 1997; 86: 316–21.

32. Yentis SM. Predicting difficult intubation-worthwhile exercise or pointless ritual? [Editorial] *Anaesthesia.* 2002; 57: 105–109.

Laryngoscopy Education, Teaching, Ocularity, and Imaging

1. Konrad C, Schupfer G, Witlisbach M, Gerber H. Learning manual skills in anesthesiology: Is there a recommended number of cases for anesthetic procedures? *Anesth Analg.* 1998; 86: 635–9.

2. Levitan RM, Goldman TS, Bryan DA, Herlich A. Training with video imaging improves the initial intubation success rates of paramedic trainees in an OR setting. *Ann Emerg Med.* 2001; 34: 46–50.

3. Levitan RM, Ochroch AE, Higgins MS. Contrary to popular belief and traditional instruction, the larynx is sighted one eye at a time during direct laryngoscopy. [letter] *Acad Emerg Med.* 1998; 5:844–6.

4. Levitan RM. A new tool for teaching and supervising direct laryngoscopy. *Acad Emerg Med.* 1996; 3: 79–81.

5. Levitan, RM. Direct laryngoscopy imaging: Teaching and research applications. Educational Synopses in Anesthesiology and Critical Care Medicine: The On-line Anesthesia Journal. Available at http://gasnet.med.yale.edu/esia/1998/june/samart.html. Reprinted in *Am J Anesthesiology.* 1999; 26: 39–42.

6. Mulcaster JT, Mills J, Hung OR, et al. Laryngoscopic intubation: learning and performance. *Anesthesiology.* 2003; 98: 23–7.

Grading Laryngeal View and the Difficulty of Intubation

1. Adnet F, Borron SW, Racine SX, Clemessy JL, Fournier JL, Plaisance P. et al. The Intubation Difficulty Scale (IDS): Proposal and evaluation of a new score characterizing the complexity of endotracheal intubation. *Anesthesiology.* 1997: 87: 1290–7.

2. Adnet F, Racine SX, Borron SW et al. A survey of tracheal intubation difficulty in the operating room: A prospective observational study. *Acta Anaesthesiol Scand.* 2001; 45: 327–2.

3. Cohen AM, Fleming BG, Wace JR. Grading of direct laryngoscopy. A survey of current practice. *Anaesthesia.* 1994; 49: 522–5.

4. Cook TM. A new practical classification of laryngeal view. *Anaesthesia* 2000; 55: 274–9.

5. Cormack RS, Lehane J. Difficult tracheal intubation in obstetrics. *Anaesthesia.* 1984; 39: 1105–11.

6. Levitan RM, Ochroch AE, Hollander J, et al. Assessment of Airway Visualization: Validation of the Percent of Glottic Opening (POGO) Scale. *Acad Emerg Med.* 1998; 5: 919–23.

7. Levitan RM, Ochroch AE, Hollander JE. A grading system for direct laryngoscopy [letter]. *Anaesthesia.* 1999; 54: 1009–10.

8. Ochroch AE, Hollander JE, Levitan RM. POGO score as a predictor of intubation difficulty and need for rescue devices [Abstract]. *Ann Emerg Med.* 2000; 36, 4 (part 2): A199.

9. Ochroch AE, Kush S, Stuart S, Hollander JE, Levitan RM. Assessment of laryngeal view in direct laryngoscopy: The percentage of glottic opening (POGO) score compared to Cormack and Lehane grading. *Can J Anesth.* 1999; 46: 987–90.

10. Yentis SM, Lee D. Evaluation of an improved scoring system for grading tracheal intubation. *Anaesthesia.* 1998; 53: 1041–4.

External Laryngeal Manipulation and Backward Upward Rightward Pressure

1. Adnet F, Racine SX, Borron SW et al. A survey of tracheal intubation difficulty in the operating room: A prospective observational study. *Acta Anaesthesiol Scand.* 2001; 45: 327–2.

2. Benumof JL, Cooper SD. Qualitative improvement in laryngoscopic view by optimal external laryngeal manipulation. *J Clin Anesth.* 1996; 8:136–40.

3. Benumof JL. Difficult laryngoscopy: obtaining the best view [editorial]. *Can J Anaesth* 1994; 41: 361–5.

4. Brunnings W. Direct laryngoscopy: Autoscopy by counterpressure. In: Direct laryngoscopy, bronchoscopy, and esophagoscopy. Balliere, Tindall, & Cox, London, 1912; pp.110–115.

5. Jackson C. Peroral endoscopy and laryngeal surgery. *The Laryngoscope Company*, St. Louis, 1915.

6. Knill RL. Difficult laryngoscopy made easy with a "BURP." *Can J Anaesth.* 1993; 40:798-9.

7. Levitan RM, Mickler T, Hollander JE. Bimanual laryngoscopy: A videographic study of external laryngeal manipulation by novice intubators. *Ann Emerg Med.* 2002; 40:30-7.

8. Roberts JT, Abouleish A, Curlin FJ, Patterson A. The failed intubation: Maximizing successful management of the patient with a compromised or potentially compromised airway. In: *Clinical management of the airway*, Roberts JT. WB Saunders, Philadelphia 1994: 201–3.

9. Roberts JT, Ali HH, Shorten GD. Using the bubble inclinometer to measure laryngeal tilt and predict difficulty of laryngoscopy. *J Clin Anesth.* 1993; 5:306–9.

10. Takahata O, Kubata M, Mamiya K, et al. The efficacy of the "BURP" maneuver during a difficulty laryngoscopy. *Anesth Analg.* 1997; 84: 419–21.

11. Ulrich B, Listyo R, Gerig HJ, Gabi K, et al. The difficult intubation: The value of BURP and 3 predictive tests of difficult intubation. *Anaesthesist.* 1998; 47: 45–50.

12. Wilson ME, Spiegelhalter D, Robertson JA, et al. Predicting difficult intubation. *Br J Anaesth.* 1988; 61:211–5.

13. Yamamoto K, Tsubokawa T, Ohmura S, Itoh H, Kobayashi T. Left-molar approach improves the laryngeal view in patients with difficult laryngoscopy. *Anesthesiology.* 2000; 92: 70–4.

14. Zeitels S. Universal modular glottiscope system: The evolution of a century of design and technique for direct laryngoscopy. *Ann Oto Rhino Laryng.* 1999: 9 (Part 2) Supplement 179:6–13.

Head Elevated Laryngoscopy Positioning, Cervical Spine Issues and Laryngoscopy

1. Adnet F, Baillard C, Borron SW, et al. Randomized study comparing the "sniffing position" with simple head extension for laryngoscopic view in elective surgery patients. *Anesthesiolog.y* 2001; 95: 836–41.

2. Adnet F, Racine SX, Borron SW, et al. A survey of tracheal intubation difficulty in the operating room: A prospective observational study. *Acta Anaesthesiol Scand.* 2001; 45:327–32.

3. *Advanced Trauma Life Support*, 6th ed. Page 97. American College of Surgeons, Chicago IL, 1997.

4. Boyce JR, Ness T, Castroman P, Gleysteen JJ. A preliminary study of the optimal anesthesia positioning for the morbidly obese patient. *Obes Surg.* 2003; 13 :4–9.

5. Brimacombe J, Keller C, Kunzel KH, et al. Cervical spine motion during airway management: A cinefluoroscopic study of the posteriorly destabilized third cervical vertebrae in human cadavers. *Anesth Analg*. 2000; 91: 1274–8.

6. Crosby E. Airway management after upper cervical spine injury: What have we learned? *Can J Anaesth*. 2002; 49:733–44.

7. Gerling MC, Davis DP, Hamilton RS, et al. Effects of cervical spine immobilization technique and laryngoscope blade selection on an unstable cervical spine in a cadaver model of intubation. *Ann Emerg Med. 2000*; 36: 293–300.

8. Hastings RH, Hon ED, Nghiem C, Wahrenbrock EA. Force, torque, and stress relaxation with direct laryngoscopy. *Anesth Analg*. 1996; 82: 456–61.

9. Hastings RH, Kelley SD. Neurologic deterioration associated with airway management in a cervical spine-injured patient. *Anesthesiology*. 1993; 78: 580–3.

10. Hauswald M, Sklar DP, Tandberg D, Garcia JF. Cervical spine movement during airway management: Cinefluoroscopic appraisal in human cadavers. *Am J Emerg Med*. 1991; 9: 535–8.

11. Hochman II, Zeitels SM, Heaton JT. Analysis of the forces and position required for direct laryngoscopic exposure of the anterior vocal folds. *Ann Oto Rhino Laryn*. 1999; 108: 715–24.

12. Horton WA, Fahy L, Charters P. Disposition of cervical vertebrae, atlanto-axial joint, hyoid and mandible during x-ray laryngoscopy. *Br J Anaest*. 1989;63:435–8.

13. Jackson C, Jackson CL. *Bronchoscopy, esophagoscopy and gastroscopy; a manual of peroral endoscopy and laryngeal surgery*. Philadelphia, London, W.B. Saunders Company, 1934: 85–105.

14. Jackson CJ. Position of the patient for peroral endoscopy, in Jackson CJ, *Peroral endoscopy and laryngeal surgery*. The Laryngoscope Company, St. Louis, 1915: 77–88.

15. Johnston RH. Extension and flexion in direct laryngoscopy: A comparative study. *Ann Oto, Rhino, and Laryn*. 1910: 19:19–24.

16. Levitan RM, Mechem CC, Ochroch EA, Shofer FS, Hollander JE. Head Elevated Laryngoscopy Positioning (HELP): Improving laryngeal exposure during laryngoscopy by increasing head elevation. *Ann Emerg Med* 2003;41: 322–30.

17. Meschino A, Devitt JH, Koch JP, Szalai JP, Schwartz ML. The safety of awake tracheal intubation in cervical spine injury. *Can J Anaesth*. 1992; 39: 114–7.

18. Ng M, Hastings RH. Successful direct laryngoscopy assisted by posture in a patient with ankylosing spondylitis. *Anesth Analg*. 1998; 87:1436–7.

19. Popitz MD. Anesthetic implications of chronic cervical disease of the cervical spine. *Anesth Analg*. 1997; 84: 672–83.

20. Scannell G, Waxman K, Tominaga G, Barker S, Annas C. Orotracheal intubation in trauma patients with cervical fractures. *Archives of Surgery*. 1993 ; 128:903–5.

21. Schmitt HJ, Mang H. Head and neck elevation beyond the sniffing position improves laryngeal view in cases of difficult direct laryngoscopy. *J Clin Anesth*. 2002;14:335–8.

22. Suderman VS. Crosby ET. Lui A. Elective oral tracheal intubation in cervical spine-injured adults . *Can J Anaesth.* 1991; 38:785–9.

23. Zeitels SM. Universal modular glottiscope system: the evolution of a century of design and technique for direct laryngoscopy. *Ann Otol Rhinol Laryngol.* 1999;108: Suppl.179: 2–24.

Laryngoscopy Techniques, Blade Design, Lighting

1. Asai T, Matsumoto S, Fujise K, Johmura S, Shingu K. Comparison of two Macintosh laryngoscope blades in 300 patients. *Br J Anaesth.* 2003; 90:457–60.

2. Benumof JL. Conventional (laryngoscopic) orotracheal and nasotracheal intubation (single lumen tube). In Benumnof JL, ed. Airway management: Principles and practice. *Mosby-Yearbook.* St. Louis, 1996: 261–76.

3. Bucx MJ, Snijders CJ, van der Vegt MH, Stijnen T. An evaluation of a modified Macintosh laryngoscope in a manikin. *Can J Anaesth.* 1998; 45(5 Pt 1): 483–7.

4. Callander CC, Thomas J. Modification of the Macintosh laryngoscope for difficult intubation [letter]. *Anaesthesia.* 1987; 42: 671.

5. Cassels WH. Advantages of a curved laryngoscope. *Anesthesiology.* 1942; 3: 580.

6. Cooper SD. The evolution of upper-airway retraction: new and old laryngoscopy blades. In Benumnof JL, ed. Airway management: Principles and practice. *Mosby-Yearbook.* St. Louis, 1996: 374–411.

7. Crosby E, Cleland M. An assessment of the luminance and light field characteristics of used direct laryngoscopes. *Can J Anaesth.* 1999; 46: 792–6.

8. Evans A, Vaughan RS, Hall JE, et al. A comparison of the forces exerted during laryngoscopy using disposable and non-disposable laryngoscope blades. *Anaesthesia.* 2003; 58: 869–73.

9. Gabbott DA. Laryngoscopy using the McCoy laryngoscope after application of a cervical collar. *Anaesthesia,* 1996; 51:812–4.

10. Galinski M, Adnet F, Tran D, et al. Disposable laryngoscope blades do not interfere with ease of intubation in scheduled general anaesthesia patients. *Eur J Anaesthesiol.* 2003; 20: 731–5.

11. Henderson JJ. Questions about the Macintosh laryngoscope and technique of laryngoscopy. *Eur J Anaesthesiol.* 2000; 17: 2–5.

12. Henderson JJ. Solutions to the problem of difficult tracheal tube passage associated with the paraglossal straight laryngoscopy technique. *Anaesthesia.* 1999; 54: 601–2.

13. Henderson JJ. The use of paraglossal straight blade laryngoscopy in difficult tracheal intubation. *Anaesthesia.* 1997; 52: 552–60.

14. Laurent SC, deMelo AE, Alexander-Williams JM. The use of the McCoy laryngoscope in patients with simulated cervical spine injuries. *Anaesthesia.* 1996; 51:74–5.

15. Levitan RM, Ochroch EA. Explaining the variable effect on laryngeal view obtained with the McCoy laryngoscope [letter]. *Anaesthesia*. 1999; 54:599–601.

16. Macintosh RR. A new laryngoscope. *Lancet*. 1943; 1:205.

17. Marks RD, Hancock R, Charters P. An analysis of laryngoscope blade shape and design: New criteria for laryngoscope evaluation. *Can J Anesth*. 1993; 40:262.

18. McIntyre JW. Laryngoscope design and the difficult adult tracheal intubation. *Can J Anaesth*. 1989; 36: 94–8.

19. Miller RA. A new laryngoscope. *Anesthesiology*. 1941; 2: 318–20.

20. Racz GB. Improved vision modification of the Macintosh larygoscope [letter]. *Anaesthesia*. 1984; 39: 1249.

21. Skilton RW, Parry D, Arthurs GJ, Hiles P. A study of the brightness of laryngoscope light. *Anaesthesia*. 1996; 51: 667–72.

22. Uchida T, Hikawa Y, Saito Y, Yasuda K. The McCoy levering laryngoscope in patients with limited neck extension. *Can J Anesth*. 1997; 44:674–6.

Bougie (Eschmann Stylet), Lighted Stylet, and Tracheal Tube Stylet Shaping

1. Agro F, Hung OR, Cataldo R, Carassiti M, Gherardi S. Lightwand intubation using the Trachlight: A brief review of current knowledge. *Can J Anaesth*. 2001; 48: 592–9.

2. Biro P, Weiss M, Gerber A, Pasch T. Comparison of a new video-optical intubation stylet versus the conventional malleable stylet in simulated difficult tracheal intubation. *Anaesthesia*. 2000; 55: 886–9

3. Cormack RS, Lehane J. Difficult tracheal intubation in obstetrics. *Anaesthesia*. 1984; 39:1105–1111.

4. Davis L, Cook-Sather SD, Schreiner MS. Lighted stylet tracheal intubation: A review. *Anesth Analg*. 2000; 90: 745–56.

5. Gataure PS, Vaughan RS, Latto IP. Simulated difficult intubation. Comparison of the gum elastic bougie and the stylet. *Anaesthesia*. 1996; 51: 935–8.

6. Hames KC, Pandit JJ, Marfin AG, et al. Use of the bougie in simulated difficult intubation. 1. Comparison of the single-use bougie with the fibrescope. *Anaesthesia*. 2003; 58: 846–51.

7. Hirabayashi Y, Hiruta M, Kawakami T, Inoue S, Fukuda H, Saitoh K, Shimizu R. Effects of lightwand (Trachlight) compared with direct laryngoscopy on circulatory responses to tracheal intubation. *Br J Anaesth*. 1998; 81: 253–5.

8. Hodgson RE, Gopalan PD, Burrows RC, Zuma K. Effect of cricoid pressure on the success of endotracheal intubation with a lightwand. *Anesthesiology*. 2001; 94: 259–62.

9. Hodzovic I, Wilkes AR, Latto IP. Bougie-assisted difficult airway management in a manikin - the effect of position held on placement and force exerted by the tip. *Anaesthesia*. 2004; 59: 38–43.

10. Hung OR, Pytka S, Morris I, Murphy M, Launcelott G, Stevens S, MacKay W, Stewart RD. Clinical trial of a new lightwand device (Trachlight) to intubate the trachea. *Anesthesiology*. 1995; 83: 509–14.

11. Hung OR, Pytka S, Morris I, Murphy M, Stewart RD. Lightwand intubation: II—Clinical trial of a new lightwand for tracheal intubation in patients with difficult airways. *Can J Anaesth*. 1995; 42: 826–30.

12. Hung OR, Stewart RD. Lightwand intubation: I—A new lightwand device. *Can J Anaesth*. 1995; 42: 820–5.

13. Latto IP, Stacey M, Mecklenburgh J, Vaughan RS. Survey of the use of the gum elastic bougie in clinical practice. *Anaesthesia*. 2002; 57:379–384.

14. Levitan RM, Rubin B, Mechem CC, Everett W, Ochroch AE. Tracheal Tube Stylet Shape and Its Effect On Target Visualization And Tip Maneuverability. [Abstract]: *Acad Emerg Med*. 2003; 10: 484 (A183).

15. Makino H, Katoh T, Kobayashi S, Bito H, Sato S. The effects of tracheal tube tip design and tube thickness on laryngeal pass ability during oral tube exchange with an introducer. *Anesth Analg*. 2003; 97: 285–8.

16. Marfin AG, Pandit JJ, Hames KC, Popat MT, Yentis SM. Use of the bougie in simulated difficult intubation. 2. Comparison of single-use bougie with multiple-use bougie. *Anaesthesia*. 2003; 58: 852–5.

17. Moscati R, Jehle D, Christiansen G, et al. Endotracheal tube introducer for failed intubations: A variant of the gum elastic bougie. *Ann Emerg Med*. 2000; 36:52–6.

18. Nocera A. A flexible solution for emergency intubation difficulties. *Ann Emerg Med*. 1996; 27: 665–7.

19. Nolan JP, Wilson ME. An evaluation of the gum elastic bougie. Intubation times and incidence of sore throat. *Anaesthesia*. 1992; 47: 878–81.

20. Soh CR, Kong CF, Kong CS, Ip-Yam PC, Chin E, Goh MH. Tracheal intubation by novice staff: The direct vision laryngoscope or the lighted stylet (Trachlight). *Emergency Medicine Journal*. 2002; 19:292–4.

21. Stasiuk RB. Improving styletted oral tracheal intubation: Rational use of the OTSU. *Can J Anaesth*. 2001; 48: 911–8.

22. Vacanti CA, Roberts JT. Blind oral intubation: The development and efficacy of a new approach. *J Clin Anesth*. 1992: 4:399–401.

23. Weisenberg M, Warters RD, Medalion B, et al. Endotracheal intubation with a gum-elastic bougie in unanticipated difficult direct laryngoscopy: Comparison of a blind technique versus indirect laryngoscopy with a laryngeal mirror. *Anesth Analg*. 2002; 95: 1090–3.

References

24. Wik L, Naess AC, Steen PA. Intubation with laryngoscope versus transillumination performed by paramedic students on manikins and cadavers. *Resuscitation*. 1997; 33: 215–8.

Nasal Intubation

1. Adamson DN, Theisen FC, Barrett KC. Effect of mechanical dilation on nasotracheal intubation. *Journal of Oral & Maxillofacial Surgery*. 1988; 46: 372–5.

2. Arya VK, Dutta A, Chari P, Sharma RK. Difficult retrograde endotracheal intubation: The utility of a pharyngeal loop. *Anesth Analg*. 2002; 94: 470–3.

3. Cameron D, Lupton BA. Inadvertent brain penetration during neonatal nasotracheal intubation. *Archives of Disease in Childhood*. 1993; 69:79–80.

4. Fassoulaki A, Pamouktsoglou P, Prolonged nasotracheal intubation and its association with inflammation of paranasal sinuses. *Anesth Analg*. 1989; 69: 50–2.

5. Fuchs G, Schwarz G, Baumgartner A, Kaltenbock F, Voit-Augustin H, Planinz W. Fiberoptic intubation in 327 neurosurgical patients with lesions of the cervical spine. *Journal of Neurosurgical Anesthesiology*. 1999; 11: 11–6.

6. Gorbach MS. Inflation of endotracheal tube cuff as an aid to blind nasal endotracheal intubation. *Anesth Analg*. 1987; 66:913–22.

7. Favaro R, Tordiglione P, Di Lascio F, Colagiovanni D, Esposito G, Quaranta S, Gasparetto A. Effective nasotracheal intubation using a modified transillumination technique. *Can J Anaesth*. 2002; 49:91–5.

8. Holdgaard HO, Pedersen J, Schurizek BA, Melsen NC, Juhl B. Complications and late sequelae following nasotracheal intubation. *Acta Anaesthesiologica Scandinavica*. 1993; 37: 475–80.

9. Hooker EA, Hagan S, Coleman R, Heine MF, Greenwood P. Directional-tip endotracheal tubes for blind nasotracheal intubation. *Acad Emerg Med*. 1996; 3: 586–9.

10. Horellou MF, Mathe D, Feiss P. A hazard of naso-tracheal intubation. *Anaesthesia*. 1978; 33: 73–4.

11. Iserson KV. Blind nasotracheal intubation. *Ann Emerg Med:* 1981; 10: 468–71.

12. Katz RI, Hovagim AR, Finkelstein HS, Grinberg Y, Boccio RV, Poppers PJ. A comparison of cocaine, lidocaine with epinephrine, and oxymetazoline for prevention of epistaxis on nasotracheal intubation. *J Clin Anesth*. 1990; 2: 16–20.

13. Kim YC, Lee SH, Noh GJ, et al. Thermosoftening treatment of the nasotracheal tube before intubation can reduce epistaxis and nasal damage. *Anesth Analg*. 2000; 91: 698–701.

14. Krishel S, Jackimczyk K, Balazs K, Endotracheal tube whistle: An adjunct to blind nasotracheal intubation. *Ann Emerg Med*. 1992; 21: 33–6.

15. Kundra P, Kutralam S, Ravishankar M. Local anaesthesia for awake fibreoptic nasotracheal intubation. *Acta Anaesthesiol Scand*. 2000; 44: 511–6.

16. Latorre F, Otter W, Kleemann PP, Dick W, Jage J. Cocaine or phenylephrine/lignocaine for nasal fibreoptic intubation?. *European Journal of Anaesthesiology*. 1996; 13: 577–81.

17. Lu PP, Liu HP, Shyr MH, Ho AC, Wang YL, Tan PP, Yang CH. Softened endothracheal tube reduces the incidence and severity of epistaxis following nasotracheal intubation. *Acta Anaesthesiologica Sinica*. 1998; 36: 193–7.

18. Marlow TJ, Goltra DD Jr, Schabel SI. Intracranial placement of a nasotracheal tube after facial fracture: A rare complication. *J Emerg Med*. 1997; 15: 187–191.

19. O'Connor RE, Megargel RE, Schnyder ME, et al. Paramedic success rate for blind nasotracheal intubation is improved with the use of an endotracheal tube with directional tip control. *Ann Emerg Med*. 2000; 36: 328–32.

20. Ovassapian A, Wheeler M. Fiberoptic endoscopy-aided techniques. In Benumof JL, ed. Airway management: Principles and practice. *Mosby-Yearbook*. St. Louis, 1996:295–6

21. Pedersen J, Schurizek BA, Melsen NC, Juhl B. The effect of nasotracheal intubation on the paranasal sinuses. A prospective study of 434 intensive care patients. *Acta Anaesthesiologica Scandinavica*. 1991; 35: 11–3.

22. Reed DB, Clinton JE. Proper depth of placement of nasotracheal tubes in adults prior to radiographic confirmation. *Acad Emerg Med*. 1997; 4:1111–4.

23. Roppolo LP, Vilke GM, Chan TC, et al. Nasotracheal intubation in the emergency department, revisited. *J Emerg Med*. 1999; 17: 791–9.

24. Rosen CL, Wolfe RE, Chew SE, Branney SW, Roe EJ. Blind nasotracheal intubation in the presence of facial trauma. *J Emerg Med*. 1997; 15: 141–5.

25. Sim WS, Chung IS, Chin JU, Park YS, et al. Risk factors for epistaxis during nasotracheal intubation. *Anaesth Intensive Care*. 2002; 30: 449–52.

26. Smith JE, Reid AP. Identifying the more patent nostril before nasotracheal intubation. *Anaesthesia*. 2001; 56: 258–62.

27. Tintinalli JE, Claffey J. Complications of nasotracheal intubation. *Ann Emerg Med*. 1981; 10: 142–4.

28. Van Elstraete AC, Pennant JH, Gajraj NM, Victory RA. Tracheal tube cuff inflation as an aid to blind nasotracheal intubation. *Br J Anaesth*. 1993; 70:691–3.

29. Van Elstraete AC, Mamie JC, Mehdaoui H. Nasotracheal intubation in patients with immobilized cervical spine: A comparison of tracheal tube cuff inflation and fiberoptic bronchoscopy. *Anesth Analg*. 1998; 87: 400–2.

Retrograde Intubation, Digital Intubation

1. Hardwick WC, Bluhm D, Digital intubation. *J Emerg Med*. 1984; 1: 317–20.

2. Hung OR, al-Qatari M. Light-guided retrograde intubation. *Can J Anaesth*. 1997; 44: 877–82.

3. Murphy MF, Hung OR. Blind digital intubation. In Benumof JL, ed. Airway management: Principles and practice. *Mosby-Yearbook*, St. Louis, 1996: 278.

4. Rosenblatt WH, Angood PB, Maranets I, Kaklamanos IG, Garwood S. Retrograde fiberoptic intubation. *Anesth Analg*. 1997; 84: 1142–4.

5. Sanchez A, Pallares V. Retrograde intubation technique. In Benumof JL, ed. Airway management: Principles and practice. *Mosby-Yearbook*. St. Louis, 1996: pp. 320–341.

6. Shantha TR. Retrograde intubation using the subcricoid region. *Br J Anaesth*. 68: 109–12, 1992.

7. Stewart RD. Tactile orotracheal intuabtion. *Ann Emerg Med*. 1984; 13: 175.

8. Vacanti CA, Roberts JT. Blind oral intubation: The development and efficacy of a new approach. *J Clin Anesth*. 1992; 4: 399–401.

Cricothyrotomy, Tracheotomy, and Percutaneous Trans-Tracheal Ventilation

1. Benumof JL. Transtracheal jet ventilation via percutaneous catheter and high-pressure source. In Benumof JL, ed. Airway management: Principles and practice. *Mosby-Yearbook*. St. Louis, 1996: 455–74.

2. Bramwell KJ, Davis DP, Cardall TV, Yoshida E, Vilke GM, Rosen P. Use of the Trousseau dilator in cricothyrotomy. *J Emerg Med*. 1999; 17: 433–6.

3. Brofeldt BT, Panacek EA, Richards JR, An easy cricothyrotomy approach: The rapid four-step technique. *Acad Emerg Med*. 1996 3: 1060–3.

4. Chan TC, Vilke GM, Bramwell KJ, Davis DP, Hamilton RS, Rosen P. Comparison of wire-guided cricothyrotomy versus standard surgical cricothyrotomy technique. *J Emerg Med*. 1999; 17: 957–62.

5. Chang RS, Hamilton RJ, Carter WA. Declining rate of cricothyrotomy in trauma patients with an emergency medicine residency: Implication for skills training. *Acad Emerg Med*. 1998; 5: 247–51.

6. Ciaglia P, Firsching R, Syniec C, Elective percutaneous dilatational tracheostomy. A new simple bedside procedure; preliminary report. *Chest*. 1985; 87: 715–9.

7. Davis DP, Bramwell KJ, Vilke GM, Cardall TY, Yoshida E, Rosen P. Cricothyrotomy technique: Standard versus the rapid four step technique. *J Emerg Med*. 1999; 17: 17–21.

8. DiGiacomo JC, Angus LD, Gelfand BJ, Shaftan GW. Cricothyrotomy technique: Standard versus the rapid four step technique. *J Emerg Med*. 1999; 17:1071–3.

9. Dulguerov P, Gysin C, Perneger TV, Chevrolet JC. Percutaneous or surgical tracheostomy: A meta-analysis. *Critical Care Medicine*. 1999; 27: 1617–25.

10. Eisenburger P, Laczika K, List M, Wilfing A, Losert H, Hofbauer R, Burgmann H, Bankl H, Pikula B, Benumof JL, Frass M. Comparison of conventional surgical versus Seldinger technique emergency cricothyrotomy performed by inexperienced clinicians. *Anesthesiology*. 2000; 92: 687–90.

11. Erlandson MJ, Clinton JE, Ruiz E, Cohen J. Cricothyrotomy in the emergency department revisited. *J Emerg Med*. 1989; 7: 115–8.

12. Fortune JB, Judkins DG, Scanzaroli D, McLeod KB, Johnson SB. Efficacy of prehospital surgical cricothyrotomy in trauma patients. *Journal of Trauma-Injury Infection & Critical Care*. 1997; 42: 832–6.

13. Gerich TG, Schmidt U, Hubrich V, Lobenhoffer HP, Tscherne H. Prehospital airway management in the acutely injured patient: The role of surgical cricothyrotomy revisited. *Journal of Trauma-Injury Infection & Critical Care*. 1998; 45: 312–4.

14. Holmes JF, Panacek EA, Sakles JC, Brofeldt BT. Comparison of 2 cricothyrotomy techniques: Standard method versus rapid 4-step technique. *Ann Emerg Med*. 1998; 32: 442–6.

15. Jaberi M, Mitchell K, MacKenzie C. Cricothyrotomy: Good, bad, or ugly? [Abstract] *Trauma Care* (Journal of the International Trauma and Critical Care Society). 2001; 11: 13.

16. Jorden RC, Moore EE, Marx JA, Honigman B. A comparison of PTV and endotracheal ventilation in an acute trauma model. *Journal of Trauma-Injury Infection & Critical Care*. 1985; 25: 978-83.

17. Metz S, Parmet JL, Levitt JD. Failed emergency transtracheal ventilation through a 14-gauge intravenous catheter. *J Clin Anesth*. 1996; 8: 58–62.

18. Okamoto K, Morioka T. Transtracheal O2 insufflation (TOI) as an alternative method of ventilation during cardiopulmonary resuscitation. *Resuscitation*. 1990; 20: 253–62.

19. Patel RG. Percutaneous transtracheal jet ventilation: A safe, quick, and temporary way to provide oxygenation and ventilation when conventional methods are unsuccessful. *Chest*. 1999; 116: 1689–94.

20. Smith RB, Schaer WB, Pfaeffle H. Percutaneous transtracheal ventilation for anaesthesia and resuscitation: A review and report of complications. *Canadian Anaesthetists Society Journal*. 1975; 22: 607–12.

21. Spaite DW, Joseph M. Prehospital cricothyrotomy: An investigation of indications, technique, complications, and patient outcomes. *Ann Emerg Med*. 1990; 19: 279–85.

22. Stothert JC Jr., Stout MJ, Lewis LM, Keltner RM Jr. High pressure percutaneous transtracheal ventilation: The use of large gauge intravenous-type catheters in the totally obstructed airway. *American J Emerg Med*. 1990; 8: 184–9.

23. Toye FJ, Weinstein JD. Clinical experience with percutaneous tracheostomy and cricothyroidotomy in 100 patients. *Journal of Trauma-Injury Infection & Critical Care*. 1986; 26: 1034–40.

24. Tran TP, Rhee KJ, Schultz HD, Carl ML. Gas exchange and lung mechanics during percutaneous transtracheal ventilation in an unparalyzed canine model. *Acad Emerg Med*. 1998; 5: 320–4.

25. Weksler N, Klein M, Weksler D, et al. Retrograde tracheal intubation: Beyond fibreoptic endotracheal intubation. *Acta Anaesthesiol Scand*. 2004; 48: 412–6.

26. Weymuller EA Jr., Pavlin EG, Paugh D, Cummings CW. Management of difficult airway problems with percutaneous transtracheal ventilation. *Annals of Otology, Rhinology & Laryngology*. 1987; 96: 34–7.

Fiberoptic and Other Optical Intubation Devices

1. Afilalo M, Guttman A, Stern E, Lloyd J, Colacone A, Tselios C, Dankoff J. Fiberoptic intubation in the emergency department: A case series. *J Emerg Med*. 1991; 11:387–91.

2. Agro F, Barzoi G, Montecchia F. Tracheal intubation using a Macintosh laryngoscope or a GlideScope in 15 patients with cervical spine immobilization. *Br J Anaesth*. 2003; 90:705–6.

3. Agro F, Cataldo R, Carassiti M, Costa F. The seeing stylet: A new device for tracheal intubation. *Resuscitation*. 2000; 44:177–80.

4. Aoyama K, Takenaka I, Sata T, Shigematsu A. Use of the fibrescope-video camera system for difficult tracheal intubation. *Br J Anaesth*. 1996; 77: 662–4.

5. Archdeacon J, Brimacombe J. Anterior traction of the tongue—a forgotten aid to awake fibreoptic intubation. *Anaesth Intensive Care*. 1994; 22:718–9.

6. Barker KF, Bolton P, Cole S, Coe PA. Ease of laryngeal passage during fibreoptic intubation: A comparison of three endotracheal tubes. *Acta Anaesthesiol Scand*. 2001; 45:624–6.

7. Bjoraker DG. The Bullard intubating laryngoscope. *Anesthesiology Review*. 1990; 17: 64.

8. Biro P, Weiss M. Comparison of two video-assisted techniques for the difficult intubation. *Acta Anaesthesiol Scand*. 2001; 45:761–5.

9. Biro P, Weiss M, Gerber A, Pasch T. Comparison of a new video-optical intubation stylet versus the conventional malleable stylet in simulated difficult tracheal intubation. *Anaesthesia*. 2000; 55: 886–9.

10. Burke LP, Osborn NA, Smith JE, Reid AP. Learning fibreoptic skills in ear, nose and throat clinics. *Anaesthesia*. 1996; 51:81–3.

11. Cohn AI, McGraw SR, King WH. Awake intubation of the adult trachea using the Bullard laryngoscope. *Can J Anaesth*. 1995; 42:246–8.

12. Cooper RM. Use of a new videolaryngoscope (GlideScope) in the management of a difficult airway. *Can J Anaesth*. 2003; 50:611–3.

13. Cooper SD, Benumof JL, Ozaki GT. Evaluation of the Bullard laryngoscope using the new intubating stylet: Comparison with conventional laryngoscopy. *Anesth Analg.* 1994; 79: 965.

14. Halligan M, Charters P. A clinical evaluation of the Bonfils Intubation Fibrescope. *Anaesthesia.* 2003; 58:1087–91.

15. Kaplan MB, Ward DS, Berci G. A new video laryngoscope-an aid to intubation and teaching. *J Clin Anesth.* 2002; 14:620–6.

16. Fuchs G, Schwarz G, Baumgartner A, Kaltenbock F, Voit-Augustin H, Planinz W. Fiberoptic intubation in 327 neurosurgical patients with lesions of the cervical spine. *Journal of Neurosurgical Anesthesiology.* 1999; 11:11–6.

17. Levitan RM, Kinkle WC, Levin W. Performance of an Optical Intubation Stylet in Simulated Difficult Laryngoscopy. Society for Airway Management meeting, Chicago IL Sept. 10-11, 2004 [Abstract].

18. Levitan RM, Kinkle WC, Levin W. The Glidescope Video Laryngoscope in the hands of novice users: Seeing the larynx does not correlate with intubation success. 2004; *ACEP Scientific Assembly, Research Forum*, San Francisco October 19th 2004 [publication pending].

19. Levin WJ, Levitan RM. The Shikani optical stylet as an adjunct for intubation: A potential rescue technique for the difficult airway. [Abstract] *Ann Emerg Med.* 2003; 42, 4 (part 2): A235.

20. Liem EB, Bjoraker DG, Gravenstein D. New options for airway management: Intubating fibreoptic stylets. *Br. J. Anaesth.* 2003; 91: 408–418.

21. Maroof M, Khan RM, Bonsu A, Raza HS. A new solution to fibreoptic intubation in the presence of blood and secretions [letter]. *Can J Anaesth.* 1995; 42:177–8.

22. MacQuarrie K, Hung OR, Law JA. Tracheal intubation using Bullard laryngoscope for patients with a simulated difficult airway. *Can J Anaesth.* 1999; 46:760–5.

23. Mlinek EJ Jr, Clinton JE, Plummer D, Ruiz E. Fiberoptic intubation in the emergency department. *Ann Emerg Med.* 1990; 19: 359–62.

24. Ovassapian A, ed . *Fiberoptic endoscopy and the difficult airway.* 2nd ed. Philadelphia: Lippincott-Raven; 1996.

25. Pfitzner L, Cooper MG, Ho D. The Shikani Seeing Stylet for difficult intubation in children: Initial experience. *Anaesth Intensive Care.* 2002; 30:462–6.

26. Reeves DS, Brown NM. Mycobacterial contamination of fibreoptic bronchoscopes. *J Hosp Infect.* 1995; 30 [Suppl]; 531–6.

27. Rudolph C, Schlender M. Clinical experiences with fiberoptic intubation with the Bonfls intubation fiberscope. *Anaesthesiol Reanim.* 1996; 21: 127–30.

28. Shaw, John D. *A colour atlas of fiberoptic endoscopy of the upper respiratory tract* . Chicago: Year Book Medical Publishers; 1987.

29. Schafermeyer RW. Fiberoptic laryngoscopy in the emergency department. *Am J Emerg Med.* 1984; 2: 160–3.

30. Shier ME. A simple technique for oral fiberoptic bronchoscopy: "No more needles, Doc" [letter]. *Anesth Analg*. 1999; 88:695.

31. Shikani AH. New "seeing" stylet-scope and method for the management of the difficult airway. *Otolaryngol Head Neck Surg*. 1999; 120:113–6.

32. Shorten GD, Ali HH, Roberts JT. Assessment of patient position for fiberoptic intubation using videolaryngoscopy. *J Clin Anesth*. 1995; 7:31–4.

33. Shulman GB, Connelly NR. A comparison of the Bullard laryngoscope versus the flexible fiberoptic bronchoscope during intubation in patients afforded inline stabilization. *J Clin Anesth*. 2001; 13:182–5.

34. Smith CE, Pinchak AB, Sidhu TS, Radesic BP, Pinchak AC, Hagen JF. Evaluation of tracheal intubation difficulty in patients with cervical spine immobilization: Fiberoptic (WuScope) versus conventional laryngoscopy. *Anesthesiology*. 1999; 91:1253–9.

35. Smith CE, Sidhu TS, Lever J, Pinchak AB. The complexity of tracheal intubation using rigid fiberoptic laryngoscopy (WuScope). *Anesth Analg*. 1999; 89:236–9.

36. Smith JE, Jackson AP, Hurdley J, Clifton PJ. Learning curves for fibreoptic nasotracheal intubation when using the endoscopic video camera. *Anaesthesia*. 1997; 52:101–6.

37. Smith JE, Mackenzie AA, Scott-Knight VC. Comparison of two methods of fibrescope-guided tracheal intubation. *Br J Anaesth*. 1991; 66:546–50.

38. Van Elstraete AC, Mamie JC, Mehdaoui H. Nasotracheal intubation in patients with immobilized cervical spine: A comparison of tracheal tube cuff inflation and fiberoptic bronchoscopy. *Anesth Analg*. 1998; 87:400–2.

39. Weiss M, Schwarz U, Gerber AC. Difficult airway management: Comparison of the Bullard laryngoscope with the video-optical intubation stylet. *Can J Anaesth*. 2000; 47: 280–4.

Special Clinical Challenges

1. Abel M, Eisenkraft JB. Anesthetic implications of myasthenia gravis. *Mt Sinai J Med*. 2002; 69:31–7.

2. Allen D, Loughnan TE, Ord RA. A re-evaluation of the role of tracheostomy in Ludwig's angina. *Journal of Oral & Maxillofacial Surgery*. 1985; 43:436–9.

3. Aufderheide TP, Aprahamian C, Mateer JR. et al. Emergency airway management in hanging victims. *Ann Emerg Med*. 1994; 24:879–84.

4. Betz P, Eisenmenger W, Frequency of throat-skeleton fractures in hanging. *American Journal of Forensic Medicine & Pathology*. 1996; 17:191–3.

5. Book WJ, Abel M, Eisenkraft JB. Adverse effects of depolarising neuromuscular blocking agents. Incidence, prevention and management. *Drug Safety*. 1994; 10:331–49.

6. Bork K, Siedlecki K, Bosch S, Schopf RE, Kreuz W. Asphyxiation by laryngeal edema in patients with hereditary angioedema. *Mayo Clinic Proceedings.* 2000; 75:349–54.

7. Brown MM, Parr MJ, Manara AR. The effect of suxamethonium on intracranial pressure and cerebral perfusion pressure in patients with severe head injuries following blunt trauma. *European Journal of Anaesthesiology.* 1996; 13:474–7.

8. Busch RF. Ludwig angina: Early aggressive therapy . *Archives of Otolaryngology — Head & Neck Surgery.* 1999; 125:1283–4.

9. Chidiac EJ. Succinylcholine and the open globe: Questions unanswered. *Anesthesiology.* 2004; 100: 1035–6; author reply 1037.

10. Culling RD, Middbaugh RE, Menk EJ. Rapid tracheal intubation with vecronium: The timing principle. *J Clin Anesth.* 1989; 1:422–5.

11. Cunningham AJ, Barry P. Intraocular pressure: Physiology and implications for anaesthetic management. *Can Anaesth Soc J.* 1986; 33: 195–208.

12. Deshpande S. Laryngotracheal separation after attempted hanging. *Br J Anaesth.* 1998; 81:612–4.

13. Fuhrman GM, Stieg FH, Buerk CA. Blunt laryngeal trauma: Classification and management protocol. *J Trauma* 1990; 30:87–92.

14. Goodie D, Paton P. Anaesthetic management of blunt airway trauma: Three cases. *Anaesth Intensive Care.* 1991; 19:271–4.

15. Gussack GS, Jurkovich GJ, Luterman A. Laryngotracheal trauma: A protocol approach to a rare injury. *Laryngoscope* 1986; 96:660–5.

16. Howell MA, Guly HR. Near hanging presenting to an accident and emergency department. *Journal of Accident & Emergency Medicine.* 1996; 13:135–6.

17. Ishoo E, Shah UK, Grillone GA, Stram JR, Fuleihan NS. Predicting airway risk in angioedema: Staging system based on presentation. *Otolaryngology- Head & Neck Surgery.* 1999; 121:263–8.

18. James R, Nasmyth-Jones R. The occurrence of cervical fractures in victims of judicial hanging. *Forensic Science International.* 1992; 54:81–91.

19. Kaki A, Crosby ET, Lui AC. Airway and respiratory management following non-lethal hanging. *Can J Anaesth.* 1997; 44:445–50.

20. Kaups KL, Davis JW. Patients with gunshot wounds to the head do not require cervical spine immobilization and evaluation. *Journal of Trauma-Injury Infection & Critical Care.* 1998; 44:865–7.

21. Kendall JL, Anglin D, Demetriades D. Penetrating neck trauma. *Emergency Medicine Clinics of North America.* 1998; 16:85–105.

22. King CJ, Davey AJ, Chandradeva K. Emergency use of the laryngeal mask airway in severe upper airway obstruction caused by supraglottic oedema. *Br J Anaesth.* 1995; 75:785–6.

23. Kovarik WD, Mayberg TS, Lam AM, Mathisen TL, Winn HR. Succinylcholine does not change intracranial pressure, cerebral blood flow velocity, or the electroencephalogram in patients with neurologic injury. *Anesth Analg.* 1994; 78:469–73.

24. Kuttenberger JJ, Hardt N, Schlegel C. Diagnosis and initial management of laryngotracheal injuries associated with facial fractures. *J Craniomaxillofac Surg.* 2004; 32:80–4.

25. Larach MG, Rosenberg H, Gronert GA, Allen GC. Hyperkalemic cardiac arrest during anesthesia in infants and children with occult myopathies. *Clin Pediatr.* (Phila). 1997; 36:9–16.

26. MacLennan N, Heimbach DM,Cullen BF. Anesthesia for major thermal injury. *Anesthesiology.* 1998; 89: 749–70.

27. Mandavia DP, Qualls S, Rokos I. Emergency airway management in penetrating neck injury. *Ann Emerg Med.* 2000; 35:221–5.

28. Marple BF. Ludwig angina: A review of current airway management . *Archives of Otolaryngology — Head & Neck Surgery.* 1999; 125:596–9.

29. Minard G, Kudsk KA, Croce MA, et al. Laryngotracheal trauma. *Am Surg.* 1992; 58:181–7.

30. Minton MD, Grosslight K, Stirt JA, Bedford RF. Increases in intracranial pressure from succinylcholine: Prevention by prior nondepolarizing blockade. *Anesthesiology.* 1986; 65:165–9.

31. Morild I. Fractures of neck structures in suicidal hanging. *Medicine, Science & the Law.* 1996; 36:80–4.

32. O'Connor PJ, Russell JD, Moriarty DC. Anesthetic implications of laryngeal trauma. *Anesth Analg.* 1998; 87:1283–4.

33. Quinn FB Jr. Ludwig angina. *Archives of Otolaryngology — Head & Neck Surgery.* 1999; 125:599.

34. Roberts JR, Wuerz RC. Clinical characteristics of angiotensin-converting enzyme inhibitor-induced angioedema. *Ann Emerg Med.* 1991; 20:555–8.

35. Schaefer SD. The treatment of acute external laryngeal injuries. *Arch Otolaryngol Head Neck Surg.* 1991; 117:35–9.

36. Schow AJ, Lubarsky DA, Olson RP, Gan TJ. Can succinylcholine be used safely in hyperkalemic patients? *Anesth Analg.* 2002; 95:119–22.

37. Shearer VE, Giesecke AH. Airway management for patients with penetrating neck trauma: A retrospective study. *Anesth Analg.* 1993; 77:1135–8.

38. Shockley WW. Ludwig angina: A review of current airway management. *Archives of Otolaryngology — Head & Neck Surgery.* 1999; 125:600.

39. Sieber TJ, Zbinden AM, Curatolo M, Shorten GD. Tracheal intubation with rocuronium using the "timing principle". *Anesth Analg.* 1998; 86:1137–40.

40. Spitalnic SJ, Sucov A. Ludwig's angina: Case report and review. *J Emerg Med.* 1995; 13:499–503.

41. Sullivan M, Thompson WK, Hill GD. Succinylcholine-induced cardiac arrest in children with undiagnosed myopathy. *Can J Anaesth.* 1994; 41: 497–501.

42. Thapa S, Brull SJ. Succinylcholine-induced hyperkalemia in patients with renal failure: An old question revisited. *Anesth Analg.* 2000; 91: 237–41.

43. Vachon CA, Warner DO, Bacon DR. Succinylcholine and the open globe. Tracing the teaching. *Anesthesiology.* 2003; 99: 220–3.

44. Vander Krol L, Wolfe R. The emergency department management of near-hanging victims. *J Emerg Med.* 1994; 12:285–92.

45. Vinik HR. Intraocular pressure changes during rapid sequence induction and intubation: A comparison of rocuronium, atracurium, and succinylcholine. *J Clin Anesth* 1999; 11: 95–100.

Confirmation of Tracheal Tube Placement

1. American Society of Anesthesiologists Policy Statement, October 16, 2002, accessed 6/6/04 via the web at: http://www.asahq.org/publicationsAndServices/Difficult Airway.pdf.

2. Andres AH, Langenstein H. The esophageal detector device is unreliable when the stomach has been ventilated. *Anesthesiology.* 1999; 91:566–8.

3. Birmingham PK, Cheney FW, Ward RJ. Esophageal intubation: A review of detection techniques. *Anesth Analg.* 1986; 65:886–91.

4. Bozeman WP, Hexter D, Liang HK, Kelen GD. Esophageal detector device versus detection of end-tidal carbon dioxide level in emergency intubation. *Ann Emerg Med.* 1996; 27:595–9.

5. Falk JL, Sayre MR. Confirmation of airway placement. *Prehospital Emergency Care.* 1999; 3:273–8.

6. Garnett AR, Ornato JP, Gonzalez ER, Johnson EB. End-tidal carbon dioxide monitoring during cardiopulmonary resuscitation. *JAMA.* 1987; 257:512–5.

7. Gentry WB, Shanks CA. Reevaluation of a maneuver to visualize the anterior larynx after intubation. *Anesth Analg.* 1993; 77:161–3.

8. Hayden SR, Sciammarella J, Viccellio P, Thode H, Delagi R. Colorimetric end-tidal CO2 detector for verification of endotracheal tube placement in out-of-hospital cardiac arrest. *Acad Emerg Med.* 1995; 2:499–502.

9. Jemmett ME, Kendal KM, Fourre MW, Burton JH. Unrecognized misplacement of endotracheal tubes in a mixed urban to rural emergency medical services setting. *Acad Emerg Med.* 2003; 10:961–5.

10. Kasper CL, Deem S. The self-inflating bulb to detect esophageal intubation during emergency airway management. *Anesthesiology.* 1998; 88:898–902.

11. Kelly JJ, Eynon CA, Kaplan JL, de Garavilla L, Dalsey WC. Use of tube condensation as an indicator of endotracheal tube placement. *Ann Emerg Med.* 1998; 31:575–8.

12. Knapp S, Kofler J, Stoiser B, Thalhammer F, Burgmann H, Posch M, Hofbauer R, Stanzel M, Frass M. The assessment of four different methods to verify tracheal tube placement in the critical care setting. *Anesth Analg.* 1999; 88:766–70.

13. Lang DJ, Wafai Y, Salem MR, Czinn EA, Halim AA, Baraka A. Efficacy of the self-inflating bulb in confirming tracheal intubation in the morbidly obese. *Anesthesiology.* 1996; 85:246–53.

14. Levin WJ, Levitan RM, and Kinkle WC. Confirming the location of previously placed tracheal tubes by direct laryngoscopy [Abstract]. *Acad Emerg Med.* 2004; 11: 491–492.

15. Levine RL, Wayne MA, Miller CC. End-tidal carbon dioxide and outcome of out-of-hospital cardiac arrest. *New England Journal of Medicine.* 1997; 337:301–6.

16. Lewis M, Keramati S, Benumof JL, Berry CC. What is the best way to determine oropharyngeal classification and mandibular space length to predict difficult laryngoscopy? *Anesthesiology.* 1994; 81: 69–75.

17. MacLeod BA, Heller MB, Gerard J, Yealy DM, Menegazzi JJ. Verification of endotracheal tube placement with colorimetric end-tidal CO2 detection. *Ann Emerg Med.* 1991; 20:267–70.

18. O'Connor RE, Swor RA. Verification of endotracheal tube placement following intubation. National Association of EMS Physicians Standards and Clinical Practice Committee. *Prehospital Emergency Care.* 1999; 3:248–50.

19. Ornato JP, Shipley JB, Racht EM, et al. Multicenter study of a portable, hand-size, colorimetric end-tidal carbon dioxide detection device. *Ann Emerg Med.* 1992; 21:518–23.

20. Pelucio M, Halligan L, Dhindsa H. Out-of-hospital experience with the syringe esophageal detector device. *Acad Emerg Med.*1997; 4:563–8.

21. Pollard BJ, Junius F. Accidental intubation of the oesophagus. *Anaesthesia & Intensive Care.* 1980; 8:183–6.

22. Salem MR, Wafai Y, Joseph NJ, Baraka A, Czinn EA. Efficacy of the self-inflating bulb in detecting esophageal intubation. Does the presence of a nasogastric tube or cuff deflation make a difference? *Anesthesiology.* 1994; 80:42–8.

23. Salem MR, Wafai Y, Joseph NJ, Baraka A, Czinn EA. Efficacy of the self-inflating bulb in detecting esophageal intubation. *Anesthesiology.* 1994; 80:42–8.

24. Salem MR, Wafai Y, Baraka A, Taimorrazy B, Joseph NJ, Nimmagadda U. Use of the self-inflating bulb for detecting esophageal intubation after "esophageal ventilation". *Anesth Analg.* 1993; 77:1227–31.

25. Wee MYK. The oesophageal detector device: Assessment of a new method to distinguish oesophageal from tracheal intubation. *Anaesthesia.* 1988; 43:27–9.

26. Williams KN, Nunn FJ. The oesophageal detector device. *Anaesthesia* 1989; 44:412–14.

27. Zaleski L, Abello D, Gold MI. The oesophageal detector device. Does it work? *Anesthesiology* 1993; 79:244–7.

Recommended Reading

1. Benumof JL, ed. *Airway management principles and practice*. Philadelphia: WB Saunders, 1996.

2. Bull TR. *Color Atlas of ENT Diagnosis*, 4th Ed. Georg Thieme Verlag, 2003.

3. Brimacombe JR. *The laryngeal mask airway: A review and practical guide*, 1997.

4. Eisele DW, McQuone SJ. *Emergencies of the head and neck*. Mosby Inc. St. Louis, 2000.

5. Gorback MS. *Emergency airway management*. Philadelphia: BC Decker, 1990.

6. Hanowell LH, Waldron RJ. *Airway management*. Philadelphia: Lippincott-Raven, 1996.

7. Norton M. *Atlas of the difficult airway*. St. Louis: Mosby Yearbook, 1996.

8. Ovassapian A, ed . *Fiberoptic endoscopy and the difficult airway*. 2nd ed. Philadelphia: Lippincott-Raven, 1996.

9. Popat MT. *Practical Fiberoptic Intubation*. Butterworth Heinemann, Oxford, 2001.

10. Roberts JT. *Clinical management of the airway*. WB Saunders, Philadelphia 1994.

Useful Web sites (accessed September 1, 2004)

1. http://www.airwaycam.com/
   Airway Cam

2. http://www.airwaycarnival.com/
   Irene Osborne, MD NYU/Mt. Sinai Medical Center Anesthesiology

3. http://www.asahq.org/publicationsAndServices/DifficultAirway.pdf
   ASA Difficult Airway Guidelines, Updated 2002

4. http://www.bartleby.com/107/
   Bartleby.com edition of Gray's Anatomy of the Human Body (1918)

5. http://www.clarus-medical.com/airwaymanagement.htm
   Clarus Medical airway management products

6. http://www.combitube.org
   Combitube

7. http://www.cookcriticalcare.com/discip/em_med/2_09/index.htm
   Cook Critical Care Difficult Airway Products

8. http://www.das.uk.com/
   Difficult Airway Society of the United Kingdom

9. http://www.entusa.com/larynx_photo.htm
   Larynx Photographs, Kevin Kavanagh, MD

10. http://groups.msn.com/DrMAGBOULAIRWAYPAGE
    Dr. Magbou's Airway Site / Department of Anesthesia, University of Iowa

11. http://www.heine.com
    Heine laryngoscopes

12. http://www.ijam.at/
    Internet Journal of Airway Management, Marcus Weiss, MD

13. http://www.lmana.com
    LMA North America

14. http://www.nellcor.com
    Nellcor Airway Products

15. http://www.olympusamerica.com/msg_section/msg_anesth.asp
    Olympus Endoscopy USA

16. http://www.parkermedical.com
    Parker Medical

17. http://www.rusch.com
    Rusch Airway Products and Laryngoscopes

18. http://www.theairwaysite.com/airway_devices.html
    Airway Management Education Center Site, John Sackles, MD

19. http://vam.anest.ufl.edu/airwaydevice/
    The Virtual Airway Device, University of Florida at Gainseville Anesthesiology Department

20. http://www.visionsciences.com
    Vision Sciences (disposable endoscopic sheaths)

Index

ACLS, guidelines recommending LMA and Combitube for cardiac arrest, 58; transtracheal jet ventilation, 62.

Adnet (author reference), 95; intubation difficulty scale, 95; comparison of laryngeal exposure in "sniffing" position versus simple head extension, 110; citations in References, 284, 296, 297, 299.

Afrin (oxymetazoline), 12, 218, 232, 233.

Airway Cam, direct laryngoscopy imaging, 89; drawing of and ease of use, 90; studying ELM, 110; studying head elevated laryngoscopy, 111; studying stylet shape, 148.

Alternative intubation devices, for awake intubation, 1,2, 8, 23–25; considerations for selection and use in the emergency setting, 26; following failed laryngoscopy, 198; different alternative devices and techniques, 225–242; adding to emergency airway kits, 280–281.

American Macintosh Design, problems using with poor Mallampati score, 34; vs. German and English designs, 185, 188, 196

American Society of Anesthesiologists, Practice Guidelines for Management of the Difficult Airway 1993, 3–4; Practice Guidelines for Management of the Difficult Airway 2002, 41; use of end-tidal CO2 detection devices throughout hospital, 275.

Angioedema, 8, 32, 33; when oral route is impossible, 45; the emergency airway, 217; flexible fiberoptic intubation, 227; as special clinical challenge, 259–261.

Articulating laryngoscope (see McCoy blade)

Aryepiglottic fold, 75–78; mistaking for epiglottis during laryngoscopy, 99; tracheal tube inducers (bougie), 152; relationship to piriform recess, 232; tracheal tube placement during retrograde intubation, 247.

Aspiration, reducing risk in elective anesthesia, 5; issues in emergency airway, 6; in RSI, 7; risk with topical anesthesia, 12; risk

with pharmacologic assisted laryngoscopy, 14; risk with mask vs. LMA and Combitube in RSI, 47; and mask ventilation technique, 49–50; and cricoid pressure, 53; and LMA, 57; and Combitube, 59, 63; and transtracheal jet ventilation, 62; and relationship to repeat laryngoscopy, 196; and relationship to esophageal intubation, 197.

Auto-PEEP (see dynamic hyperinflation)

Awake laryngoscopy, in cooperative patent in elective anesthesia vs. emergency patient, 5; risks in emergency airways, 12, 13–14; use in patients who are obtunded, 26.

Bag mask, need for ventilation prior to onset of neuromuscular blockade, 49; checking prior to RSI and laryngoscopy, 96.

Beck Airflow Airway Monitor (BAAM whistle), 221, 222, 279.

Benumof JL (author reference), critical desaturation and succinylcholine, 43; transtracheal ventilation, 63; interpretation of CL grades, 93; comparison cricoid vs. thyroid manipulation, 109; optimal external laryngeal manipulation, 110; references, 283, 287, 293, 296, 299, 304, 314.

Berman airway (for fiberoptic oral intubation), 234.

Bevel of trachea tube, intubation through LMA, 65; passing tube over bougie or introducer, 150, 152; and nasal intubation, 220; and nasal intubation with a fiberscope, 233;

Bimanual laryngoscopy, historical origins, 83–83; and external laryngeal manipulation 106-107, 114, 123, 126, 129, 135, 144, 179, 194; as part of laryngoscopy strategy, 195, 196, 198; pediatric laryngoscopy, 202, 205.

Binocular suppression and laryngoscopy, 86.

Biomechanics of laryngoscopy, 88.

Blast injuries to face, case example and decision making 17; intubation, 261.

Blind nasotracheal intubation, as an option in combative patient, 5; in overall approach, 8; bypassing problems about the mouth, 16, 25, 26; case example in morbid obesity, 22; case example in mandible fracture, 217; technique and overview 217-224.

Blind orotracheal intubation with neck palpation, 240–241.

Bonfils Intubating Stylet, 155.

Bougie, 30, 37; with the ILMA, 68; stylet shaping, 147; recommended use, 151-154; tube placement and stylet shaping, 164; in laryngoscopy strategy, 195–199; nasal intubation using flexible fiberscope, 233; in airway equipment kit, 279, 281.

Bronchoscope (see intubating fiberscope)

Brunning's counterpressor attachment, 83.

Bullard laryngoscope, 24; versus optical stylets, 158; alternative intubation devices, 225; and other rigid fiberoptic devices, 236.

Cervical spine, and surgical airways, 17; and thyromental distance, 34; neck mobility testing, 35; precautions in ED intubated patients, 36; and ventilation position, 50; intubating LMA, 68; historical origins of positioning for laryngoscopy, 77, 80, 84; laryngoscopy with in-line stabilization, 97, 98; ; head elevated positioning, 196; fiberoptic intubation and fractures, 227.

Children, and short thyromental distance, 34, 161, 198; straight blades used in, 35, 164; laryngoscopy position and head size, 51; pediatric laryngoscopy and intubation 201–216; digital intubation, 241; succinylcholine and cardiac arrest in, 270.

Cocaine, for topical anesthesia, 218.

Cold Sterilization, cleaning fiberoptic equipment, 155, 158, 188, 227, 235.

Combitube, 6; cardiac arrest, 7; in overall approach to emergency airway, 8; as back-up in RSI, 44, 46, 47; rescue ventilation, 55, 59–62,; laryngoscopy with Combitube in place, 64; transition to rescue intubation, 63–65; preparation for RSI, 96; role in angioedema and facial trauma, 259, 261;

avoidance in laryngeal fracture and intrinsic lesions of the larynx, 265, 267.

Cormack RS and Lehane J (author reference), grading system for laryngeal view, 93–94.

Counter-pressor attachment, 82, 83.

Cranwall, straight blade design, 190-191.

Cricoid pressure, pros and cons, 53-54; effects on LMA insertion and performance, 58; preparation for laryngoscopy, 97; versus ELM and BURP 109-110; efficacy of, 196.

Cricoid ring, downward pressure with Sellick maneuver, 53; as complete circular structure 76; location of, 78; Gray's Anatomy illustration, 248; and the rapid 4-step technique, 253.

Cricothyrotomy, vs. tracheotomy in emergency settings, 17; time requirement and as back-up in RSI, 45; declining use, 46; traditional and rapid 4-step, 248–255; percutaneous (Melker), 255–258.

Curved blade laryngoscopy, 99-142; equipment variables, 29; problems with manikin training, 72; illumination, 79; mechanics of vs. straight blade 161–162; pediatric, 201.

Czermak, Johann, pioneer of indirect laryngoscopy, 81-84.

Dental gaps, 41; problems with the Macintosh blade, 161, 198.

Determinants of laryngoscopy success or failure, 27–31.

Digital intubation, 241.

Difficult airway prediction, 27–41.

Displacement space (see thyromental space)

Direct laryngoscopy imaging (see Airway Cam)

Dynamic hyperinflation, 272.

ELM (see external laryngeal manipulation)

Ear to sternal notch positioning, for ventilation, 51; for laryngoscopy, 96–97.

Endoscopic sheath, 158-159, 235.

Endotrol tube, in nasal intubation, 218, 220, 222, 224; in the airway equipment kit, 279.

End-tidal CO2, 3, with Combitube, 60, with ILMA, 66; preparation for laryngoscopy and RSI, 95, 98; nasal intubation, 224; colormetric and other devices, 275–277.

English Macintosh design, 185–186.

Epiglottic tubercle, 73, 76, 80, 114, 145.

Epiglottis identification, 99, 101-102; in straight blade laryngoscopy, 161.

Epiglottis first approach (epiglottoscopy), 102-103.

Epiglottis-only view, incidence with optimal laryngoscopy technique, 29; Cormack and Lehane grading and POGO score, 94-95; external laryngeal manipulation, 110; stylets, 147, 197; and tracheal tube introducers, 151, 153-154, 156, 196; and ELM, 198.

Epiglottitis, 227, 267–268.

Eschmann stylet, 151-154.

Esophageal intubation, (see also end-tidal CO2 detection); esophageal intubation detectors, 95, 98; consequences of esophageal intubation even when recognized, 197; overview, 273-277; verification of tube placement by direct laryngoscopy, 277.

External laryngeal manipulation (ELM), 29, 77, 106–107, 114, 123, 126, 129, 135, 144, 179, 194; historical perspectives, 83–83; and direct laryngoscopy, 83-85; intubation difficulty scale, 95-96; versus cricoid pressure and BURP, 110; improving laryngeal view, 163; as part of laryngoscopy strategy, 195, 196, 198; pediatric laryngoscopy, 202, 205.

Eye dominance and laryngeal sighting during laryngoscopy, 86-87.

Eye injury and succinylcholine, 271.

False vocal cords, 73, 79, 80, 81, 129, 166, 194.

Fiberoptic augmentation of direct laryngoscopy, 155–159.

Fiberoptic intubation, in anticipated difficult intubation in OR, 3; in emergency airways, 4; cooperative patient in elective setting, 5, technical challenges of and need in emergency airways, 6; in emergency patients for awake intubation, 24; through LMA, 46, 65; through ILMA, 68; following failed laryngoscopy in OR setting, 69; Parker Flex-tip tracheal tube and ease of intubation over fiberscope, 150–151; in patients with cervical spine immobilization, 224; technique of nasal intubation 227–233; technique of oral intubation, 234–235; in Ludwig's angina, 260; in blunt laryngo-tracheal injury, 265; in obstructing intrinsic lesions, 267; airway equipment kits, 280.

Flexion-flexion positioning, 110.

Frerk CM(author reference), thyromental distance, 34; citations in References, 288, 294.

Frova introducer, 151, 154.

Gag testing, 10.

German Macintosh laryngoscope design, 185–186, 188, in the pre-planned step-wise approach, 196; airway equipment kits, 279.

Glidescope video laryngoscope, for use in awake patients, 24; demonstrating laryngeal inlet and posterior structures, 76, 78; comprehensive overview, 237–238.

Glutaraldehyde, for cleaning fiberoptic instruments 155, 225.

Gray, Henry (author reference), illustrations from Gray's Anatomy 1918 text, 73, 81, 248.

Grandview blade, 186.

Guedel blade, 180, 190, 191.

Guillain-Barré Syndrome, contraindication to using succinylcholine, 271.

Gunshot wounds to face and neck, 19, 261, 262; cervical spine precautions, 264.

Hanging, 269.

Head elevated laryngoscopy position, historical origins, 84; laryngeal exposure, 103, 110-111; laryngoscopy technique, 198.

Head extension, in surgical airways, 17; in laryngoscopy positioning, 110; in oral fiberoptic intubation, 234; in digital intubation, 241; in retrograde incubation, 243.

Heath ML(author reference), intubation through LMA technique, 65; citation in References, 288.

Heine German Blade Design, 185.

Heine XP disposable blade, 188.

Henderson blade, 191–194.

Hochman I (author reference), 110; citation in References, 298.

Holding the laryngoscope, 87–88.

Huffman prism, 188.

Hyoepiglottic ligament, inability to externally assess, 27-28; and curved blade laryngoscopy, 72, 76, 78, 83, 88, 103, 108–110; location of, 76; illustration of, 78; and mechanics of curved and straight blade laryngoscopy, 161–162.

Hyoid bone, in blast injury, 17; in gunshot wound, 21; and submandibular lift with mask ventilation, 52; location and relationship to other structures, 74, 76, 78, 102; and external laryngeal manipulation, 110; and surgical landmarks, 248; and penetrating trauma, 261; and hanging, 269.

Hyperkalemia, and succinylcholine, 270.

Improved-vision Macintosh blade, 134–137, 186–187, 189.

In-line stabilization, and neck mobility, 35; preparation for laryngoscopy, 96, 98; ad oral intubation vs. nasal intubation and flexible fiberoptic rhinolaryngoscopy for cervical injury, 217, 227.

Interarytenoid notch, 75–81, 102–105, 107, 117, 120, 123, 124, 126, 128, 129, 131, 135, 137, 138, 139, 141, 143; as landmark using straight-to-cuff shaping of stylet, 148; and straight blade laryngoscopy, 163, 166, 168, 170, 175, 179, 180, 183, 193; and laryngoscopy strategy, 196, 199; and pediatric laryngoscopy, 203, 205, 206, 209, 210, 212; and rhinolaryngoscopy, 230, 231; and Glidescope, 238; and esophageal intubation, 273, 274.

Interdental gap, and difficult laryngoscopy, 32.

Intubation difficulty scale, 94–95.

Introducer (see bougie, Eschman stylet, Frova)

Jackson, Chevalier (author reference), external laryngeal manipulation, 83; progressive visualization of landmarks, 84; comparison of head and neck positions, 85; and finding epiglottis using midline approach, 99; and head elevation, 110; citations in References, 297, 298.

Johnston, R (author reference), supine laryngoscopy, 84; citation in References, 298.

Killian's suspension laryngoscope, 82, 83.

Kirstein, pioneer of direct laryngoscopy, 81, 82, 84.

Laerdal Trachlight, 154, 239.

Laryngeal carcinoma, 267.

Laryngeal fracture, 265–266.

Laryngeal inlet, and fit of LMA, 56, 57, 62, 65, 68; structures about, 71–73, 75–77, 102, 103; and passing the tracheal tube, 147, 148, 152; and bougie, 153; and straight blade, 161, 163; as seen during rhinolaryngoscopy, 231; passing tube during fiberoptic intubation, 233, 235; and Glidescope view, 237–238; and tube passage with retrograde intubation, 247; and esophageal intubation, 273.

Laryngeal vestibule (ventricle), 79, 81.

Laryngeal mask airway, 2, in the OR, 3; as backup to RSI, 44; in rescue ventilation, 55; comprehensive overview, 56-58; efficacy in unanticipated difficult airway, 63; possible role in Ludwig's angina, 260; in airway equipment kits, 279.

Laryngo-tracheal injury, contraindication to RSI, 7–10, 44; avoidance of blind nasotracheal intubation with, 16; indication for surgical airway, 16, 65; blunt injury to, 265–266.

Laryngoscope, gripping handle, 87–88; spatula designs, 186–189, ; lighting and bulb position, 29, 72, 73, 78, 79, 91–93, 119; Bulb position and blade design, 95, 185, 188, 191; force vector of laryngoscope during procedure, 72, 87, 100–101, 103; flange, 29, 34, 86, 87, 92, 100, 101, 108, 161, 163, 164, 165, 172, 178, 185–192, 196–198; articulating or levering tip (see McCoy); disposable versions, 188.

Laryngoscopy education and training, 71–75, 84, 90, 201.

Laryngoscopy equipment variables, as a contributor to intubation success or failure, 29–30.

Laryngoscopy preparation, 95–98.

Laryngoscopy strategy, 195–198.

Laryngoscopy with sedation only, 13–15 (i.e., Pharmacologic Assisted Laryngoscopy, PAL, as opposed to RSI including use of a neuromuscular blocker).

Laryngoscopy with topical, injected, and nebulized anesthesia, 11–13.

Lidocaine, 11–13; for nasal intubation, 218–220, 232; surgical airways, 248; head injury, 271; toxicity, 11, 218.

Lighted stylet, 24–25; with Combitube, 65; with LMA, 68; as laryngoscopy adjunct, 154–155; in laryngoscopy strategy, 197; as independent intubation device, 225, 226, 239–240; with retrograde intubation, 243; in airway kit, 281.

Lingual tonsillar hyperplasia, as a cause of failed laryngoscopy, 28; straight blade laryngoscopy, 161.

Ludwig's angina, 2, 9, 33, 45; Mallampati scoring, 33; impossible oral route, 45, 217; fiberoptic intubation, 227; presentation and management, 260.

Mallampati scoring, 31–36, 38, 40–41.

Malleable stylet, equipment variables, 29; use with LMA, 56-57; preparation for laryngoscopy, 97; stylet shaping, 147; withdrawal from tracheal tube, 151.

Mandible fracture, 17, 18, 20, 21, 33, 217.

Manikin training for laryngoscopy, problems with, 71-72, 89, 90, 163; in pediatric laryngoscopy, 201.

Mask ventilation, 2, 6, 8, 49–56; case examples or problems with, 21, 22; and patient safety in RSI, 45, 47; oral and nasal airways, 51; positioning for, 51; submandibular lift 52; two person technique, 52; pre-oxygenation and, 96; problems with specific clinical pathology, 259–263, 265–268.

McCoy blade, 112–114, 120–124, 128–129; 130–133, 136–137; 186–187.

Melker percutaneous cricothyrotomy, 69, 255–257; in airway kit, 279.

Miller blade, 29, 108, 161; tube placement with, 164; 168–173, 182–184; 185, 189–191, pediatric sizing, 202; 204–207, 210–215.

Mort T(author reference), 196-197; 273; citation in References, 285.

Muscle relaxants, 3, 7, 12–15; and laryngoscopy success or failure, 30; in mask ventilation, 49; and repeat administration, 55; and Combitube, 63; use after nasal intubation technique, 218, 224; and safety in specific situations, 270–271, and hypotension post-intubation, 271.

Myasthenia gravis, pathology of, 271; and use of succinylcholine, 271; and use of non-depolarizing agents, 271.

Nasal intubation, historical use of, 3; bypassing problems about the mouth, 16; in case examples of RSI decision making, 17–22; 25, 26; use in ED case series, 36; tracheal tube tip design, 150; 217–224; with fiberscope, 232–234; angioedema, 259; Ludwig's, 260.

Nasal trumpet, illustration, 12; nasal intubation technique, 218–223.

Nasal turbinate, 16, 74; injury to during intubation, 219–221; appearance of during rhinolaryngoscopy, 228–229.

Neck mobility, evaluation for difficult laryngoscopy, 5, 22, 31, 35, 36, 37, ; case examples of problems with, 22, 97, 269.

Neck wounds, 9, 261–264.

Neosynephrine (phenylephrine), proper topicalization and prevention of bleeding, 218.

Non-rebreather mask, 47, administering oxygen via, 49.

Ocularity of laryngoscopy, 84–86.

Operator positioning and posture, 85, 86.

Optimal external laryngeal manipulation, as described by Benumof, 110.

Oral airways, determining need for RSI, 7, 9, 11; proper technique for mask ventilation,51–52; specialized for fiberoptic intubation through the mouth, 65, 234–235.

Ovassapian A(author reference), lingual tonsillar hyperplasia, 28; fiberoptic intubation with intrinsic lesion, 267; citations in References, 294, 303, 397, 314.

Ovassapian airway, 65, 234–235.

Oxymetazoline, nasal intubation technique and prevention of bleeding, 12, 218; use in rhinolaryngoscopy, 228, 233.

Paraglossal straight blade technique, 161–184, 192; in laryngoscopy strategy, 195, 197–199; in Ludwig's angina, 260.

Parmet JL (author reference), LMA vs. TTJV for rescue ventilation in unanticipated difficult airways, 63; fiberoptics after failed laryngoscopy, 69;citation in References, 289.

Parker Flex-tip tracheal tube, 150–151, 218, 221, 233.

Parker TrachView fiberoptic scope, 156–158.

Pediatric intubation, and short thyromental distance, 34, 161, 198; straight blades used in, 35, 164; laryngoscopy position and head

size, 51; pediatric laryngoscopy and intubation 201–216; digital intubation, 241; succinylcholine and cardiac arrest in, 270.

Penetrating trauma to face and neck, 9, 19, 261–264.

Percentage of Glottic Opening (POGO) score, 93–94, 102, 111, 147.

Pharmacologic Assisted Laryngoscopy (PAL), 13–15.

Phenylephrine, in prevention of bleeding, 218.

Phillips blade, 178–180, 190, 191; airway equipment kits, 279.

Piriform recess, 81, 223, 232.

Positioning of patient, predictive tests of difficult laryngoscopy, 33–35; mask ventilation, 50–53; laryngoscopy, 96–98, 110–111; in laryngoscopy strategy 196, 198; pediatric laryngoscopy, 201; nasal intubation, 221, 224; fiberoptic intubation, 233; surgical airways, 243; cervical halo and fixed kyphosis, 269.

Practical Approach to Emergency Airway Management, algorithm, 7-10.

Progressive visualization of landmarks, 45, 83-85, 104–105; key to determining tip of blade placement, 101; pediatric laryngoscopy, 201.

Rapid Sequence Intubation (see RSI)

Rapid 4-step cricothyrotomy, 249, 253.

Rescue intubation, 3, 8, 45, 46; with Combitube in place, 64–65; with LMA 65–66; with ILMA, 66–67; surgical airway as rescue intubation, 68–69; considerations in choosing technique, 68–69; specific alternative techniques and devices, 225–241, devices in emergency airway kits, 279–282.

Retrograde intubation, 25, 69; time requirements, 45–46; following Combitube 65; with ILMA, 68; tube passage in, 151–152; technique, 243-247; in emergency airway kit, 281.

Rhinolaryngoscopy, skill acquisition, 6; technique, 227–232.

Rigid fiberoptic devices, 24, 225–226, 236.

Roberts JT (author reference), 108-109; citations in References, 297.

RSI, in emergency airway management, 1-2; decision making, 7–10; when unnecessary, 11; case examples , 17–23; prediction of laryngoscopy failure with RSI in ED setting, 35–41; patient safety, 43–48; mask and rescue ventilation, 49–70; preparation for laryngoscopy with, 95–97; laryngoscopy strategy with, 195–200; RSI pharmacology, 270–271.

Rusch, Emerald series, 185; ViewMax 188–189.

Scalpel, designs for cricothyrotomy, 252, 253.

Schmitt HJ (author reference), combining head elevation with ELM, 29, 111; citation in References, 299.

Scissor technique opening the mouth, 99, 112, 115, 122, 125, 134, 164, 168, 172, 178, 182, 204, 206.

Sellick BA (author reference), cricoid pressure, 53-54; citation in References, 286.

Shiley tracheostomy tube, 249, 251–254.

Shikani Seeing Optical Stylet, alternative devices, 24; laryngoscopy with fiberoptic augmentation, 155-158; as independent intubation device, 225–227; in emergency airway kit, 280, 281.

Siker blade, 188.

Statistical aspects of difficult airway prediction, 36–40, examples of sensitivity, specificity, and prevalence on positive predictive value, 39.

Steris, 155, 225.

Stroboscopic imaging of larynx, 79–80.

Storz Bonfils Intubating Stylet, 155.

Storz Henderson laryngoscope blade, 191–194.

Straight blade laryngoscopy, in poor Mallampati score and short thyromental distance, 34–35; around Combitube, 64; technique, 151–184; mechanics of, 161–162; improving laryngeal view with ELM and head elevation, 163; tube passage, 164; straight blade paradox, 161, 190–191.

Straight-to-cuff stylet shape, 96, 121, 147–151; 154; 156, 164; as part of laryngoscopy strategy, 195, 198, 199.

Stylet shaping, and passing the tracheal tube during laryngoscopy, 147-151; with lighted stylet, 154, 225; with Shikani as laryngoscopy adjunct, 155-158; with Shikani as independent intubation device, 225–227; with Glidescope, 237; with blind technique and neck palpation, 240.

Succinylcholine, recovery of spontaneous respiration, 43; repeat laryngoscopy, 55; burns, 265; hyperkalemia and exaggerated hyperkalemic response, 270–271.

Sun Med Greenline, Greenline D, 185, 188.

Sun Med Prism View, 188-189.

Surgical airways, as rescue airways, 9, 16–17, 44–46; rescue intubation, 68–69; techniques, 243–258.

Tracheotomy, 8, 10, 17; case example, 18; 248, 258; Ludwig's, 260; facial and neck trauma, 261; laryngeal trauma, 265–266; intrinsic laryngeal lesions, 267–268.

Trans-illumination (see lighted stylet), 239–240, with optical stylet, 226–227.

Trans-tracheal jet ventilation, 62–63; vs. LMA as rescue device in unanticipated difficult airway, 63, avoidance in blunt laryngo-tracheal injury, 265.

Trigger tube (see Endotrol)

Tracheal hook, 249, 250, 252, 253.

Trousseau dilator, 249, 251, 252.

Upsher scope, 225, 236.

Vacanti CA (author reference), 240–241, citation in References, 301.

Ventricular fold (also called the false vocal cord or vestibular fold), 79, 81.

Vestibule of larynx, 79, 81.

Video laryngoscope (see Glidescope)

Video optical intubating stylet (VOIS), 157.

ViewMax laryngoscope blade, 188–189.

Vocal cords, 72–81; in CL grading, 93; in POGO score, 94; in Intubation Difficulty Scale, 95; curved blade laryngoscopy, 105, 113, 114, 121, 126, 129, 132, 133, 135, 141, 144, 146; visualization with straight blades, 161; straight blade laryngoscopy, 166, 167, 169, 173, 175, 176, 179, 181, 183, 184, 194; not the narrowest point of pediatric airway, 201; pediatric laryngoscopy, 203, 205, 209, 211, 213, 215; nasal intubation, 220, 223, 224; optical stylet, 226; rhinolaryngoscopy, 231; fiberoptic intubation, 233; retrograde intubation, 243; esophageal intubation, 273, 275, 277.

Vocal fold (true vocal cord), 73, 81.

Wisconsin blade, 164-165; 174, 178, 191, 203, 208; straight blade designs, 190; in the pediatric airway, 202.

Williams airway, 234.

Wu scope, alternative oral intubation devices, 24; 155, 225, 236.

Yankauer suction, preparation for laryngoscopy, 96, 197.